PHARMACEUTICAL PRODUCTS

PHARMACEUTICAL PRODUCTS

By

Dr. S.K. Prasad

School of Studies of Zoology & Biotechnology

Vikram University

Ujjain (India)

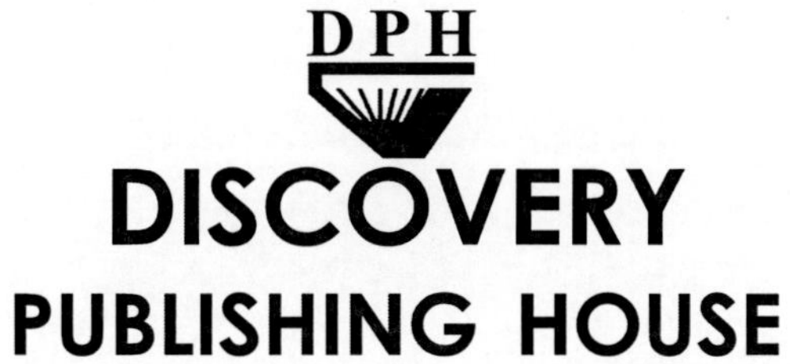

Published by:

DISCOVERY PUBLISHING HOUSE
4383/4B, Ansari Road, Darya Ganj
New Delhi-110 002 (India)
Phone : +91-11-23279245; 23253475; 43596065
E-mail : discoverybooksindia@gmail.com
discoverypublishinghouse@gmail.com
namitwasan9@gmail.com
web : www.discoverypublishinggroup.com

***First Edition:* 2011**
***Reprinted:* 2025**

ISBN: 978-81-8356-734-3

Pharmaceutical Products

Printed at:
Infinity Imaging Systems
Delhi

Preface

The present title "Pharmaceutical Products" has been written for those in the pharmaceutical research and those responsible for the education and training in pharmaceutical science and technology of graduate and undergraduate students. Medicine is an ever changing science. As new research and clinical experience broaden our knowledge, changes in treatment and drug therapy are required. This branch of life science has progressed enormously in recent years and the significant advances in therapeutics and an understanding of the need to optimize during delivery in the body have brought about an increased awareness of the valuable role played by the dosage forms. This statement is as true as it was back in ninteenth century and perhaps more so, given the increasing emphasis being placed on discovery, development, and use of large molecular entities as therapeutic and diagnostic agents. Development of these abilities requires an integration of knowledge, skills, attitudes, and values that can be acquired only through structured learning process including independent study, hands on practice and the availability of advanced literature. This tittle has designed to meet such needs of learners in the health professions.

In the last two decades, the pharmaceutical industry has experimented and successfully adopted several integrated and multidisciplinary approaches in the research areas of dring compound screening, toxicological evaluation, and pharmaceutical product development. The book is written in a concise style that facilitates an in-depth level of understanding of the essential concepts. The objectives of the present title are three folds: (i) to serve as a useful tool to help guide scientists in research and development by out-lining the theory and successful practice of in vitro - in vivo correlation, (ii) to help formulators apply the tool in designing and developing prototypes that enable selection of clinical formulations, and (iii) to help formulate strategy(ies) for product life-cycle management.

To make the work more comprehensive and informative, the author has consulted many authoritative books, research journals, abstracts, monographs etc., so there can be no claim to originality except in the manner of treatment.

The author expresses his thanks to his friends and colleagues whose continue inspirations have initiated him to bring out this book.

The author expresses his gratitude to Mr. Wasan and staff of M/s Discovery Publishing House Pvt. Ltd. for their whole hearted co-operation in the publication of this book.

Author

CONTENTS

1

INTRODUCTION

Biotechnology and biotechnology-based methods are increasing in importance in medical therapies and diagnostics as well as in the discovery, development, and manufacture of pharmaceuticals. Biotechnologically manufactured pharmaceuticals will soon reach a market volume of more than $100 billion USD and, thus, some 20% of the total pharmaceutical market. The key step in their manufacture is the conversion of the genetic information into a product with the desired pharmacological activities by an appropriate selection, design, and cultivation of cells and microorganisms harboring the corresponding biosynthetic pathways and physiological properties.

The intention of this chapter is to give insights into the typical issues and problems encountered in the manufacture of biopharmaceuticals, to mediate general ideas and current strategies on how to proceed in the design and development of biotechnological processes, and to deliver the immediate theoretical backgrounds necessary for comprehension rather than to give detailed experimental instructions like a manual does. In focusing on gene recombinant proteins and peptidic antibiotics, the biotechnologically produced pharmaceuticals with the highest market share, representative aspects will be discussed (1) for process development and optimization approaches to increase product yield and process rentability and to ensure a consistent product quality, (2) for experimental approaches to design and to modify the molecular structure of compounds to meet specific medical needs, (3) for the replacement of chemical procedures by economically and ecologically advantageous biotechnological processes, (4) for critical issues of product purification, and (5) for specific demands in pharmaceutical production to conform to regulatory requirements. Finally, the advantage of an integrative biotechnology is emphasized, which designs the biosynthetic steps of the product in accordance with the requirements of product purification procedures already during early development stages.

PRODUCTION ORGANISMS AND EXPRESSION SYSTEMS

Design and development of all microbial production processes start with the selection of appropriate organisms, strains, and expression systems enabling high yields and high quality of a desired product with defined pharmacological properties.

Industrially Established Recombinant Expression Systems

Industrially established expressions systems for production of the marketed compounds are, besides inclusion, body-forming *Escherichia coli* strains, the yeast *Saccharomyces cerevisiae* and mammalian cells like CHO- and BHK-cells. These systems were the genetically and physiologically most advanced and therefore mostly applied when recombinant production processes were starting to be developed in the mid-1980s and are now widely accepted by regulatory bodies. *E. coli* and *S. cerevisiae* can be grown cheaply and rapidly, are amenable to high cell density fermentations with biomasses of up to

130 g/L, possess short generation times, have high capacities to accumulate foreign proteins, are easy to handle, and are established fermentation organisms.

However, because gene recombinant pharmaceuticals continuously gain an increasing importance in medicine and are expected to help curing diseases that are not yet treatable today, new expression systems have to be exploited enabling the production of such pharmaceuticals with innovative properties that simultaneously meet key criteria like consistent product quality and cost effectiveness. Of particular interest in this regard are expression systems enabling the secretion of correctly glycosylated and folded proteins into the culture broth. Such secretory systems offer advantages in terms of simple and fast product purification procedures and the avoidance of costly cell rupture, denaturation, and refolding processes and thus conform to the requirements of an integrated production process.

Even though animal and plant systems (molecular pharming) and secretory plant cell culture systems have received a great deal of attention, their commercial feasibility is still under investigation, particularly with respect to their slightly different posttranslational modification modus leading to an altered pharmacological behavior and to allergenic properties. Established in the pharmaceutical industry as production organisms are, besides the above-mentioned systems, further prokaryotic and yeast species as well as filamentous fungi, which are already employed for the manufacture of natural products.

The suitability of the most prominent secretory systems among these organisms from the viewpoint of an integrative process design for the manufacture of recombinant proteins will be evaluated in the next section by discussing their potential productivity and their physiological properties.

Evaluation of Secretory Expression Systems for Pharmaceutical Purposes

Escherichia coli

As *E. coli* lacks fundamental prerequisites for efficient secretion, the marketed pharmaceuticals manufactured by *E. coli*-systems are mostly produced as inclusion bodies. Due to the membrane structure, the low chaperone and foldase level and the high periplasmatic protease concentration *E. coli*-secretion systems allow only comparably low product yields, making them suitable only for compounds marketed in small quantities like orphan drugs. Genentech, for instance, has patented a secretory *E. coli*-system for the preparation of human growth hormone. The secretory potential of *E. coli* is indicated by exceptional high product titers in the range of several grams per liter, which were reached in a system developed for secretion of hirudin using the alpha-cyclodextringlykosysl-transferase signal sequence as a leader und secretor mutants deficient in their membrane structure. Titers of human-insulin-like-growth-factor or human-epidermal-growth-factor were reported to be as high as 900 mg/L and 325 mg/L, respectively.

Most of the reached and published data, however, refers to processes leading to a periplasmatic product concentration (e.g., 2 g/L of a human antibody fragment, 700 mg/L of a monoclonal antibody) or stays below 100 mg/L, a value that generally is not considered to be in a competitive and economic range. Efforts are thus undertaken to condition *E. coli*-strains to efficient secreters. The main strategies to enhance secretion efficiency comprise (1) employment of well-characterized secretion pathways like the alpha-hemolysin system or components of such pathways like efficient signal sequences from efflux proteins or outer membrane proteins, for instance, the maltose binding protein or the TolC-protein; (2) variation of the signal peptide; (3) cocloning of and coexpression of chaperones and foldases; (4) enhancement of gene expression by employment of strong promotors and efficient transcription termination sequences; (5) generation of protease deficient mutants; (6) generation of cell wall lacking or cell wall deficient mutants; and (7) modulation of the protein primary structure that was found to exert a strong influence on productivity and secretion efficiency by influencing protease resistance, folding efficiency, and the tendency to form inclusion bodies.

Alternative prokaryotic expression systems

In addition to conditioning *E. coli*-strains to efficient secreters, alternative species, which are considered to inherently possess a superior secretion capacity, are tried to be established as expression systems. Comparably high product yields of 2 g/L and 1 g/L were reported for production of human calcitonin by *Staphylococcus carnosus* and of proinsulin by *Bacillus subtilis*, an organism that is continuously characterized and improved as a cell factory for pharmaceutical proteins. *Bacillus megaterium*, which is thought to be as efficient as *B. subtilis*, is currently developed as a secretory expression system by a Collaborative Research Center (SFB) of the German Research Community (DFG). For *Ralstonia eutropha* (formerly *Alcaligenes eutrophus*), employed at ICI and Monsanto for polyhydroxyalkanoate production at a scale of several 100 m^3 and genomically completely sequenced, 1,2 g/L of secreted organophosphohydrolase, a model enzyme proned to form inclusion bodies in *E. coli*, were reported. *R. eutropha* displays a more efficient carbohydrate metabolism than *E. coli* and is easily amenable to high cell density fermentations with biomass concentration of more than 150 g/L dry weight. This permits a lower specific productivity that in turn reduces the inclinement to form inclusion bodies and thus enables a more efficient secretion. *Rhodococcus*, *Corynebacterium*, *Mycobacterium*, actinomycetes, and streptomycetes are also considered to be potentially suitable for the development of efficient secretion systems.

A comparative study with recombinant alpha-amylase demonstrated that final yields as well as enzyme activity were considerably higher when produced by *Streptomyces lividans*, by which it was completely secreted than by *E. coli* in which it was concentrated periplasmatically. The yields reported so far, however, are still below costefficient ranges. A system developed by Hoechst/Aventis for insulin production yielded around 100 mg/L, and the yields of correctly folded human CD4-receptor sites are in the range of 200 mg/L. Attached as signal proteins were the prepeptide of the alpha-amylase inhibitor from *S. tendae* (tendamistat) and the signal sequence of a protease inhibitor (LTI) from *S. longisporus*. In the course of these studies, it was found that the choice of the linker and its length strongly influences secretion efficiency. The comparably low yields, however, demonstrate that still a lot of fundamental research is necessary to render streptomyces systems competitive. A general focus of research will be the detailed exploration of the twin arginine translocation (TAT) pathway, which has been recently discovered in addition to the conventional prokaryotic secretory (sec) pathways and enables the export of proteins with cofactors in a fully folded conformation. It evidently plays a more important role in *Streptomyces* species but might also be useable in other species.

As the potential and capacity of prokaryotes for prosttranslational modification appear to be quite limited and the knowledge about the pathways is quite scarce, the employability of most of the known prokaryotes usually is restricted to the preparation of proteins that are naturally not glycosylated, such as insulin, hirudins, or somatotropins, or to natively glycosylated proteins that are pharmacologically also active without glycosylation, like various cytokines (tumor necrosis factor, interleukines, interferones). For production of proteins that are pharmacologically active only with an appropriate modification pattern, eukayotic cell systems are more suitable.

Yeasts

Besides possessing complex posttranslational modification pathways, they offer the advantage to be neither pyrogenic nor pathogenic and to secrete more efficiently. Species established in industrial production procedures are *Saccharomyces cerevisiae*, *Kluyveromyces lactis*, *Pichia pastoris*, and *Hansenula polymorpha*, which will be dealt with more in detail in this section. Whereas *S. cerevisiae* is the best genetically characterized eukaryotic organism at all and still is the prevalent yeast species in pharmaceutical production processes, *P. pastoris*, first employed by Phillips Petroleum for single-cell-protein production, is currently the most frequently used yeast species for heterologous protein expression in general. Whereas only just a few proteins were expressed by *Pichia* species at the beginning of the last decade, the expression of more than 400 proteins have been meanwhile reported now. *P. pastoris* is considered to be superior to any other known yeast species with respect to its secretion efficiency and permits the production of recombinant proteins without intense process development.

The highest yields were reported for murine collagen (15 g/L), tetanus toxin fragment C (12 g/L compared with 1 g/L in *S. cerevisiae*), human serum albumin (10 g/L compared with 3 g/L in *K. lactis* and to 90 and 150 mg/L in *S. cerevisiae*), and human interleukin 2 (10 g/L). The highest reported yields for *H. polymorpha* relate to phytase (13,5 g/L) and to hirudin (g/L range) and for *K. lactis* to human serum albumin (3 g/L). Even though *S. cerevisiae* offers a high secretory potential as evidenced by some 9-g/L secreted *Aspergillus niger* glucose oxidase, such data document a general inferior secretory capacity, the reasons for which are numerous. For the methylotrophic species *Hansenula* and *Pichia* and the lactose using *K. lactis*, natively strong promoters are available that derive from the methanol and lactose assimilating pathways and their enzymes (e.g., alcohol- and methanol oxidase, lactose permease, galactosidase).

As the enzymes of these pathways account for up to 30% of the total protein content, the metabolic efficiency with respect to the secreted protein is significantly higher as documented by Buckholz and Gleeson: Only one or a few gene copies are sufficient in *P. pastoris* to gain the same yields as with 50 gene copies in *S. cerevisiae*. Furthermore, proteins with a molecular mass of above 30 kD are retained in the cytoplasma of *S. cerevisiae*, whereas *H. polymorpha* efficiently secretes proteins with a molecular mass of up to 150 kD, like the glucoamylase of *Aspergillus niger*. Further reasons for the differing secretion rates among the species are the specific proteolytic activities and the specific degrees and patterns of glycosylation. Besides having an impact on the protein's final pharmacological activity, glycosylation also exercises an influence on the folding and secretion efficiency. Among the discussed species, *S. cerevisiae* was shown to possess, besides a higher enzymatic activity in the secretion vesicles that leads to a reduced portion of intact secreted proteins, also the highest glycosylation capacity leading to a hyperglycosylation of the protein and a reduced secretion rate. Both the degree and the pattern of glycosylation are dependent on the genetic background of the species and strains employed as well as on the sequences of the expressed protein and adjacent regions.

By employment of the natively highly glycosylated alpha-mating type factor as a secretion signal, the extent of the glycosylation of the product can be diminished or completely avoided as shown for human interleukin 6. NovoNordisk reported leader sequence-dependent insulin yields in *S. cerevisiae* and in *S. cerevisiae* and *P. pastoris*: The sequence and therewith the degree of glycosylation of the leader influences the efficiency of the multistage cleavage and folding processes as well as the insulin glycosylation rate and secretability. Further enhancement of the secretion efficiency can be achieved by (1) mutating secretion enhancer genes, (2) suppressing secretion blocking functions, and (3) reducing proteolytic activities in secretion vesicles. So-called supersecreter strains of *S. cerevisiae* have, for instance, been generated by inactivation of the PMR1 (SSC1) function and suppression of the secretion blocking ypt1-1 gene: the yields of non-glycosylated human pro-urokinase, of human serum albumin, and of human plasminogen-activator have been augmented to a factor of up to 10. The traditional approaches pursued for enhancement of gene expression are gene amplification, employment of strong promoters, and enhancement of the transcription and translation rate.

A high amplification of the gene copy number usually is achievable with episomal vectors, which however do not reach the mitotic stability of integrative systems like the transposon (e.g., Ty-element) mediated embedment of reiterative, dispers repetitive sequences in *S. cerevisae*. Transcription rates were reported to be enhanced up to 100 times through cotransformation with transcription activators and enhancers, which evidently are limiting factors for overexpression of foreign proteins. Translation efficiency can be enhanced by preventing an accelerated degradation of transcripts and the yeast typical random transcription termination through modulation of the recognition sequences. Prevention of the random transcription termination led to an increase of tetanus toxin fragment C yields in *S. cerevisiae* by a factor 2000–3000 to 1 g/L and 3% of the total soluble protein fraction.

Table 1.1. Typical sequence of biotechnological production process steps

Step	*Method/approach*
Selection/design/engineering/development of an appropriate species/strain/expression system	*Criteria*: pharmacological activity and properties of the compound, productivity, process behavior, suitability for downstream processing steps, spectrum and and pharmacological activity of side products to be removed, experimental experience with the respective system, biological and medical safety, acceptance by regulatory bodies
Strain improvement	Mutation/selection, strain recombination (e.g., breeding/protoplast fusion), directed genomic alteration/ metabolic engineering/enhancement of gene expression rates
Biosynthetic product structure modification	Amino acid exchange/combinatorial biosynthesis/precursor directed biosynthesis
Fermentation optimization	Empirical optimization of culture conditions (media components, pH, oxygen supply), clarification of the influence of process parameters on growth, productivity and side product formation
Fermentation scale-up	Detailed process characterization for reduction of stress exposure, insurance of homogenized reaction conditions, and identification of suitable scale-up parameters (e.g., with the help of chemometric modeling, computational fluid dynamics)
Downstream processing	
Cell separation and harvest, removal of particulate matters	Centrifugation (decanter, disk-stack separator, (semi) continuous centrifuges), filtration (dead-end, tangential flow filtration)
Cell rupture	High-pressure homogenization, bead mills, sonication, enzymatic treatments
Product capture	Filtration (micro-, ultra-, nano-filtration), precipitation, solvent extraction, ion exchange, size exclusion, affinity chromatography
Product purification/polishing	Hydrophobic interaction/reversed-phase chromatography
Clearance of contaminant agents (e.g., viruses, endotoxins)	Nano-filtration, heat, pH, chemical inactivation, ultraviolet, gamma irradiation
Drying	Heat, freezing, vacuum
Galenic preparation/filling	Addition of galenic excipients, supplements, stabilizers, and adjuvants

Despite their physiologically advantageous properties and natively high expression and secretion capacity, just one industrial application is reported for each of the alternative yeast species: *H. polymorpha* is employed for hepatitis B vaccine production at Rhein-Biotech, *K. lactis* for bovine prochymosin production in a 40-m^3 scale at Gist-Brocades, and *P. pastoris* for production of recombinant carboxypeptidase B and trypsin at Roche. For pharmaceutical application, it has to be considerered that the methylotrophic yeasts in contrast to *S. cerevisiae* and *K. lactis* are not used in the production of foodstuffs and therewith have no GRAS (generally regarded as safe) status according to the U.S. Food and Drug Administration (FDA) criteria and have to be grown in expensive explosion-proofed equipments when the above- mentioned native induction systems are used. The employ-ability of yeasts in some cases however might reach a limit, particularly when the pharmacological activity of the product is impaired by the glycosylation pattern. In *K. lactis*, for instance, which usually does not hyperglycosylate, an exceptional high glycosylation of human interleukin 1â has been observed, reducing the biological activity to 5%. In such cases, a postsynthetic chemical modification has to be considered or the employment of higher developed organisms.

Filamentous fungi

Filamentous fungi are higher organized than yeasts and consequently have a more complex posttranslational modification apparatus more similar to mammals. Some proteins like t-PA in *Aspergillus nidulans* are produced with the natural human glycosylation pattern. For recombinant protein production, species are prefered, which are broadly employed in industry for production of enzymes, acids and antibiotics and thus possess GRAS-status: *A. nidulans*, *A. niger*, *A. sydowii*, *A. awamori*, various *Fusarium* and *Trichoderma* species, *Penicillium chrysogenum*, and *Acremonium chrysogenum*. Their productivity and secretion potential, which is in the range of 30–40 g/L for homologous enzymes like cellulases and amylases, is considered to be superior to any other system, but unfortunately could not be converted into corresponding yields of recombinant products, even when these were fused to such homologous enzymes. The highest yields are still obtained with heterologous fungal enzymes: 4-g/L *Fusarium* protease in *A. chrysogenum* and 4.6-g/L *A. niger* glucoamylase in *A. awamori*. The highest yield of a mammalian protein was reported for human interleukin 6 in *A. sojae* in a range of 300 mg/L. The yields of most human proteins like t-PA and various interferons, however, were reported to be below 1 mg/L.

Possible reasons for these incompetitive yields are restrictions in posttranslational metabolic steps like intracellular transport, folding, and processing. Even though filamentous fungi are industrially used now for decades, they are not adequately characterized on the physiological and genetic level. Little is known about details of the modification and secretion metabolism, and efficient gene transformation is hampered by degradation of foreign DNA, low transformation rate, and therefore, low copy numbers of the transferred genes and random genomic integration. Expression rates are restricted by a high RNA turnover, incorrect processing of the foreign messenger, and incomplete folding and secretion, which are, as in yeasts, both influenced by the glycosylation pattern. Proteins not completely or incorrectly glycosylated and excreted are rapidly degraded as shown for human interleukin 6. Currently, filamentous fungi cannot be regarded as a serious alternative for the production of pharmaceuticals. To fully exploit the potential of filamentous fungi, their physiology, particularly the glycosylation metabolism, thus has to be investigated and clarified in more detail.

Insect and mammalian cell cultures

Animal cell cultures are the systems with highest similarity to human cells with respect to the pattern and capacity of posttranslational modifications. However, their cultivation is more complicated and costly and usually yields lower product titers. Among the known systems, insect cells transformed by baculovirus vectors have reached a comparable popularity as *Pichia* among yeasts because they are considered to be more stress resistant, easier to handle, and more productive compared with mammalian systems and are thus frequently employed for high-throughput protein expression. The highest reported yields refer to human collagenase IV in *Trichoplusia* (300 mg/L). Yields reported for non-insect cultures were 80 mg/L for human apolipoprotein A1 in chinese hamster ovary (CHO)-cells and 1 mg/L for human laminin in human embryonal kidney cells.

For commercial application scale-up, related questions have to be clarified, particularly concerning oxygen supply and carbon dioxide accumulation, stability of the cell line, and the bioreactor type to be employed. Further deficiencies of insect cells are observed in (1) an inefficient processing and an impairment of the folding and secretion capacity due to the baculovirus infection; (2) the high, in part baculovirus encoded, protease activity and the resulting necessity to routinely employ protease inhibitors in the culture media or to develop protease deficient vectors; (3) an insufficient expression strength; and (4) deviations of the posttranslational modification pattern, which could act immunogenic. For optimization, the construction of new innovative vectors and the coexpression of chaperones, foldases, and folding factors such as canexin have been suggested as has been the broader development and application of alternative systems like *Drosophila*. Preferably applied in pharmaceutical production processes are mammalian systems like CHO- and baby hamster kidney (BHK)-cells. These systems are generally considered to be genetically more stable and easier to transform and to handle in scale-up processes, grow faster in adherent and submerged cultures, and are more similar to human cells and more consistent in their complete spectrum of modification, which minimizes the risk of the formation of structurally altered compounds with immunogenic properties.

In some cases, mammalian systems can be the only choice for the preparation of correctly modified proteins. Studies of Tate et al. comparing the expression of a rat serotonin transporter in various expression systems demonstrate that biologically active transporter was only synthesized in mammalian cells, whereas it was partially degraded in *E. coli*, not correctly folded in *Pichia* and not correctly glycosylated in insect cells. CHO- and BHK-cells further have the advantage to be recognized as safe regarding infectious and pathogenic agents and therefore to have a higher acceptance by regulatory bodies, which accelerates or at least does not delay approval procedures.

Criteria for the Choice of Recombinant Expression Systems

In summary, the criteria for the choice of an expression system in pharmaceutical production are the existing expertise, the available physiological and genetic know-how and tools, the patent situation, and to avoid delays of product launch and commercialization, regulatory aspects like the acceptance by the approving authorities.

The overall decision criteria, however, is the pharmacological activity profile of the yielded protein in context with the posttranslational modification pattern followed by rentability.

For production of non-glycosylated proteins and proteins that are natively glycosylated but pharmacologically active also without glycosylation, prokaryotes, which usually lack metabolic pathways for glycosylation, theoretically are the most suitable organisms, offering two alternatives: Either *E. coli*-strains are conditioned to efficient secreters, or efficient native secreters like *Bacillus*-species are accordingly developed. To fully exploit the secretion capacity of fungal species, a deeper understanding of their posttranslational modification physiology will be necessary to steer the degree and pattern of glycosylation, which influences both folding and secretion efficiency. Insect and mammalian cells display posttranslational modification patterns more similar or identical to humans, but in view of the entailed expenditures, their employment can only be justified if their modification machinery is required to ensure a desired pharmacological activity.

E. coli, *P. pastoris*, and Baculovirus-based systems are currently preferred in fundamental research for structural and functional analysis of proteins and are employed as high-throughput-expression systems but will certainly find their ways into production processes in the near future. None of the systems, however, can be considered to be generally superior to any other. For each product, the most suitable expression system has to be identified and optimized individually both on the genetic and on the fermentative level by taking into account the properties of the product, the organism, and the expression cassettes, which suggests to always have a set of accordingly developed expression systems available.

Table 1.2. Features and characteristics of expression systems

Property	*Bacteria*	*Yeast*	*Insect and mammalian cell cultures*
Growth	Fast	Fast	Slow
Nutrient demand	Minimal	Minimal	Complex
Costs of media	Low	Low	High
Possible product yield	High	High	Low
Secretory capacity	Limtited	High	Medium
Glycosylation capacity	Limited	High	High
Modification capacity	Limited	High	High
Risk of retroviral Contamination	Low	Low	High
Risk of pyrogens	High	—	—
Scalability	Good	Good	Low
Process robustness	Good	Good	Low

Once an expression system has been selected, the respective strains are continuously submitted to improvement programs to render fermentation processes more efficient by increasing strain productivity and by modifying physiological properties and process behavior to enhance process economy. This does not only apply to the fermentation process, but also to parts of downstream processing, thus requiring an integrated strain selection and process design.

Enhancement of Productivity

Secretory Recombinant Expression Systems

In terms of downstream processing efficiency, secretory expression systems indeed offer potential advantages for production of recombinant proteins compared with inclusion body-forming cytosolic systems, but most of the potentially available secretory systems are not yet fully competitive for high-volume therapeutics like insulin and therefore still require intensive improvement efforts.

Current strategies to improve productivity and secretion efficiency comprise (1) enhancement of gene expression rates, (2) optimization of secretion signal sequences, (3) coexpression of chaperones and foldases, (4) creation of protease deficient mutants to avoid premature product degradation, and (5) subsequent breeding and mutagenesis.

Natural Products

Completely different is the situation faced in the production of the so-called natural products, which are mostly secondary metabolites and therewith the endproducts of complex biosynthetic pathways of filamentous bacteria and fungi and thus require different approaches. With few exceptions like the antidiabetic drug acarbose or the chosterol-lowering drug lovastatin, such fermented pharmaceuticals of natural origin currently belong for the most part to the class of antibiotics.

Enhancement of the productivity is achieved at first by rounds of random mutation and selection and, if possible, by breeding, and/or by DNA injection or fusion techniques like protoplasting and at further stages, after a com prehensive characterization of the usually complex biosynthetic pathways, directed genomic alterations and metabolic engineering. These approaches, developments, and states in industrial strain improvement and pathway characterization will be illustrated for some of the best characterized organisms, namely the two fungal species mainly employed in industrial β-lactam antibiotic production, the penicillin producing *Penicillium chrysogenum*, and the cephalosporin C producer *Acremonium chrysogenum*.

Characterization of biosynthetic pathways

The productivity of *Penicillium chrysogenum* could have been augmented impressively during the last decades: Penicillin titers have been increased by a factor of 50,000 from a very few milligrams/ Liter in the 1940s to more than several 10 g/L by now and also some several 10 g/L cephalosporin are currently gained. This development, however, has come to a halt during the last couple of years. As these titers have been reached through conventional mutation and selection and no further significant increase in productivity could be noted, the tools of genetic engineering were more and more included into the improvement programs. To gain a profound basis for directed genomic alterations, studies were conducted at various corporations and universities to elucidate the mechanisms and genes involved in β-lactam biosynthesis to characterize the respective biosynthetic pathways.

Cephalosporin C synthesis in acremonium chrysogenum

Biosynthesis starts with the polymerization of L-α-aminoadipic acid, L-cysteine, and L-valine to the linear tripeptide L-α-aminoadipyl-L-cysteinyl-D-valine (ACV-peptide). This reaction is catalyzed by the ACV-synthase (MW about 420 kD) through the following steps: (1) the ATP-dependent activation of these amino acids to bind them as thiolesters, (2) the epimerization of L-valine, and finally (3) the condensation by a thiotemplate mechanism.

Cyclization of the ACV-peptide to the bicyclic isopenicillin N (IPN) occurs under oxygen-, Fe^{2+}-, ascorbate-, and α-ketoglutarate-dependent action of the IPN-synthase (IPNS), which has an MW of about 38 kD. Inhibitory to IPNS activity are cobalt ions and glutathione.

Further pathway reactions are as follows:

1. IPN-epimerization to penicillin N (IPN-epimerase).
2. Penicillin N conversion to deacetoxycephalosporin C (DAOC) by expansion of the five-membered thiazolidine ring to a 6 C-dihydrothiazine-ring (DAOC-expandase).
3. Formation of deactylcephalosporin C (DAC) by dehydroxylation and oxidation of the methylgroup in C3-position (DAC-hydroxylase).
4. The acylation of DAC to cephalosporin C (DAC acetyltransferase).

DAOC-expandase and DAC-hydroxylase activities in *A. chrysogenum* are exerted by the same enzyme (MW 41 kD), which like the IPNS belongs to the group of α-ketoglutarate-dependent dioxygenases.

The first two enzymes, ACV- and IPN-synthase, are encoded by the *pcbAB*- and the *pcb C* gene, respectively. Both genes are linked to each other on chromosome VI by a 1.2-kb intergenic region carrying the putative promotor sequences from which they are divergently transcribed. The *pcb C*-promotor seems to be about five times stronger than the one of the *pcbAB*-gene. The *cefEF*-gene and the *cefG*-gene encoding for the bifunctional expandase/hydroxylase and the DAC-acetyltransferase, respectively, are located adjacent to each other on chromosome II. Again the genes are separated by an intergenic region of 938 bp, which is supposed to harbor the promotors from which they are transcribed in opposite directions. The *cefG*-gene has been proven to contain two introns. Due to an extreme *in vitro* lability, no information is yet available on the epimerase converting IPN to penicillin N as well as its putative *cefD* gene. Until recently, the structure of the *cefD* gene could have not been elucidated. Meanwhile, data could have been obtained indicating the existence of two reading frames (*cefD1* and *cefD2*) containing all characteristic motifs of mammalian acyl-CoA ligases and a-methylacyl-CoA racemases. Regulatory studies demonstrated that the early functions are expressed simultaneously, whereas the later pathway genes *cefD* and *cefEF* seem to be induced sequentially. In contrast, the penicillin biosynthesis genes in *P. chrysogenum* are considered to be expressed completely concomitantly.

Penicillin formation by penicillium chrysogenum

The first reactions of the penicillin biosynthetic pathway are identical to the ones in *A. chrysogenum*. IPN, however, is not epimerized to penicillin N; instead it is converted to 6- aminopenicillanic acid (6-APA) by removal of the L-α-aminoadipic acid side chain, which is substituted by a hydrophobic acyl group. Both steps are catalyzed by the same enzyme, the acyl coenzyme A: IPN acyltransferase (IAT). The enzymatic activity of IAT is believed to be the result of the processing of a 40-kD monomeric precursor into a dimeric form consisting of two subunits with MWs of 11 and 29 kD. Due to the broad substrate specifity of IAT, various penicillin derivatives are synthesized naturally by attachment of different acyl-CoA derivatives to the 6-APA-core. For industrial purposes, to facilitate extraction by organic solvents, synthesis usually is directed to the less hydrophilic penicillin V or penicillin G. This is by addition of phenoxyacetic acid or phenylacetic acid, respectively, as precursors to the culture broth. The IAT encoding *penDE*-gene (also named *aatA*) is located on chromosome I and organized as a cluster together with the ACV-synthase and IPN-synthase encoding genes *pcbAB* (also named *acvA* in *Penicillium*) and *pcbC* (*ipnA*).

The enzymes involved in penicillin biosynthesis are distributed at different sites of the cell: ACV-activity was found to be bound to vacuole membranes, IPN-synthase occurs dissolved in the cytoplasm and IAT-activity is microbody associated.

Approaches and Goals for Further Strain Improvement

Analysis and comparison of strains

To get hints for more rational strain improvement approaches, (1) highly mutated production strains were gene tically and physiologically compared with their less-productive ancestors, (2) concentrations of pathway intermediates were determined to identify potential pathway bottlenecks, and (3) regulatory mechanisms were investigated.

In the course of such studies, high-performance strains of *P. chrysogenum* turned out to possess amplified copies of single genes like the *pcbC* gene or even copies of the whole cluster as well as increased steady-state transcript levels of pathway genes. In some strains, the amplifications were shown to be organized in tandem repeats, which presumably were generated by a hot-spot TTTACA hexanukleotide. Comparison of promotor strengths of these genes from high and low productive strains did not reveal any differences. This indicates the involvement of additional unknown trans-acting factors, as the amounts of increased mRNA did not correlate with the degree of gene amplification. Also a high specific activity of IPN synthase was reported in a more evolved *Penicillium* strain, which was independent from transcript amounts and probably due to a higher enzyme stability.

In *A. chrysogenum*, no amplification of the relevant genes could be detected. Nevertheless, transcript amounts in production strains are significantly increased. Also chromosome rearrangements could be detected in high titer strains, but their causative influence on productivity remains unclarified for the moment.

Directed genomic alterations

Enhancement of gene expression

Considering these findings, the experiments conducted so far to improve productivity mainly concentrated on enhancing the pathway gene dosages and on enhancing promotor strengths to remove presumed pathway bottlenecks. For instance, the *cefEF*-activity was generally believed to constitute a potential rate-limiting step in view of the high accumulation of penicillin N in various strains of *A. chrysogenum* and accordingly amplified. Such approaches resulted in partially significant increases of productivity in low and medium titer strains: Improvements of the final yields by 50% have been reported. However, all improvements achieved so far with high-performance production strains remained with a 5% maximum in the range of normal statistical deviations.

Also more exotic approaches like the (presumed) improvement of the intracellular oxygen supply through cloning and expressing of a bacterial hemoglobin gene from *Vitreoscilla* failed to increase productivity in high titer strains.

The reasons for these failures are manifold:

1. As both direction and site of integration of the imported DNA cannot be controlled sufficiently and transformation efficiency is still quite low, the probability of finding new, higher producing mutants even in a large-scale screening is rare.
2. Most of the data available are from studies performed at academic institutions with original strains. Even when sharing the same ancestral strain, the high-performance strains employed in industries have an individual genealogy and mutation-selection history, so that their physiological behavior and properties differ drastically. Data and knowledge obtained with a particular strain thus cannot always be generalized and transfered to other strains. Even among industrial strains, significant differences have been revealed. For instance, the expression of the *cefG*-gene and the acetyl transferase activity was reported to constitute a possible rate-limiting step in Panlabs-strains. Studies conducted on other industrial strains, however, could not confirm this observation.
3. The genetic instability and drift rises with the degree of genomic alterations, particularly during long-term vegetative propagation with numerous generation cycles in industrial large-scale fermentations.
4. The complex interdependence with other metabolic areas is not yet completely investigated. Consequently, after removal of an obvious β-lactam pathway bottleneck, unknown reaction steps of the linked and preceding pathways might become flux limiting. To overcome such flux limitations, one of the most exciting recent discoveries in molecular biology, namely RNA interference (RNAi), might play a major role in the future.

Possible impact of RNAi in strain improvement

The mechanisms of post-transcriptional gene silencing, generally summed up as RNAi offer potential approaches for the specific shut down of any gene of interest: Native genes can be silenced by triggering the RNAi cascade through introduction of homologous genetic sequences. As a result of these possibilities, RNAi has already revolutionized fundamental research in molecular biology, particularly in functional genomics, and will substantially contribute to novel therapeutic approaches in medicine. For fungi, which evidently were among the first organisms in which RNAi and associated phenomena were observed, this RNAi triggered cosuppression phenomenon has been termed "quelling" and bears an enormous potential with respect to the study of biosynthetic pathways and the improvement of metabolic productivity. On the one hand, the implication of RNAi may supply an explanation for observations made in the course of strain improvement programs of *Penicillium chrysogenum* and *Acremonium chrysogenum*, according to which antibiotic productivity can decrease drastically upon amplification of genes involved in antiobiotic biosynthesis.

The characterization and inactivation of these cosuppression mechanisms thus might help to overcome such limitations as does an application of fungal RNAi tools for silencing of pathway blocking or metabolic flux limiting genes, e.g., by the use of a novel vector system consisting of dsRNA viruses.

To fully realize the potential for further enhancement of productivity, which is generally assumed to be in the range of some 300% and to fully exploit the potential of RNAi, current and future studies thus aim at filling the actual gaps of knowledge and will be focused on

1. The exploration of regulatory mechanisms and circuits on the transcriptional, translational, and posttranslational level.
2. The determination of the specific intermediate turnover rates resulting from specific enzyme activities, enzyme titers, and enzyme stabilities.
3. The detailed investigation of linked and preceding pathways.
4. The investigation of product secretion mechanisms.

However, as no great leaps in productivity are currently reached, strains emerging from the development programs are also selected for beneficial alterations of genetic, physiological, and morphological properties that contribute to an enhanced process economy.

Improvement of process behaviour

Among the desired alterations are:

1. A decrease of side products, which (i) consume metabolic energy at the expense of the desired main product, (ii) hamper the final product purification, or (iii) even can be inhibitory to the production organism. For instance, a significant reduction of DCPC concentrations has been reached through knocking out esterases that hydrolyze cephalosporin C to DCPC during fermentation. Esterase inactivation was by conventional mutagenesis as well as through gene-disruption and by introduction of anti-sense genes.
2. Increase of the tolerance toward toxic side products and fed precursors like phenyl- or phenoxyacetic acid.
3. Further reduction of feedback inhibition by endproducts and metabolites (see below).
4. Further reduction of catabolite repression.
5. Enhancement of genetic stability.
6. Enhancement of viability, stress resistance, and life span.
7. Accelerated product formation and enhancement of time-specific productivity to shorten fermentation time.
8. Enhancement of the strain-specific productivity to reduce the amount of biomass to be processed and disposed.
9. Increase of product secretion rate.
10. Improvement of the fermentation behavior like (1) higher efficiency of substrate/precursor consumption, (2) diminished oxygen demand, and (3) diminished shear sensitivity.
11. Improvement of filterability.

The in-depth characterization of physiological properties and biosynthetic pathways not only aims at improving process behavior and process economy, but also it relates to modifications of the inherent biosynthetic pathways (pathway engineering) to create innovative, novel products with improved properties and enhanced therapeutic values, e.g., to overcome the antibiotic resistance problem, a major global health-care problem of today.

Biosynthetic Structure Modification

Although the metabolic engineering of beta-lactams by combining β-lactam encoding genes from various sources is still in an explorative state, the study of polyketide pathways and the creation of polyketide antibiotic derivatives is more advanced.

Combinatorial Biosynthesis

Compounds emerging from the polyketide pathways are the classic subject of metabolic engineering and for creation of novel structures. To create novel antibiotics, the natural biodiversity of polyketides is trying to be enhanced artificially by modifying and newly combining the biosynthetic pathway steps and enzymes involved. Polyketide synthases are multienzyme systems, which due to their modular structure and the occurrence of their encoding genes as clusters, are considered to be most amenable for directed alterations, genetic intervention, and heterologous expression in foreign hosts with different metabolic pathways. Concepts and strategies that are currently being pursued for creating novel and un-natural polyketides comprise (1) creating block mutants at various biosynthetic levels to accumulate intermediate metabolites; (2) elimination of unwanted groups; (3) modification of polyketide synthases to further broaden substrate range, eventually combined with a precursor-directed biosynthesis; (4) formation of new structures by deleting or intro ducing additional modules; (5) modification, addition, or elimination of postsynthetic modification steps like glycosylation, lactonization, and amidation; (6) the cloning and combination of various polyketide synthase genes in heterologous hosts to construct hybrid pathways and antibiotics; and (7) linking and combining routes of polyketides with pathways of nonribosomal peptide synthesis to create hybrid peptide–polyketide compounds.

As the microbial nonribosomal peptide synthases share many structural and catalytic properties with polyketide synthases like their organization into catalytic modules and domains, they are also envisaged as ideal subjects for metabolic engineering by creating large sets of modules and subsequently combining them artificially. The rapidly growing body of patents makes evident that an increasing number of companies are working on the field of combinatorial biosynthesis. However, it also becomes evident that, despite their promising prospects, these strategies of combinatorial biosynthesis are still in an initial state and need further intense research to elucidate the required genetic and physiological details.

This is just in contrast to another approach of modifying the molecular structure of peptidic compounds on the biosynthetic level, namely the directed biosynthesis of the desired compound structures by feeding of appropriate biosynthetic precursors or stimulating agents during fermentation, as it is routinely performed for production of penicillin V und G by the addition of phenoxyacetic acid or phenyl- acetic acid, respectively, as precursors to facilitate penicillin extraction from the culture broth.

Precursor Directed Biosynthesis

Microbial peptidic compounds can be modified not only in their peptide structure by direct incorporation of amino acids supplemented during fermentation but also, if present, in their fatty acid moiety. The possibilities of precursor-directed derivatization of cyclic peptides cores and fatty acid moieties by amino acids will be illustrated for three compound complexes with unique modes of action and outstanding spectra of activity against multidrug resistant germs, which were developed by Aventis, Eli Lilly, and Cubist Pharmaceuticals. The complex A1437 of Aventis is synthesized by *Actinoplanes friulensis*, which originally produced a mixture of altogether eight lipopeptides, classified according to the exocyclic amino acid position and the type of their fatty acid chains. Through addition of L-valine and asparagines, the biosynthesis could be directed toward the production of the desired D-peptide, which exhibited superior pharmacological properties in preclinical trials and is characterized by an exocyclic asparagine and an iso-C14 fatty acid moiety. The A54145 complex from Eli Lilly exhibits the noteworthy characteristic, that a built-up resistance was immediately lost in the absence of this compound. It consists of eight lipopeptides produced by *Streptomycesfradiae* containing four similar peptide nuclei in combination with three different fatty acid acyl side chains. The nuclei differ in their valine/isoleucine and glutamate β-methylglutamate substitutions at one or both of two locations of the peptide ring.

The composition of the peptide nucleus as well as the percentage of branched-chain fatty acid acyl substituents could be directed by supplementation of either valine or isoleucine. Likewise, the complex A21978 from *Streptomyces roseosporus*, also developed at Eli Lilly, can be influenced in its composition by modification of the fatty acid chain. Precursing with valine results in an enhanced formation of the compound C2, whereas the compound C1 was preferably built upon feeding of isoleucine. Compound C1 was inlicensed as daptomycin by Cubist Pharmaceuticals for clinical development. However, due to rhabdomyolytic activities and a slight haemolytic potential, it has been approved by the U.S. Food and Drug Administration in 2003 as Cubicin salve for topical use only. Despite such disadvantageous properties, peptides in general, including those that are from nonmicrobial sources and ribosomally synthesized, are currently considered to be among the most promising compound classes for development of novel antibacterials.

However, it has to be taken into account that amino acid and precursor incorporation as well as regulation mechanisms of biosynthetic pathways also depend on growth phases, on environmental influences, and thus on the conduction of the fermentation process during which the cells are propagated.

A prerequisite for a successful fermentation are controlled and homogenous environmental conditions for the cellular reactions. However, the ensurance of controlled reaction conditions, particularly in large production scales, has been turned out to be one of the most critical issues of industrial biotechnology, as will be illustrated in the next section.

Fermentation Optimization and Scale-Up

The scale-up of fermentation processes as a central problem in biotechnology was first recognized and described during industrial penicillin production at the beginning of the 1940s and has been studied in more detail in *E. coli* and recombinant protein production.

Reduced Mixing Quality and Enhanced Stress Exposure

Fermentation scale-up is aimed at the manufacture of larger product quantities, if at all possible, with a simultaneous increase or at least consistency of specific yields and product quality. The changed geometric and physical conditions in larger scales, however, has lead to a less favorable mixing behavior and to impaired physiological reaction conditions, which in turn may lead to a decreased process constance and reproducibility, to reduced specific yields, to an increase of unwanted side products, and thus ultimately, to a diminished batch-to-batch consistency and product quality, which are all key issues in industrial production processes.

The problem of reduced mixing quality in larger scales is aggravated with increasing vessel sizes: The opposite substrate and oxygen gradients along the vessel height that are formed as a result of the conventional fermenter design, according to which substrate feed usually occurs from the top and aeration from the bottom, are more pronounced in larger reactors due to (1) longer distances to be covered leading to larger substrate and oxygen depletion zones, (2) larger volumes of culture broth to be stirred and therewith longer mixing times, and (3) stronger hydraulic pressure gradients influencing the oxygen transfer rate. Cells at the fermenter top are exposed to excess glucose concentrations and simultaneously suffer from oxygen limitations, whereas those at the bottom are exposed to glucose starvation. Excess glucose concentrations (threshold value for *E. coli* at 30 mg/L) result in acetate overproduction (overflow-metabolism), and a simultaneous oxygen limitation further induces the formation of ethanol, hydrogen, formiate, lactate, and succinate (mixed acid fermentation). The produced acids can become reassimilated in oxygen-rich zones but in any case first lead to a temporary acidification of the microenvironment and later eventually of larger regions. Combined with a decreased transportation and elimination of carbon dioxide, detrimental metabolites, and surplus heat generated by agitation and metabolic processes, resulting in zonal overheating, the lower mixing rates in large scales thus lead to the formation of zones with enhanced stress conditions. The subsequent activation of stress genes only partially protects the cell against detrimental stress effects. For instance, despite activation of heat stress genes like *E. coli* dnaK and clpB, reducing misfolding and aggregation of heat-sensitive proteins, metabolic changes and damages such as translocation of proteins and membranes have been observed upon heat exposure. The evidently unavoidable detrimental effects of the repeated and cyclic passing of different stress zones and the subsequent continuous activation and shut down of the corresponding stress genes are believed to lead to a completely altered physiology with metabolic shifts, which ultimately reduce growth and productivity and increase byproduct formation.

Altered physiology

Changes in respiratory states like the switch from aerobic to anaerobic conditions and the imposed stress conditions, increased by induction and overproduction of the recombinant protein, lead to shifts in the coupled amino acid biosynthesis, an altered composition of the amino acid pools and changes in the protein biosynthesis machinery. Even though translation processes are considered to be generally performed precisely, the resulting shifts in the amino acid pool in turn lead, due to the inherent inaccuracy of the translation machinery (unspecificity of aminoacyl-tRNA-synthases, "wobbling" of tRNA), to aminoacid misincorporations in freshly synthesized proteins, particularly in phases of high protein production rates, which are characterized by amino acid shortages. Muramatsu et al. report the incorporation of β-methylnorleucin instead of isoleucin into recombinant *E. coli* hirudin in positions 29 and 59. A misincorporation of norvalin instead of leucin and methionine into human recombinant hemoglobin in *E. coli* has been published by Apostol et al. and Kiick et al. Amino acid misincorporations are thus a cause for an increase of byproducts at the expense of the desired main product yields.

Reduced plasmid stability

An essential prerequisite for high product yields particularly in larger scales, in which cultures pass a higher number of generations due to larger culture broth volumes and longer inoculation chains from the cell bank to the production stage, is the stable propagation of plasmids to daughter cells. Plasmid stability is influenced by the plasmid properties, including size and nucleotide sequence; by the genetic background of the host; as well as by process parameters like temperature, growth rates, and substrate concentrations. Lin and Neubauer show that rapid glucose oscillations favor plasmid stability and recombinant protein production rate, whereas high glucose concentrations diminish plasmid stability. Plasmid stability and plasmid numbers are thus negatively influenced, more difficult to control, and less easy to be maintained in larger scales.

A concept to render plasmid stability and expression rates more independent from such physiological influences is the application of runaway-plasmids, the replication of which can be induced separately from growth in the desired fermentation phase, enabling copy numbers of up to 1000 in the expression phase and, due to the separation of their replication and expression from the growth phase, simultaneously a more precise replication and amino acid incorporation. Further possible measures to enhance the accuracy of metabolic processes are a reduction of the generation time and numbers throughout the process and a deceleration of the metabolic speed, e.g., through reduction of temperature, and the development of more stress-resistant microbial strains.

A prioritized goal of process optimization and scale-up thus consists of an appropriate process design that improves the physiological conditions and the metabolic accuracy by minimizing microbial stress exposure.

Process Characterization

To identify process-specific stress factors and to understand the physiological responses to the vessel-specific physical conditions, the mutual influences and interactions of the various physical and physiological parameters have to be analyzed in detail. An overview on the analytical methods currently applied and yet in development is given in the following.

Analytical methods

Among the physiologically most relevant parameters are, besides the pH as discussed, biomass, cell viability, the concentrations of substrates, metabolites and products, the partial oxygen and carbon dioxide pressures in culture broth, and the composition of the exhaust gas, giving information about respiratory states as indicated, e.g., by the respiratory quotient. Established analytical methods and tools are colorimetric procedures, chromatography, mass spectroscopy, enzymatic and electrophoretic methods, hybridizing techniques, biochips, or flow cytometry. Multiparameter flow cytometry permits, in addition to the analysis of usual metabolites, also the analysis of the cellular DNA-, RNA-, and protein content, cell viability, membrane potential, intracellular pH, cell size, and cell development stages. In general, the data are, if possible, preferably captured as real-time values by in situ online measurements as occurring for physical parameters to avoid falsified or gappy data due to time differences between sampling and analysis. *Ex situ* methods can be designed as real-time procedures in combination with robust automated sampling and sample preparation methods like ultra-filtration and flow injection analysis (FIA). An online FIA glucose analysis method of the native culture broth without prior sampling and filtration has been presented by Arndt and Hitzmann and Kleist et al. For their robustness, *in situ* measurements of biological parameters are preferably performed by optical probes (optodes), working either on a physical base, e.g., by refractional or spectroscopic measurements, chemically as by ion exchange reactions or enzymatically by gel-embedded biocatalysts, the activity of which can be measured by means of pH-changes or by fluorophores (chemo- and biosensors). The hitherto employed enzymes have restricted their application mostly to the analysis of sugar compounds, whereby the most frequent applications are reported for glucose. However, despite intensive research, only a few concepts practically applicable for industrial purposes could have been developed.

Broader applications are physical optodes enabling the simultaneous measurement and quantification of several parameters and metabolites through continuous scans or excitations and subsequent absorption and scattering measurements within defined wavelength ranges like (1) 2-D-fluorescence spectroscopy as shown for the determination of NAD (P)H concentrations through excitation at 350 nm and the fluorescence measurements at 450 nm; (2) near-infrared-spectroscopy (NIR), which has been employed as a 700–2500-nm scan in the antibiotic fermentation at Pfizer for the measurement of nutrient and product as well as side product concentrations; or (3) measurements in infrared, ultraviolet, or visible wavelength spectra. By means of capacitance measuring electrodes, viable cell counts can be performed by seizing the electric capacitance and conductivity of cells with intact membranes in a generated electric field.

To gain a picture as comprehensive as possible by enhancing the amount of analyzable substances, multichannel arrays with parallel employment of various analytical procedures monitoring several parameters simultaneously have been established and new concepts like artificial noses and electronic tongues currently being integrated into fermentation technology, allowing the analysis of a large number of analytes by cross-talking semi-specific sensors that act in analogy to the human olphactory sensoric system. The realization of this concept will be facilitated by a further miniaturization of the sensors and chips employed as it has been achieved with biochips developed for the pharmaceutical natural product screening, onto which the needed number of reactants is fixed in smallest space or is brought together in microchannels and the analytes are separated in microcapillars (lab-on-a-chip-technology).

Process Optimization

For analysis, interpretation and correlation of the obtained signals and data through chemometric modeling, neural network—tools—seem to have gained an increasingly important role. Despite inherent limitations, adequately trained neural networks are capable of recognizing and revealing nonlinear, highly complex, and even nonobvious, hidden relations among a multitude of various physical, biochemical, and physiological process parameters and to design the according process models. Hooked up to expert systems, they allow immediate and short-term reactions to process deviations by anticipating physiological drifts and their influences on product yield and quality and to change the according set points and process profiles. In this way, neural network tools help to optimize process control and to facilitate the identification of suitable strategies for process optimization and scale-up, e.g., with respect to an optimized glucose–oxygen equilibrium.

As the maximum glucose and oxygen uptake rates are not constant but depend on growth phases and rates and get reduced by induction of product synthesis, Lin et al. established an integrative kinetic model combining these parameters with the aid of the simulation program SCILAB (Inria, F) enabling the determination of the maximum glucose and oxygen uptake rates through determination of the time that passes between glucose pulses and subsequent changes of partial oxygen pressure (pO_2) and biomass concentration. Such a model thus allows the alignment of the glucose feed meeting the maximum uptake capacity and therefore avoiding overflow metabolism. The observed pattern of glucose oscillation even can serve as a key parameter condition in later scale-up stages. The equilibration of carbohydrate and oxygen supply thus constitutes a key component of process control and optimization.

Further strategies aiming at the avoidance of oxygen limitation and glucose overflow metabolism consist of the employment of alternative carbon sources like glycerol or galactose and of a drastic glucose restriction. Wong et al. report that minimal concentrations of glucose and yeast extract yielded the highest concentrations of 0.5 and 1 g/L of a recombinant K99 antigen. Yim et al. achieved constant yields of 4.4 g/L of human granulocyte colony stimulating factor during scale-up from 2.5 to 30 L by limiting glucose feed and keeping the growth rate at the minimum (μ = 0.116 h^{-1}). Besides the above-mentioned parameters like the maximum uptake capacities, the various different physiological or directly measurable physical process parameters like pH, ammonium consumption, pO_2, OTR, or the growth parameters can be applied as a reference parameter for glucose feed in a closed-loop design. Dantigny et al. describe a biomass controlling feed depending on the ethanol formation rate and RQ for *S. cerevisiae*. To achieve a more uniform glucose distribution in large-scale tanks, Larsson et al. and Bylund et al. suggested a glucose feed at the dynamic zones of the fermenter bottom together with the injected air. A step ahead in this regard would be a further enhancement of the mixing quality by a reactor and process design permitting a multilevel injection of both air and substrates into high turbulence zones.

A supportive approach for comprehension of the large-scale hydrodynamic and reaction conditions to ensure homogenous reaction conditions and to reduce both the size of stress zones and the zonal residence times is the depiction of these zones through transfer into small reactors (scale-down) or through high-performance computing computational fluid dynamics (CFD). Whereas the sort and amount of parameters that can be simulated by the scale-down approach appear to be restricted, CFD is meanwhile broadly applied, e.g., the flow modeling software tools of Fluent Inc., Lebanon, NH. A simulation of the trajectories and distributions of gas bubbles and mass transports enables the determination of zonal pO_2 values and oxygen transfer rates. The combination with parameters like substrate concentrations and gradients, the residence times in the respective zones, population dynamics, and metabolic fluxes (structured metabolic models) leads to integrative models (integrated fluid dynamics, IFD), which permit the prediction of physiological effects and reactions. Even though it is emphasized that the integration of CFD and structured biokinetics currently requires a deeper understanding of the dynamics of metabolic and regulatory networks and cascades of signal transduction triggered by microenvironmental fluctuations and thus further research, it will most likely contribute long term to a realistic modeling of the interplay between physics and physiology and thus will facilitate the identification of key parameters influencing product yield and quality the most and therewith of suitable scale-up parameters and strategies.

Physical Scale-Up Parameters

Suitable for employment as physical scale-up parameters are all known process parameters and coefficients exerting known physiological effects, particularly those affecting oxygen supply; heat transportation and mixing, such as power input, aeration, and agitation rate; mixing time; pO_2; OTR; oxygen mass transfer coefficient; and biocalorimetric variables like heat fluxes and heat transfer coefficients. Biocalorimetric measurements were found to be in definite correlation with metabolic activities and with OTR and are employable as growth phase indicators; the calculations, however, require a precise measurement and knowledge of heat fluxes and sources, energy inputs, and the temperature distribution in the vessel. In most cases, however, it is, depending on the scale-up factor, not, or only restrictedly, possible from the physical viewpoint to keep physical parameters constant throughout the scale-up. Constance of even a single specific parameter mostly leads to an uncontrolled and unpredictable change of other variables into dimensions that are technically not realizable. Classic examples are (1) the mixing time, which inevitably increases in larger vessels due to the larger volumes to be stirred and that cannot be unlimitedly compensated and kept constant by increasing stirrer speeds and energy inputs, and (2) the volumetric energy input P/V. A constant volumetric power input has indeed been successfully applied as a scale-up parameter for the early industrial penicillin fermentations (1 hp per gallon, equivalent to 1.8 kW per 1 m^3) and in fermentations with low energy inputs, but it is limited in fermentations requiring high energy inputs, like recombinant *E. coli* cultures.

For this reason, mathematically driven approaches are pursued for both process and reactor scale-up by forming dimensionless coefficients, which are kept constant by an appropriate choice and adjustment of the relevant influencing process and fermenter parameters. Well-established examples are, among many others, the dimensionless power number, Reynolds number, gassing number, and the modified dimensionless power number and the modified dimensionless mixing time. The comparison of the latter two coefficients and of the corresponding curves enables the identification of appropriate types of stirrers capable of exerting the desired mixing performance at a given stirrer speed with a minimum of energy consumption and therewith to compensate the above-mentioned limitations of volumetric energy inputs at larger scales. (A quantum leap in stirrer technology in this regard seems to be the Visco-Jet of Inotec, which possesses cone-formed short tubes instead of blades and pretends to exhibit the best mixing performance with a minimum of power input and shear stress without foam generation.) The performance of further various types and designs of stirrers is presented and discussed by Junker et al. Stirrer performance coefficients and curves are thus crucial scale-up aids.

Furthermore, any of these parameters and coefficients can be combined with other variables to set up and create new, process-specific parameter correlations, coefficients, terms, groups, and characteristic curves. This relates also to the k_La—value, which currently is the most applied physical scale-up variable because it includes the relevant parameters influencing oxygen supply like agitation (via energy input) and aeration as superficial gas velocity and that, as a component of dimensionless terms, is also frequently employed for reactor scale-up.

Taking into account the limitation of a k_La-oriented scale-up in the form of a limited power input, OTR, and tolerable shear stress, Flores et al. integrated the backpressure *p* by maintaining the product of $k_La \times p$ constant through a variation of pressure, agitation, and aeration for scale-up of *Bacillus thuringiensis* fermentations. Although the specific growth was reduced and the biomass production and sporulation efficiency remained constant, fermentation time could be shortened and toxin yields were increased. Wong et al. successfully scaled-up *E. coli* fermentations from 5 L to 200 L by keeping constant the product of k_La and aeration rate (vvm) under variation of power input, working volume, and aeration according to the Wang–Cooney equation, which reflects these parameters in dependence of the fermentation scale. Diaz and Acevedo argue that the oxygen transfer capacity, indicated by the k_La value, is not the most process-relevant parameter, but the effective oxygen transfer rate as a product of k_La and mass transfer potential is, i.e., the difference between the pO_2-values in the gas and the liquid phase, and suggest an OTR-based scale-up strategy. A common, simple and robust method is the maintenance of a constant pO_2 in the culture broth by variation of stirrer speed and aeration rate. To avoid shear stress and to keep the energy input (P) at the lowest possible level, the pO_2 is steered at the minimum limit. Riesenberg et al. employ a stirrer speed and glucose-feed steered pO_2 of 20% for interferon α–*E. coli*-fermentations in 30-L and 450-L scales. These examples demonstrate that, for each process, appropriate variables and coefficients and therewith scale-up strategies have to be identified individually.

Development of Fermentation Models and Strategies

Despite the central role of the scale-up issue in biotechnology and the comparably large body of literature, no common, generally applicable strategy seems to be established. For each product, process, and facility, a suitable scale-up strategy has to be elaborated. A wholistic scale-up strategy consists of a comprehensive and detailed process characterization to identify key stress factors and key parameters influencing product yield and quality the most, and of an appropriate process control and process design ensuring optimum mixing and reaction conditions, supported by appropriate knowledge and data-driven models as well as computational tools. It should be kept in mind, however, that any approach and any model will always be approximative and that a compromise in the process-related knowledge will always be gappy and that the known mathematical methods and relations cannot completely reflect the highly complex interactions and relationships of the physical conditions governing the fermentation process. As a matter of fact, it seems, that, in view of the high complexicity of the fermentation parameters influencing each other and the only rudimentary and fragmentary reflection of the reality any model can deliver and finally the different layouts of vessels and facilities that rarely are designed according to strict scale-up criteria, successful scale-up in most cases will not be the result of a conclusive and straight-lined experimental strategy but will be the outcome of an independent optimization on each scale that highly depends on the experience, skill, and last, but not least, intuition of the experimentalist. To a lesser extent, this also holds true for the design of procedures aimed at the isolation and purification of the compounds from the culture broth. As these purification steps follow upon the biosynthetic steps and the upstream processing in the bioreactor, they are usually referred as "*downstream processing.*"

Downstream Processing

Product Recovery and Purification

Biopharmaceutical products consist of a multitude of compounds and structures with most having different physical and chemical properties and derive from a large variety of sources like human and animal tissues, body fluids, plant material, and as illustrated above, microbial fermentations. Accordingly, purification strategies have to be developed individually and empirically that reflect the physicochemical properties of the product, of the product source, and of potential contaminants by finding appropriate sorts, sequences, combinations, and operation modes of the respective downstream processing steps to finally achieve high purities and high recovery rates while maintaining the pharmaceutical activity of the molecule. Traditionally, downstream processing steps are roughly subgrouped into operations related to cell harvest, cell rupture in case of intracellularly occurring products, product capture, product purification, and product polishing to manufacture a drug ready for galenic preparation and consist of a sequence of solid–liquid separation and solvent and solid-phase extraction steps. Large-scale cell harvest usually occurs by preparative centrifugation, e.g., in a decanter or in disk stack separator or by filtration to simultaneously separate existing suspended particles from the surrounding broth. Fragile mammalian cells are usually separated by filtration methods only.

If the value product occurs intracellularly, the slurry is taken up in washing buffers of appropriate ionic strength for preparation of the cell rupture, which occurs, e.g., by high-pressure homogenization, sonification, bead milling, or enymatic procedures.

Product capture is defined as the first product extraction and purification step aimed at a product concentration by volume reduction and partial purification, whereas polishing constitutes the final purification step, which removes persistent residual minor impurities like denatured, aggregated, or nonfunctional isoforms of the product, and which follows the preceding (intermediate) purification steps aimed at the removal of contaminating solutes like host cell proteins, DNA, and media components. Product capture usually starts with precipitation, solvent extraction, and/or a cascade of ultra-filtration and nano-filtration steps before the first ion exchange or size exclusion chromatography. Antibodies and antibody derivatives, which account for about 20% of the biopharmaceutical products currently in development, are preferably bound to affinity matrices by natural immunoglobulin-binding ligands such as the *Staphylococcus aureus* membrane and cell wall protein A or the streptococci surface protein G. To broaden the availability of specific structures with suitable binding properties, synthetic ligands with enhanced stability and resistance to chemical and biochemical degradation are continuously attempting to be developed, supported, e.g., by computer-aided design. The development of synthetic ligands with enhanced selectivity and stability, tailored to specific biotechnological needs and product structures, will lead to more efficient, less expensive, and safer procedures not only for purification of antibodies but also for other proteins at manufacturing scales. Also, antibodies can be employed as a means for protein purification in the form of immunoaffinity chromatography. A novel emerging technology is the use of synthetic single- stranded nucleic acid molecules (aptamers) as affinity ligands, which fold up into unique three-dimensional structures specifically binding to the desired target structure as it has been shown for the purification of thyroid transcription factor or selectin receptor globulin.

The subsequent purification steps including polishing are mostly performed on hydrophobic interaction resins and/or on reversed-phase matrices.

Downstream Processing Optimization and Economization

Mostly due to the tremendous costs of sometimes several thousand per liter for chromatographic resins and production scales of up to several hundred liters column volume and due to the prices for the columns themselves of up to hundreds of thousands of U.S. dollars, downstream processing expenses account for the largest part (50–90%) of the total production costs and are therewith a focal area for process economization attempts. One of the many criteria for the choice of a resin is its shelf life. Bearing in mind that every downstream processing step coincides with a minimum product loss of 5–10%, the removal of a particular step not only helps to save the respective capital investment, but concomittantly to increase the final product yields, and thus to render the whole production process more economical in several respects. To reduce the number of required steps, a selection has to be made for resins exhibiting excellent separation, resolution, and yield with respect to a given product and the contaminants, i.e., for resins exhibiting excellent product binding selectivity and capacity. Likewise, the operation mode of the column has to be optimized with respect to the specific product load, adjustment of the physico-chemical operational conditions like pressure, temperature, pH(- shift), ionic strength, and sort of buffers and eluents (e.g., evaluation of continuous vs. step gradients).

A further approach is the combination of the solid–liquid separation and product recovery into a single step, e.g., by expanded bed adsorption, which permits the direct initial purification from culture broths without the need of prior removal of suspended solids. In contrast to the conventional column operation, the mobile phase is pumped upward through the column bed from beneath. The bed thus starts to expand at a liquid flow rate above a critical value, and the gaps between the sorbent beads expand. The controlled distribution of bead size and bead weight results in a stable expanded bed in which the beads oscillate around a steady position and thus avoid clogging of the column. Whereas preparative liquid chromatography methods have become a well-established separation and purification method in the pharmaceutical industry, techniques like two-phase system partitioning and its variant reverse micellar extraction, which also potentially offer advantages like the possibility of a direct extraction from the culture broth through partitioning of the compounds into two immiscible phases, need further developmental activities for economic large-scale applications in the production of biopharmaceuticals and are less common. A further criterion for the choice and design of a downstream processing procedure is thus its scalability.

Downstream Processing Scale-Up

Comparable with the scale-up of fermenters and fermentation processes, the scaleup of downstream processes, particularly of column and column operation, is not simply a matter of increasing size. Increasing column diameters, reducing the stabilizing wall effects, and increasing resin bed heights may lead to an altered settling behavior of the beads, to channel formation through shrinking and swelling of the packed matrix, to column clogging with a concomittant reduction of the flow rates and an increase of the column back pressure, to altered hydrodynamic behavior and residence times of the process fluids, and to an altered pattern for the product/ contaminants adsorption/desorption pattern. To avoid the resulting quality impairments and deviations, resins with a suitable scale-up behavior have to be selected and the resin bed height is tried to be kept constant as far as possible as is the flow rate as key scale-up parameters, which requires an appropriate experimental design in early laboratory development stages. As this, however, is only possible to a limited extent, downstream processing scale-up also is the result of an optimization of the respective operation conditions on each scale. A procedure that has been optimized for decades and scaled-up to dimensions of several cubed meters is the commercial β-lactam purification.

Downstream Processing of β-Lactam Compounds

As most of the product is secreted and is thus concentrated in the culture broth, the recovery process starts with filtration, usually with a rotary vacuum filter, followed by a cascade of solvent and solid-phase extraction steps.

Common penicillin extraction solvents are amyl- and butyl-acetate or methylisobutylketone. As penicillin is extracted as a free acid at pH 2–2.5 and the molecule is instable at this pH, extraction occurs in a counter-flow using Podbielniak- and Luwesta-centrifugal extractors to shorten the contact time with the solvent and to prevent product decomposition. Purification is through subsequent and repeated crystallization from an aqueous solution after alkalization.

In contrast to penicillin, the hydrophilic cephalosporin is more suitable fo solid- phase extraction. For high yield and purity extraction, a combination of several, different chromatographic steps is used.

Hydrophobic interaction chromatography on neutral polyaromatic resins like Amberlite XAD4, 16, 1180, or Diaion HP20 is widely used in combination with weak basic anion exchangers like Diaion WA-30 or strong acidic cation exchangers like Amberlite XAD 2000 and Diaion SK-1B. The mentioned resins are recognized for their high sorption capacity and their long shelf life.

Whereas the improvements on the extraction level are less spectacular, significant progress over the last few years can be noticed with respect to side-chain cleavage to 6-aminopenicillanic acid (6-APA) and 7-aminocephalosporanic acid (7-ACA) in switching from chemical to enzymatic procedures.

Postsynthetic Structure Modification

Most antibiotics in therapeutic use are synthesized or modified exclusively by the means of chemistry and are derived from the established compound classes, which have been known for decades. Chemical derivatization thus has also been applied to substances that are of microbial origin and that therefore are termed semi-synthetic.

Among the most recent semi-synthetic antimicrobials are Aventis' streptogramin derivative Synercid and the erythromycin derivatives clarithromycin (Klacid) from Abbott and roxithromycin (Rulid) and the brand new ketolide telithromycin (Ketek), both from Aventis.

Despite these recent successes and increasing efforts, the yields of therapeutically useful entities emerging from such chemical derivation programs are continuously decreasing.

For this reason, large-scale derivation methods (combinatorial chemistry) are integrated in the search for innovative antibiotics as are biotechnological approaches for structure modification. Biocatalytic procedures, which have been shown to be useful for generating novel antibiotic structures like Loracarbef, a novel β-lactam compound from Eli Lilly highly active against various β-lactamase producing species, are also about to replace continuously chemical production processes. At several universities and corporations, screening studies have been initiated to find appropriate enzymes for compound conversions, as it has been successfully established in production processes for penicillin and cephalosporin.

β-Lactam Side-Chain Cleavage

6-APA and 7-ACA as the key intermediates for the production of semisynthetic penicillins and cephalosporins are obtained by removal of the acyl side chains.

There is a large body of patents existing for chemical and enzymatic splitting procedures, but enzymatic processes have been more successful for economical as well as for ecological reasons.

Enzymatic 7-ACA splitting procedures have been developed and commercialized by companies like Asahi Chemical, Hoechst, and Novartis. The replacement of the hitherto employed chemical deacylation processes like the imino ether or the nitrosyl chloride method resulted in a cost reduction of 80% and a decrease of the waste volume by a factor 100 from 31 t to 0.3 tons per 1-ton 7-ACA. Chlorinated hydrocarbons like dimethyl aniline and methylene cloride as well as heavy metal ions can be completely avoided. Instead of zinc salt formation, multiple silylation, formation of the imino chloride, imino ether, and finally an imino ether hydrolysis, the side chain is removed in two enzymatic steps.

Cephalosporin C is first oxidized and deaminated by a D-amino acid oxidase (DAO), which can be obtained from various fungal species, like the yeasts *Trigonopsis variabilis* and *Rhodotorula gracilis* or the ascomycete *Fusarium solani*. The resulting α-keto-adipyl-7-ACA, upon decarboxylation, is converted into glutaryl-7-ACA (G-7-ACA). DAO is a flavoenzyme containing flavin adenine dinucleotide as the prosthetic group and catalyzes oxidation of D-amino acids to their corresponding keto acids. In a second step, the glutaryl side chain of G-7-ACA is deacylated by a glutarylamidase from *Pseudomonas diminuta*. The molecular data of other potentially suitable enzymes and genes from various sources are given by Isogai. It is noteworthy that the enzymatic splitting process could have only been rendered economical and therefore commercially employable through a significant increase of glutarylamidase yield on the fermentation level by using a gene-recombinant *E. coli*-strain.

A recombinant amidase from *E. coli* is also the most commonly employed enzyme for 6-APA production by deacylation of penicillin G, a process that has been established now for decades. With an annual turnover of 30 tons, the *E. coli* penicillin amidase is one of the most widely used biocatalysts, despite the discovery of further similar acting enzymes from various microbial sources, including penicillin V acylases from the basidiomycetes *Bovista plumbea* and *Pleurotus ostreatus*; from the ascomycete *Fusarium*; or from the yeast *Cryptococcus*.

A significant milestone in economization of enzymatic β-lactam production has been reached by enzyme immobilization permitting a preservation and multiple use of the cleavage enzymes. The currently most employed resins in industries for this purpose are epoxyacrylic acids and silica gel derivatives. The general economic criterion for the preparation of a biocatalyst is production costs in relation to yield, turnover rate, storage stability, and operational/mechanical stability. Further criteria are outlined in the *Guidelines for the Characterization of Immobilized Biocatalysts* by the European Federation of Biotechnology. Application criteria are filterability, sedimentation velocity, and particle firmness. Operational and storage stability as well as the activity of this biocatalyst and the quality of 6-APA with respect to color are improved by sulfur reducing compounds. As pointed out, the ensurance of product quality and drug safety is a key issue in pharmaceutical production processes.

Quality Issues

According to regulatory requirements, pharmaceutical production facilities and processes have to be proven to function properly across the entire range of process critical parameters by a qualification of the facilities and equipment, which consists of the steps design qualification (DQ), installation qualification (IQ), operational qualification (OQ), and performance qualification (PQ) and which results in a validation of the production process to substantiate that the complete system is capable of manufacturing the respective product reproducibly in a consistent quality as expected within preset specifications and in compliance with all laws and guidelines, like the cGMP (current good manufacturing practice) regulations, among others, issued by regulating authorities like the FDA and European Medicines Agency (EMEA).

The products have to be sterile and free of any contaminations that might derive from process material, residues of preceding production campaigns (cross-contaminations) in the case of product changes, and of the agents used for facility cleaning. To restrict the introduction of such contaminations into the repective production steps, the production facilities, equipments, and solutions are usually cleaned according to validated cleaning procedures (e.g., with 1 M NaOH) and sterilized by heat or filtration before their use. Product sterility is achieved by aseptical performance of the last manufacturing steps and by micro-filtration (0.2 μm) or, if possible, by terminal heating of the product before filling. Residues of chemical cleaning agents are removed according to validated procedures by rinsing with purified water.

As biopharmaceuticals are potentially contaminanted with possibly harmful viruses and allergenic and pyrogenic acting endotoxins as residual components of their host cell, guidelines and directions have been issued by the FDA's Center for Biologics Evaluation and Research (CBER) requesting validated procedures for virus and endotoxin removal and inactivation.

Virus and Endotoxin Removal

Endotoxins, which consist of the lipopolysaccharide fraction present in the cell wall of gram negative germs and which tend to adhere to equipment surfaces and to persist in products and product solutions, as do viral contaminants deriving from cell culture processes or from starting plasma or tissue material, can also be efficiently removed by final filtration steps. Whereas ultra-filtration with a cut-off of or below 10 kDa is sufficient for endotoxin removal, viruses need to be removed by nano-filtration steps complemented by a variety of inactivation measures like pasteurization, pH inactivation, solvent/detergent treatment, or ultraviolet and gamma ray irradiation. Usually, endotoxins and viruses are already deconcentrated to a significant extent by the chromatographic steps and the solvent exposure in the course of the normal purification procedures.

Marching in step with the technical and methodological progresses, biotechnology is gaining in increasing importance in pharmaceutical production processes by replacing chemical production procedures for economical and ecological reasons and in the development and commercialization of novel therapeutic principles.

To fully exploit the potential of biotechnological production methods, an integrated process design will be necessary considering the downstream processing requirement during the design of upstream operations and vice versa. As the fate of a compound as a pharmaceutical also depends on the prospective production costs already estimated in the development phase and production processes cannot be significantly changed after approval without running the risk of having to perform ad-ditional clinical trials, it is of utmost importance to choose and design production organisms, strains, vectors, expression cassettes, and fermentation procedures as early as possible in compliance with the prospective harvest and purification methods also to be chosen and designed according to cost criteria. Integrative biotechnology thus is not only a key prerequisite for the development of competitive and economical production processes to relieve the downward price pressure applied by generic drug makers after patent expiration and for the acceleration of market approval for new drugs in the highly competitive environment of the biopharmaceutical industry, but also it is a key technology to save and liberate capital for the development of novel drugs for the benefit of mankind.

2

MICROMOLECULES

Regulation is the logical consequence of the search from health institutions and governments to ensure public protection from unsafe products. The regulation of drugs emerged first in developed countries. The first initiatives of regulation appeared in 1862 with the Bureau of Chemistry in the Department of Agriculture of the United States, lead by Harvey Wiley, trying to regulate food, drug, and biological products. At that time, adulterated food and drugs as The Great Blood Purifier System (Peter's specific) and Mrs. Winslow's Soothing Syrup for teething and colicky babies (which was related with morphine, without a label indication) were the main targets of regulation.

The Bureau of Chemistry enforced a 1906 law until 1927, when it was reorganized to form the Food, Drug and Insecticide Administration, later renamed, in 1931, as the Food and Drug Administration. The 1906 Act prohibited the sale of adulterated or misbranded drugs and prohibited interstate transport of disallowed food and drugs. It also mandated that a variety of information be stated on the drug package. Changes to labeling requirements and a provision to label certain dangerous ingredients led many patent medicine makers to reformulate their products because many of the products contained harmful chemicals.

After an event in 1937, when a marketed anti-infective called Elixir Sulfanimide caused over 100 deaths regulators were forced to change the law to require that drugs meet certain safety requirements before being marketed. A new 1938 Act called for evidence of drug safety, prohibited false therapeutic drug claims, and also included cosmetics and therapeutic devices under FDA regulation. The 1938 Act established a listing of active ingredients on the drug label and required that drugs be labeled with adequate directions for safe use.

Even after all these efforts to ensure the safety of drugs were implemented, many incidents (included the thalidomide tragedy) occurred and the U.S. Congress had to pass major amendments to the Act in 1962. In addition to safety issues, for the first time drug manufacturers were required to prove the effectiveness of their drug products before marketing.

In parallel with the development of drug regulations, biological regulations were historically developed in connection to safety concerns. The 1902 Biologics Control Act enacted by the U.S. Congress established the initial concepts used for the regulation of biologicals. These provisions were revised in 1944 and expanded in the 1950s. Attention to regulation of vaccines and toxins was enforced until a major tragedy occurred in the United States, and only then were actions taken by the federal government to ensure public protection from unsafe products. The incident occurred in 1901, in St. Louis, Missouri, when 20 children became ill and 14 died after administration of an equine-derived diphtheria antitoxin (prepared from horse serum) contaminated with tetanus toxin. The serum had been manufactured in local establishments designed without any of the current knowledge of Good Manufacturing Practices, particularly without procedures that guarantee the product's safety and potency. This event forced legislation to regulate the sale of biologicals. In July 1902, Congress passed the Biologics Control Act also known as the "*Virus-Toxin*" law, which is the first time that the United States' government took control over biologicals' production, consequently with the responsibility to ensure their safety for the public. In this act, the need to include the control of the manufacturing establishments and facilities was recognized, as assurance of purity could not be demonstrated if control was limited to inspection and testing of a final product. This act settled the essential concepts for ensuring the safety of biologicals. These ideas are used as the basis for ensuring safety and effectiveness of biologicals throughout the world.

The history of vaccine control and regulation in developed nations has been one of increasing complexity. By 1955, many biologicals, including blood products and vaccines, had been licensed and the need for appropriate regulation was evident. In the United States, the use of inactivated polio vaccines from different manufacturers, licensed in the country, provoked a number of children to develop poliomyelitis, and some of the children died. The reason was incompletely inactivated vaccines. This incident led to the expansion of the biologicals control function to the establishment of the Division of Biological Standards (DBS) within the National Institutes of Health. Later, in 1972, the DBS was transferred to FDA and became the Bureau of Biologics. In 1982, the Bureau of Biologics was renamed the Office of Biologics Research and Review (OBRR) and combined with the Office of Drugs Research and Review (ODRR) formed the Center for Drugs and Biologics. In 1987, the OBRR was separated and renamed the Center for Biologics Evaluation and Research (CBER).

The need to develop and institute an independent evaluation of medicinal products before they are allowed into the market for public consumption was reached at different times in different regions, generally associated with the level of technological development. In Japan, government regulations requiring all medicinal products to be registered for sale started in the 1950s. In many countries in Europe, the thalidomide tragedy of the 1960s was the trigger. This tragedy revealed that the new generation of synthetic drugs, which were revolutionizing medicine at the time, had the potential to harm as well as to cure.

Between 1960 and 1970, important developments transpired regarding laws, regulations, and guidelines for reporting and evaluation of data on safety, quality, and efficacy of new medicinal products. At the same time, the industry was becoming more international and seeking new global markets, but still the registration of medicines remained a national responsibility.

The urgent need to rationalize and harmonize regulation has been forced by the need of countries to have access to drugs and biologicals to cure, treat, and prevent diseases according to the development of important technological advances in science and responding to the effort of manufacturers to gain access to more and new markets. For the purpose of this review, drugs will be classified as small molecules, biologicals, and biotech products:

1. Small molecules are most medicines or drugs chemically synthesized with molecular weights of typically less than 500 Da applicable to prevention, treatment, or cure of diseases or injuries in man.
2. Biologicals are any virus, therapeutic serum, toxin, antitoxin, vaccine, blood component or derivative, allergenic extract, or analogous product applicable to the prevention, treatment, or cure of diseases or injuries in man, generally with molecular weights larger than thousands of Daltons.
3. Biotechnological products are any biological or pharmaceutical product made using recombinant DNA techniques and intended to prevent, treat, or cure diseases or injuries in man. This group includes mainly proteins of high molecular weight.

Issues Related to Regulation for Biologicals (Vaccines) Compared with Regulation for other Medicinal Products

WHO has established that effective drug regulation promotes and protects public health by ensuring that:

1. Medicines are of the required quality, safety, and efficacy;
2. Health professionals and patients have the necessary information to enable them to use the medicines rationally;
3. All premises, persons, and practices engaged in the development, manufacture, importation, exportation, wholesale, supply, dispensing, and promotion of drugs comply with approved standards, norms, procedures, and requirements;
4. Product information is unbiased, accurate, and appropriate;
5. Illegal manufacturing and trade are detected and adequately sanctioned;
6. Promotion and advertising are fair, balanced, and aimed at rational drug use; and
7. Access to medicines is not hindered by unjustified regulatory work.

National drug budgets, as a proportion of total health budgets, currently range from 7% to 66% worldwide. The proportion is higher in developing countries (24–66%) than in developed countries (7–30%). People and governments willingly spend money on drugs because of the role they can play in saving lives, restoring health, preventing diseases, and stopping epidemics. However, to accomplish these goals, drugs must be safe, effective, and of good quality and used appropriately, which means, in turn, that their development, production, importation, exportation, and subsequent distribution must be regulated to ensure that they meet prescribed standards.

In the search of implementing regulations for drugs, biologicals, and all medicines to guarantee the protection and benefit of the users, governments have established the national drug regulatory authorities (DRAs). These institutions must be developed with a clear mission, solid legal basis, realistic objectives, appropriate organizational structure, adequate number of qualified staff, sustainable financing, access to technical literature and information, and with the capacity to exert effective market control. DRAs must be accountable to both the government and the public and their decision-making processes should be transparent. Monitoring and evaluating mechanisms should be built into the regulatory system to assess attainment of established objectives.

Regulatory authority is generally based on laws, which represent policy choices. This authority is assigned to designated organizations, generally part of the bureaucratic institutions, with the mission to carry out drug regulation. Several factors regarding the authority and the capacity for exercising such authority affect the operation and drug regulatory activities. Among the most important are:

1. Availability of standards, procedures, and guidelines to be used as guidance in performing the authorized functions;
2. Consideration of strategies to overcome structural and resources constraints, including financial adequacy and sustainability;
3. Establishment of clear strategies for planning, monitoring, and evaluation;
4. Availability of appropriate human resources including number, qualifications, remuneration, and human resources development; and
5. Definition of the scope of regulatory authority, in relation to type and extent of the activities carried out to implement legal provisions, including sanctions for noncompliance.

The value of drug regulatory activities depends on whether they produce the intended outcomes in terms of the following:

1. The quality of pharmaceutical products marketed;
2. The proportion of licensed pharmaceutical facilities meeting international standards in Good Manufacturing Practices, Good Laboratory Practices, Good Clinical Practices, and so on;
3. The number of illegal products on the market; and
4. The number of illegal facilities marketing pharmaceutical products.

In addition to effectiveness, policy makers must also address regulatory efficiency, transparency, and accountability when evaluating regulatory policies. The cost effectiveness of drug regulation; the cost for pharmaceutical businesses and consumers of regulatory delays; political and commercial influence over regulatory decisions, public access to regulatory procedures and decision-making criteria; communication among the regulatory authority, its clients, and the consumer; and the accountability for the results of regulatory actions are performance indicators that must be assessed in the evaluation of regulatory agencies.

Regulation of Small Molecules

Since the mid-1930s, many new pharmaceutical products have emerged, and trade in the pharmaceutical industry has taken on international dimensions. At the same time, however, the circulation of toxic, substandard, and counterfeit drugs on the markets has increased, mainly because of ineffective regulation of production and trade of pharmaceutical products in exporting and importing countries. Problems relating to drug safety and efficacy are generally caused by the use of drugs containing toxic substances or impurities, drugs whose claims have not been verified or that have unknown severe adverse reactions, as well as substandard preparations or counterfeits drugs. All these problems can be tackled effectively only by establishing an effective drug regulatory system.

The development process stages for a small molecule drug that are relevant to the regulatory scrutiny are as follows:

(a) Drug discovery,
(b) Drug purification,
(c) Preclinical research, and
(d) Clinical trials.

When the dossier of a drug is submitted to the DRA, an exhaustive review of the medical/clinical, chemistry/manufacture, pharmacology/toxicology aspects, and their statistical validity is conducted. The main element of the evaluation is to certify its safety and, during this stage of the approval, the manufacturer can be required to submit additional information to ensure the safety of the product. When safety is acceptable, the DRA proceeds with complete reviews to ensure efficacy, stability, and all other specifications that guarantee the product complies with the required norms. At any stage of the trial, the DRA of the country where the trial is being conducted should have the authority to put it on hold if deficiencies or safety issues appear and until they are resolved. If results of clinical trials demonstrate that the drug is safe and efficacious over existing treatment drugs, an application is made in most of the regulatory agencies to seek approval for marketing the drug.

As part of the new drug approval process, the DRA conducts inspection for Good Manufacturing Practices (GMP inspection) of the facilities where the drug is being manufactured. GMP is a quality concept and consists of a set of policies and procedures for manufacturing processes to guarantee that drugs are pure, consistent, safe, and effective. These policies and procedures describe the facilities, equipment, methods, and controls for producing drugs with the intended quality. The guiding principle for GMP is that quality cannot be tested in a product, but must be designed and built into each batch of the drug product throughout all aspects of its manufacturing processes.

Regulation of Classic Vaccines and Biologicals

Well-managed programs of vaccination have brought about profound reductions in the impact of diseases in terms of morbidity and mortality in the majority of countries of the world. One major disease, smallpox, has been totally eradicated largely as a result of vaccination and another, poliomyelitis, is absent from large areas of the world and on target for eradication during the next few years, and the incidence of measles has been greatly reduced. Vaccines provide one of the most cost-effective public health interventions and are among the safest medicinal products.

Table 2.1. Classification and characteristics of vaccines

- *Classic vaccines*: products of a whole or part (subunit) of a microorganism. They can be attenuated or inactivated vaccines, subunits, or toxoids products of the microorganism's metabolism, for instance, Diphtheria-Tetanus-Pertussis (DTP), Measles–Mumps–Rubella (MMR), oral polio vaccine (OPV), inactivated polio vaccine (IPV), smallpox, rotavirus, and so on.
- *Recombinant vaccines*: obtained as products of gene modification of different organisms (yeast or bacteria) with posterior purification to get the immunogenic protein (example Hepatitis B vaccine).
- *Synthetic vaccines*: Part or the whole antigen is a product of chemical synthesis, proteic nature (peptides and oligopeptides), or carbohydrates (saccharides and oligosaccharides) (polyribosylribitol phosphate (PRP) synthetic antigen conjugated to tetanus toxoid).
- *Combined vaccines*: including different combination of classic, recombinant, or synthetic vaccines (DTP-HepB-Hib).
- *New approach of vaccines*: DNA vaccines and plant-derived vaccines, under development but still not licensed.

These enormous achievements have been possible in part because inter nationally agreed principles and procedures are in place to secure high levels of safety, efficacy, and quality of vaccines. Vaccines differ from therapeutic medicines first because of the biological and thus inherently variable nature of the products themselves, the raw material used in their production, and the biological methods used to test them. Thus, special expertise and procedures are needed for their manufacture, control, and regulation. The use of appropriate standard materials and reference preparations, whenever they exist, is fundamental to the standardization and control of vaccines.

Vaccines are unique in the fact that they are usually administered to very large numbers of healthy people, mostly infants, in national immunization programs. Thus, safety and quality are of high relevance. Although vaccines have a key role in preventive medicine, recent history of their use has shown a general high level of safety compared with their benefit. In most cases, minor adverse reactions may occur, but these reactions do not challenge the risk-benefit advantage of vaccination. A number of potential and theoretical risks are implicit in their use. They include, in particular, the presence of adventitious agents derived from the source materials or introduced during manufacture or, as is the case of live vaccines, the presence of virulent organisms caused by reversions of the vaccine virus or bacteria to its virulent form. In these cases, a possible risk to the community at large may exist in addition to the vaccinees.

A remarkable difference between vaccines and biologicals and other synthetic pharmaceutical drugs consists of the difficulty of evaluating the activity for those biological products, and thus the differences among them in their control and regulation. In general, for synthetic drugs and medicinal products, the active ingredient is totally defined and the activity can be evaluated by quantitative methods. They are synthesized in the laboratory in a precisely controlled way by a defined sequence of chemical reactions, and the nature of these molecules is such that, once they are made, their exact structure and composition can be determined by laboratory tests. Today, technology allows the modeling of small drug-receptor interactions that can be studied using computational chemistry (*in silico*) methods and extraction of valuable data and information from databases (bioinformatics). The modeled drug is then synthesized using combinatorial chemistry. The application of technologies such as X-ray crystallography and Nuclear Magnetic Resonance are standard procedures for the 3D structural determinations and drug-receptor interactions.

For biologicals, the biological activity and its consequences must be evaluated in an integrated way before starting clinical trials. The complexity and challenge that regulators face with vaccines can be exemplified with the case of combined vaccines, where different epitopes are being introduced in the human body, inducing different responses to the regulatory mechanisms of the immune system, while not causing interference in the responses between them. New vaccines challenge regulators with the development of novel procedures for the proper evaluation of their efficacy and safety. It is important that the standardization and control of vaccines by the national regulatory authority and the manufacturer are continually reviewed and modified so as to reflect the current state of science and technology incorporating an improved understanding of quality and safety issues. Regulatory authorities must thus be proactive and maintain an acute awareness of scientific developments in the vaccine field.

Regulation of Biotechnology Products

Recombinant insulin was the first biotechnology product, which emerged in 1982. Today, biopharmaceutical products have diverged to encompass not only recombinant forms of natural proteins and biologicals derived from natural sources, including recombinant plant-derived pharmaceutical proteins, but also monoclonal antibody (mAb)-based therapeutics. All these products require special consideration from a regulatory point of view. In the past, microbial and animal cell culture was the most common method of producing recombinant proteins. Currently, the interest is focusing increasingly on transgenic animals because of their apparent ability to produce complex proteins at a high volume and a low cost. Many of these products are now in different phases of clinical trials, although some of them without encouraging results.

During 2002 and 2003, regulators in North America and Europe approved a total of 64 biopharmaceuticals for human use. These approved drugs included hormones, blood factors, thrombolytics, vaccines, interferons, monoclonal antibodies, and therapeutic enzymes. Data published by Walsh suggest that during the past three years, over a quarter of all new drug approvals were biopharmaceuticals, taking into account that these numbers do not reflect duplication for products with different formulations and different commercial names for the same active ingredient. All of the new biopharmacuticals approved in United States in 2003 are protein-based drugs (rather than nucleic acid-based drugs). According to estimates at that time, around 500 biopharmaceuticals were undergoing clinical trials.

To date, no gene therapy drug has gained marketing approval as a direct consequence of the technical, manufacturing, and regulatory difficulty that still beset this class of therapeutic compounds. Besides, it is important to consider that a bad reputation on these products exists as a consequence of reported incidents of adverse reactions after their use. Monoclonal antibody therapeutics have been hit particularly hard regarding warnings mainly related to hypersensitivity or anaphylactic reactions or cytokine storms.

The major target indications of biopharmaceuticals currently undergoing clinical trials include cancer, cardiovascular, and infectious diseases, the major killers within the developed world. Although in excess of 30 nucleic acid-based drugs are currently being evaluated for gene therapy, vaccines, and other applications, the majority remain in the early stages of clinical development (phase I/II).

Another kind of biotechnological product that is acquiring interest as a therapeutic agent is the biopharmaceuticals derived from plants. As a result of the limited production capacity of many pharmaceutical products, the production in plants represents an innovative tool that can expand the yields of active principles because the large volume of biomass that can be developed at the fields. An extra advantage is that these products are free of human diseases and mammalian viral vectors. In products derived from bacteria, the bacterial endotoxin content of the final product has always been of concern, which is not an issue in products derived from plants.

To date, only proteins have been developed through genetically modified plant, including mammalian antibodies, blood components, coagulation factors, vaccines (edible vaccines), hormones (insulin, somatotropin, and erythropoietin), various interferons, and other therapeutics agents such as enzymes and interleukins.

Monoclonal antibodies for therapeutic and diagnostic use seem to be the best potential successful products produced in plants, but they currently have not reached the marketplace. Tobacco plants are the most commonly used plant in these developments. Hepatitis B surface protein and rabies virus glycoprotein are examples of advances in edible vaccines.

In the production of biopharmaceuticals derived from genetically modified plants, several steps are part of the process, and they commonly include:

1. Selection of host plant;
2. Selection of the gene expression system;
3. Location of gene expression within the plant (green matter, the seed, or other tissues);
4. Production of biomass; and
5. Implementation of purification systems for the protein.

Several of these steps will require new and special regulatory developments. The products obtained from genetically modified plants must be carefully studied by regulators focusing on some main issues such as the development of Good Manufacturing Practices appropriate for the use in the fields that can guarantee the consistency of production during the manufacturing process. Environmental issues also exist that must be taken into account. Potential effects on nontarget species such as butterflies, honeybees, and other wildlife at or near the growing sites are important to be considered. The possible transgene escape through pollen or seed dispersal, the potential for recombinant molecules to enter the food chain, and the proper evaluation of the impact that the introduction of virus from plants into the human body can cause are issues that have to be resolved for the success of this modern biotechnology tool.

Main Regulatory Agencies

Food and Drug Administration (FDA)

FDA is recognized as the strongest regulatory agency in the world. Although the agency has limited its regulatory functions to products to be used in the United States, this agency has been the pioneer in the development of the regulation for drugs, including vaccines, blood products, and a lot of new biotechnology products emerging in the field that are used worldwide by other regulatory agencies.

Since 1962, the key elements of product safety and efficacy have not changed, although the agency's level of participation, collaboration, and transparency has increased as demonstrated with review goal dates, meetings with industry, guidance documents, and public and private partnerships. Today, according to FDA estimates, 10,510 approved drugs and more than 100,000 over-the-counter drugs are on the market. As discussed by Ray and Stein, "the current regulatory process does not have systematic provisions for obtaining important data needed to guide clinical practice. Planned data collection happens almost exclusively during pre-marketing testing. The FDA approves medications on the basis of studies of limited duration that include relatively small numbers of patients who are often healthier than the target populations for the new drug. Although many important effects of a new medication almost certainly will be unknown at the time of licensing, there are no systematic provisions for post-marketing studies."

This problem is common for regulatory agencies around the world. The lack of information presented by manufacturers regarding the safety during the use by populations at large, the identification of the best indicators for efficacy, and the differentiation that manufacturers try to obtain between products with the same active ingredient, frequently make the regulation function difficult to perform. In addition, in developing countries, the lack of expertise in the different areas of regulation, particularly on clinical trial evaluation and interpretation of statistical results, increases the high uncertainty of the regulatory agencies' results.

European Medicines Agency (EMEA)

The European Medicines Agency (EMEA) is a decentralized body of the European Union created with the objective to harmonize regulatory activities in Europe. EMEA began its activities in 1995, when the European system for authorizing medicinal products was introduced, providing for a centralized and a mutual recognition procedure. Its main responsibility is the protection and promotion of public and animal health through the evaluation and supervision of medicines for human and veterinary use.

Before 1995, the legal framework in Europe for drugs was 25 independent national regulatory authorities and thus 25 parallel national review processes, with the same number of independent marketing authorizations. The consequence was poor resource utilization, divergent scientific opinions, and confusion by physicians, nurses, and health workers in general when decisions had to be made. At the present time, EMEA coordinates the evaluation and supervision of medicinal products throughout the European Union. The Agency brings together the scientific expertise of the 25 European Union Member States in a network of 42 national competent authorities. It cooperates closely with the international partners, reinforcing the European Union contribution to global harmonization.

At the beginning, the EMEA set up two procedures for product authorization in Europe, the centralized and decentralized procedures. The centralized procedure is as follows:

1. Submission of the marketing authorization application to EMEA;
2. A unique evaluation is carried out through the Committee for Medicinal Products for Human Use (CHMP);
3. If the committee concludes that the product has proven its quality, safety, and efficacy, it adopts a positive opinion; and
4. The positive opinion is sent to the commission to be transformed into a single market authorization valid for the whole of the European Union.

The decentralized procedure establishes a mutual recognition between Member States. Briefly, this procedure is based on:

(a) a marketing license application is submitted to one Member State;
(b) if the national regulatory authority concludes that the product has proven its quality, safety, and efficacy, it grants a marketing authorization to the product; and
(c) the marketing authorization is extended to one or more additional Member States.

Today, EMEA uses both procedures, but is primarily involved in the cen tralized procedure. The regulation 2309/93 has defined a mandatory centralized procedure for medicinal products developed by means of one of the following biotechnological processes: recombinant DNA, controlled expression of genes coding, hybridoma, and monoclonal antibody methods. In addition, after 2005, the regulation establishes the mandatory centralized procedure for medicinal products containing new active substances for AIDS, cancer, diabetes, and neurodegenerative diseases, including orphan designated medicinal products. The regulation still allows the mutual recognition procedure for generic centralized products or for medicinal products with a significant therapeutic benefit, products of scientific or technical innovation, or products answering the interest of patients or animal health at the community level.

The fact that more and more products are being included in the mandatory centralized procedure is indicative of a general reliance on this procedure more than on the mutual recognition procedure; it can also reflect that not all national regulatory authorities have developed the same regulatory capabilities to authorize the marketing of new products for the whole European Community.

Although European countries have faced many challenges in the establishment of regulatory activities of the agency, mainly because the diverse conflicting priorities between the Member States, the centralized procedure has generated harmonization in the scientific opinion in Europe, getting one marketing authorization valid in the European Community, one common name, and, most important for the impact on health professionals and users (potentially 370 million), one common product information.

After 10 years of been established, EMEA is a good example of harmonization, with both centralized and mutual recognition procedures, that can be extrapolated to other regions of the world, mainly in the developing world where the few countries that have developed strong regulatory systems can share technical knowledge and expertise in the different areas of regulations with those countries in the corresponding regions with limited resources to the benefit of the whole region.

International Committee for Harmonization (ICH)

The ICH is not a regulatory agency, it is a unique project that brings together the regulatory authorities of Europe, Japan, and the United States and experts from the pharmaceutical industry in the three regions to discuss scientific and technical aspects of product registration.

The purpose is to make recommendations on ways to achieve greater harmonization in the interpretation and application of technical guidelines and requirements for product registration to reduce or obviate the need to duplicate the testing carried out during the research and development of new medicines. The objective of such harmonization is a more economical use of human, animal, and material resources and the elimination of unnecessary delay in the global development and availability of new medicines while maintaining safeguards on quality, safety, and efficacy and meeting regulatory obligations to protect public health. The guidelines established by ICH are followed by many countries around the world, sometimes as the only guide available to establish harmonized standards on quality, safety, and efficacy for their products. However, its impact in classic vaccine regulation is limited, being more developed regarding biotechnological products. Six founding members of ICH are directly involved in the decision-making process. They represent the regulatory bodies and the industry in the European Union, Japan, and the United States. They are the European Commission and the European Federation of Pharmaceutical Industries and Associations (EFPIA) in Europe; the Ministry of Health Labor and Welfare and the Japan Pharmaceutical Manufacturers Association (JPMA) in Japan; the FDA and the Pharmaceutical Research and Manufacturers of America (PhRMA); and a group of observers including WHO, The European Free Trade Area, and Canada represented by Health Canada.

Global Role of WHO in Drugs and Biologicals Regulation

Although WHO is not a regulatory agency, it provides guidelines for acceptability of products taking in consideration the specifications needed in regions where the regulatory institutions have not fully developed. With the responsibility to guarantee the quality, safety, and efficacy of products all around the world, WHO develops guidelines joining efforts from experts in the most diverse regions, getting a generalized opinion about the best way to establish technical guidelines. WHO provides relevant expertise ant technical assistance through such activities as guidelines development; workshops and training courses; coordination and promotion of anti-counterfeiting measures; prequalification of medicines for priority diseases; pharmacovigilance for global medicine safety, regulatory, and other information exchange; and review of narcotic and psychotropic substances for scheduling within the 1961 Convention on Narcotic Drugs and the 1971 Convention on Psychotropic Substances.

WHO Procedure for Assessing Drug Regulatory Authorities

As WHO establishes, the overall objective of a DRA is to ensure that medicinal products (pharmaceuticals, biologicals including vaccines, blood products, and other biologicals) are of acceptable quality, safety, and efficacy and that they are manufactured and distributed in ways that ensure their quality until they reach the patient/consumer and their commercial promotion is accurate.

According to WHO, the main functions of a DRA are as follows:

- Registration (licensing) of products,
- Inspection and licensing of manufacturers,
- Inspection and licensing of distributors,
- Post-marketing surveillance, and
- Regulation of claims that can be made for commercial promotion of products as well as authorization of clinical trials.

A DRA can be effective only if it has the following:

1. A legal basis for all its functions in legislation and regulations,
2. Sufficient human and financial resources,
3. Access to appropriate scientific expertise, and
4. Access to a quality control laboratory.

Particularly for vaccines and biologicals, in comparison with medicines, because the inherent variability of these products caused by the biological nature of their starting materials, their manufacturing processes, and their test methods, WHO has identified six essential regulatory functions to evaluate a regulatory system as effective. These functions are as follows:

1. A published set of clear requirements for licensing,
2. Surveillance of vaccine field performance (safety and efficacy),
3. System of lot release,
4. Use of laboratory when needed,
5. Regular inspections of manufacturer for Good Manufacturing Practices compliance, and
6. Evaluation of clinical performance in clinical trials.

An extra function not included in the six established by WHO must be considered during the evaluation of regulatory authority for vaccines. This function must include the distribution and vaccine's shipment mechanisms; it must be able to guarantee the delivery of vaccines to all points of use with an acceptable level of quality.

Finally, research in the regulatory agencies, looking to have experts in each function updated in all relevant aspects involved in the regulation activities, is an aspect that must be considered during the implementation of regulatory systems in the countries. The difference of the regulatory activities that WHO performs in comparison with the activities of other regulatory institutions is the impact that WHO guidelines, norms, and procedures have all over the world. The documents are developed looking for consensus with globally recognized experts. They are a reflection of the activities that are being developed in the world, and it facilitates their implementation.

Other Initiatives for Harmonized Regulation

The Pan American Network for Drug Regulatory Harmonization (PANDRHA) is an initiative to support the process of drug regulatory harmonization throughout the Americas, with the mission to promote drug regulatory harmonization for all aspects of quality, safety, and efficacy of pharmaceutical products as a contribution to the quality of life and health care of the citizens of the member countries of the Americas. It includes the participation of all regulatory authorities in the region along with representatives of academia, industries, and other experts. The main forum for developing the PANDRHA activities is the Pan-American Conference on Drug Regulatory Harmonization, where there is also participation from other organizations such as the Caribbean Common Market (CARICOM), the Southern Countries Common Market (Mercado Comun del Sur, MERCOSUR), the North American Free Trade Agreement (NAFTA), and the Central American Integration System (Sistema de Integracion Centro Americano, SICA) and constitutes a way to disseminate the decision on drug regulatory harmonization of global initiatives such as the ICH. The network functions through working groups assigned to different areas including: good manufacturing practices, bioequivalence, good clinical practices, combat to drug counterfeiting, pharmacopoeia, drug classification, medicinal plants, pharmacovigilance, good laboratory practices, vaccines, and drug registration.

Other initiatives around the world exist that are incorporating, among many objectives, the harmonization of drug regulation. Although not all of these organizations have been developed exclusively for regulation, such initiatives can be found in the Association of South-East Asian Nations (ASEAN), Andean Community of Nations (CAN), the Collaboration Agreement of Drug Regulatory Authorities in European Union Associated Countries (CADREAC), the European Union, the Gulf Central Committee for Drug Registration (GCC-DR), the Southern Common Market (MERCOSUR), and the Southern African Development Community (SADC).

Future Prespective of Regulation

Regulators must be prepared to face challenges resulting from the fast scientific, technological, and methodological development of drugs, biologicals, and biotechnological products. This effort will require that DRAs establish stronger alliances with the research community, universities, and academia in general so as to have available experts in all fields. Still, much remains to be done in the development of clinical trials with products derived from new technologies, mainly focusing on those that target the immune system's natural control mechanisms, including therapeutic monoclonal antibodies, interleukins, and some vaccine's adjuvant, to avoid the recent disastrous example in Europe with the use of a monoclonal antibody.

Regulatory authorities have been receiving important pressure from industry to decrease approval times. Some agencies are trying to reduce approval times by making changes to the review system such as: improving communication and consultation by applicants, which leads to better preparation of dossiers; eliminating unnecessary administrative time loss; interacting with similar regulatory agencies; and increasing the number of employed reviewers with appropriate expertise. The latter has impacted through the accumulation of experience, know-how, and proficiency within the regulatory agency. However, it must be clear that from the point of view of society and improving public health, approval times alone are not the only goal. It is more critical to make the best decision to secure safety, efficacy, and effectiveness of the new drugs.

At the same time, for product developers, the recommendation to integrate regulation in the very early stages of their research and development work exist. This strategy can contribute as a success factor instead of a bottleneck at the later stages of licensing and market authorization. Incorporating a regulatory perspective will have a positive effect on the cost and time frame of product development. Furthermore, having a good understanding of regulatory requirements will also assist the developer in identifying nonviable projects at an early stage, thus reducing the risk of the loss of investment.

Regulation of drugs must balance the extreme efforts to regulate and control the presence of adverse effects while trying to address health care needs of the population in general. New products are costly to develop and produce. To guarantee their safety, specifically for possible rare events associated to its use, the need of designing and conducting large clinical trials to show statistical significance exist.

This cost will be included in the product's price. As a recent example, in the vaccine area, large clinical trials had to be conducted to demonstrate safety for two new rotavirus vaccines. Over 60,000 children were involved in trials for each vaccine. These regulatory requirements add not only onto the cost of development but also onto the timing for the products to access the markets.

Post-marketing surveillance activities follow programs based in passive collection of spontaneous reports for ensuring safety using voluntary reporting of adverse reactions from physicians and other health workers is a common practice in developed countries, in many cases without or with poor participation from the regulatory agencies. This procedure shows deficiencies such as underreporting, difficulty in calculating rates because incomplete numerator data along with unreliable denominators, and limited ability to establish cause and effect.

Recent withdrawals from the market of high-profile drugs are more often being carried out by the manufacturer who proceeds to withdraw the product before the regulatory agency does so, in principle to protect the public from further harm, but, at the same time, the manufacturer avoids the drastic consequences of penalties that the law establishes if the recall is done by the regulatory agency. Although much has been done to strengthen quality and safety during the development and production processes, post-marketing surveillance involvement by the regulatory authorities is still a pending issue.

The strongest regulatory agencies are still looking for reforms on drug regulation focused to improve the current regulatory process. Modifications proposed for the regulation in developed countries generally are focused on solving the particular problems in terms of the country or region that is involved, and, in general, are not applicable to regulation in developing countries. To be able to address the enormous challenges faced by regulation of new products, regulatory agencies in developing countries will have to urgently strengthen their networks and establish new harmonized regulatory and methodological procedures.

3

PHARMACEUTICAL INDUSTRY

In the pharmaceutical industry, identification of a development drug candidate (preclinical lead profile, PLP, or early candidate notification, ECN), filing of investigational new drug application (IND), and new drug application (NDA) are important milestones before the launch of a new drug. The IND and the NDA are the events where the industry interacts with the Food and Drug Administration (FDA) prior to launching. Various governmental departments play specific roles in furthering drug development programs. The medicinal or discovery chemists identify the new drug candidates to treat or prevent a particular medical indication, whereas the process chemists are responsible for devising a synthesis and supplying the active pharmaceutical ingredient (API) or bulk drug substance (BDS) in multigram quantities for various studies needed to file the IND and support other drug development programs. On approval of the IND, the compound can be administered to humans for the first time as part of the phase-I clinical studies, also known as first-in-man (FIM) trials. Studies that are reported in an IND include synthesis, animal toxicology, pharmaceutics and formulation, drug substance and drug product stability and safety, and metabolic and pharmacokinetics.

The clinical development is the most expensive and resource-intensive segment of the process. Process research and development play a key role in shortening the overall timeline from candidate identification to drug launch. On an average, it takes about 10–15 years from discovery to launch a drug into the market at a cost in excess of $400 million. The paradigm shift (in the 1990s) of increasing the number of compounds entering development has made a tremendous impact on chemists responsible for preparing supplies of these new drug candidates. Early and effective interaction of process research personnel with medicinal chemists and early innovations in process development are believed to shorten the IND and NDA timelines, respectively. These overall reduced timelines would allow for an early launch of the drug into the market.

PHARMACEUTICAL DRUG DEVELOPMENT EVENTS

Genomics to Lead Development Candidate (PLP)

During the past decade, the pharmaceutical industry has seen a paradigm shift in the drug discovery process. The driving force for such change, arguably, was propelled by a variety of factors, including:

1. Generation of new targets (for human diseases) from advances in genomics and functional genomics.
2. Advances in combinatorial chemistry methods to increase the number of compounds for high throughput screening (HTS), and
3. Advances in automation and high-throughput screening techniques for rapid identification of lead compounds.

Although these approaches promise to provide an increased number of novel drug candidates for evaluation in the treatment of a greater number of diverse diseases, successful realization of the potential benefit of these compounds is very much dependent on the ability of the pharmaceutical industry to develop suitable manufacturing processes.

PLP Development Candidate to IND and the Kilo Lab

The IND studies require relatively large amounts of the drug substance, substantially more than what was prepared during the course of the medicinal chemistry programs. Generally, it becomes the responsibility of the process research group to produce this material within the shortest feasible time frame. Most of the major pharmaceutical companies have kilo-lab facilities as an interface between the process research labs and the pilot plants. Pharmaceutical process groups are organized in different ways. In some companies, process research is responsible for providing the supplies of BDS required for an IND filing, including the initial clinical batch (or batches). Typically, the initial supplies are prepared by the combination of modified medicinal chemistry synthesis and new, alternative synthetic processes more suitable for scale-up. In some companies, the chemists in process research labs and kilo labs share this responsibility. Kilo-lab scale-up work typically is performed in 22-L glassware and small reactors (50–100 L). The process development group, on the other hand, is responsible for further optimization and scale-up in the pilot plant and interfaces with the manufacturing.

Clinical Phase, NDA, and Launching of the Drug

The clinical phase (phase I) of the drug development begins after the IND where humans are subjected to the clinical trials. After a successful phase-I trial, efficacy of the drug is tested on a large number of patients as part of the phase-II/III clinical trials. Once the phase-II/III clinical trials are completed, the NDA is filed with the FDA. Clinical trials and NDA are prerequisites for launching the drug.

Process Research and Development

The goal of the medicinal or drug discovery chemist is to identify a new lead to treat or prevent some particular medical indication and define a synthetic strategy to allow for the preparation of as many analogs as possible. The focus of process chemistry differs from routine organic chemistry. It emphasizes optimization and defines the controls to make the sequence of chemical reactions amenable to scale-up. A viable process should reliably yield a high-purity product made by a process unencumbered by a patent. In short, the overall thrust of the scientists engaged in process chemistry is to develop the shortest, least expensive, safest, and most environmentally friendly processes to produce the API in multi-kilogram quantities.

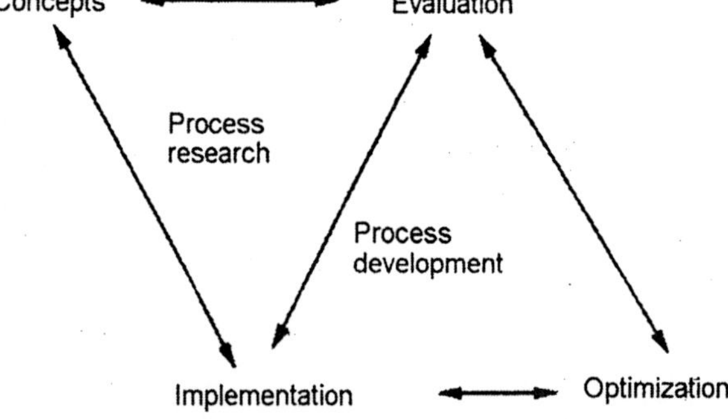

Fig. 3.1. Algorithm for process research and development.

The term "process" is, in general, misinterpreted as scale-up work by the overwhelming majority of the scientists and technologists involved with drug discovery and development programs in the pharmaceutical industry. Scientists and engineers engaged in the various aspects of pharmaceutical process research and development have a highly refined appreciation for the challenges of large-scale synthesis and the purification of the API. The mission of process chemistry in the pharmaceutical industry is to provide documented, controlled synthetic processes for the manufacture of the supplies to support the development programs and future commercial requirements of the API. The science and technology

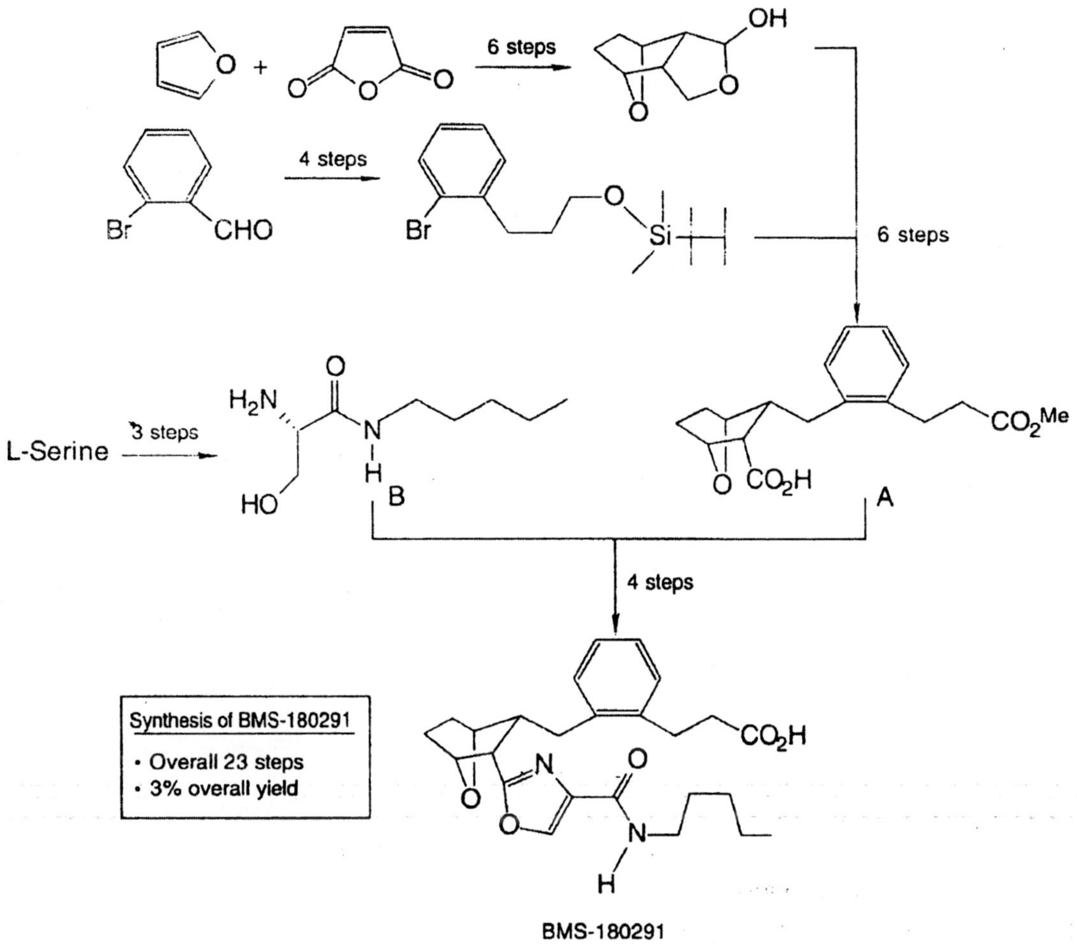

Fig. 3.2. Original synthesis of BMS-180291.

associated in accomplishing this mission provide a tremendous challenge to the individuals or the group of individuals for the drug supply progress from milligram to metric ton quantities.

Route Scouting

As the development drug candidate moves from discovery to process, a workable synthesis is available, which, however, may not be scalable. Route scouting plays a key role in identifying synthetic transformations that are safe, practical, scalable, cost effective, and environmentally friendly, thus setting the stage for eventually delivering a manufacturing synthetic process. An integral part of route scouting is to identify key intermediates that could be easily out-sourced.

An example of route scouting and process improvements

Figure 3.2 depicts the medicinal chemistry approach to the synthesis of BMS- 180291 (Ifetroban). A condensed schematic of the overall alternative- synthesis of BMS- 180291 (Ifetroban) is provided in Figure 3.3. The synthesis of the key acid ester intermediate A has been reduced dramatically from 16 to 4 steps, and the yield has been increased 10-fold from 5 to 52%. The overall synthesis of Ifetroban has been cut virtually in half (from 23 to 12 steps) and the yield (via the longest linear sequence) improved from 3 to 28%.

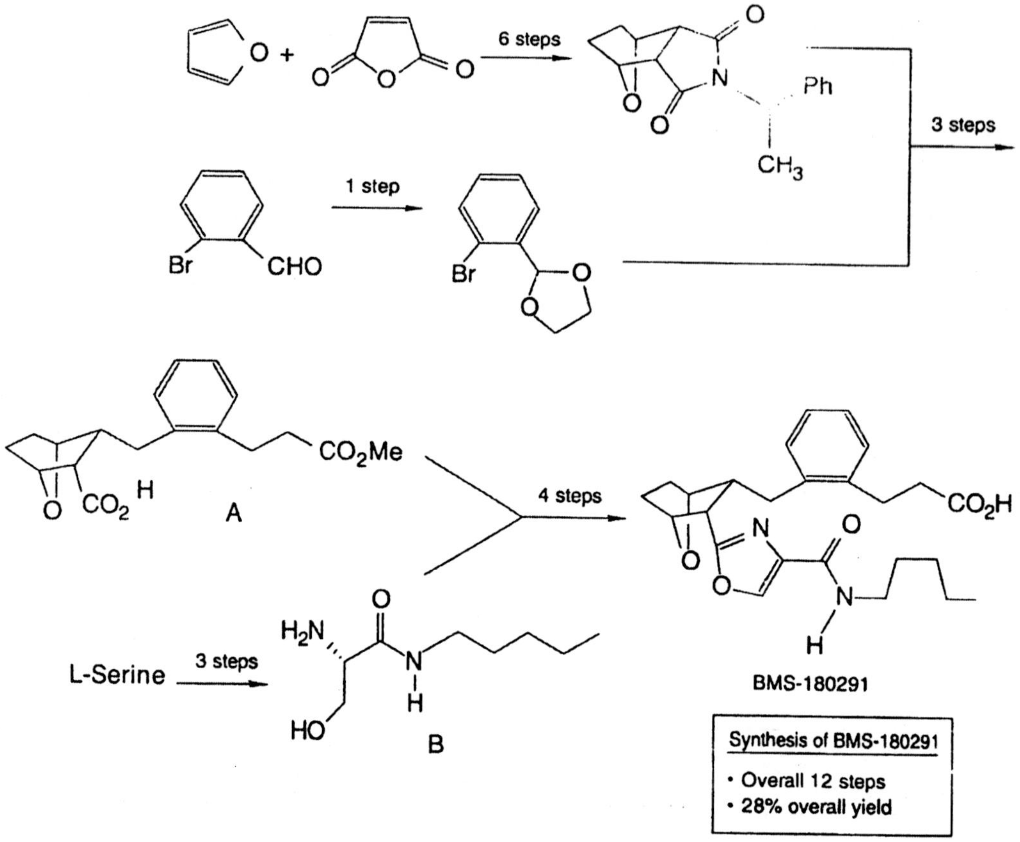

6 steps

Ph

CH_3

3 steps

1 step

Br CHO

Br

CO_2Me

CO_2H

A

4 steps

CO_2H

L-Serine 3 steps

H_2N

HO

B

BMS-180291

Synthesis of BMS-180291
• Overall 12 steps
• 28% overall yield

Fig. 3.3. Alternative synthesis of BMS-180291.

Process Development and Optimization

Human safety is the first priority when developing a process, followed by quality (purity, crystallinity of the product, etc.) and product yield. In addition, the process chemist takes into account the following factors:

1. Hazards associated with the chemical step (human and equipment safety).
2. Waste generated (disposal cost, environmental concerns).
3. Cost and availability of raw materials, reagents, and solvents (cost of goods, sourcing issues).
4. Ease of performing the reaction on-scale (savings in capital and labor).
5. Ease of product isolation (crystallization), and
6. Opportunity to combine two or more chemical steps with no intermediate isolation (telescoping to increase throughput).

Once a route has been selected, the next step is to understand the effect of interactions of variables with each other on the reaction yield and quality for each and every step of the synthetic scheme and to define the limits for these process variables. This requires designing appropriate experiments including controls. This is important because as the scale of the reaction increases, every unit operation, such as addition of reagents, solvents, distillation, phase splits, etc., takes a considerably longer time. Mixing begins to play a major role as the size of the vessel increases. Due to uneven mixing, localized differences in variables such as temperature and concentration are expected, which may have an adverse effect on the reaction.

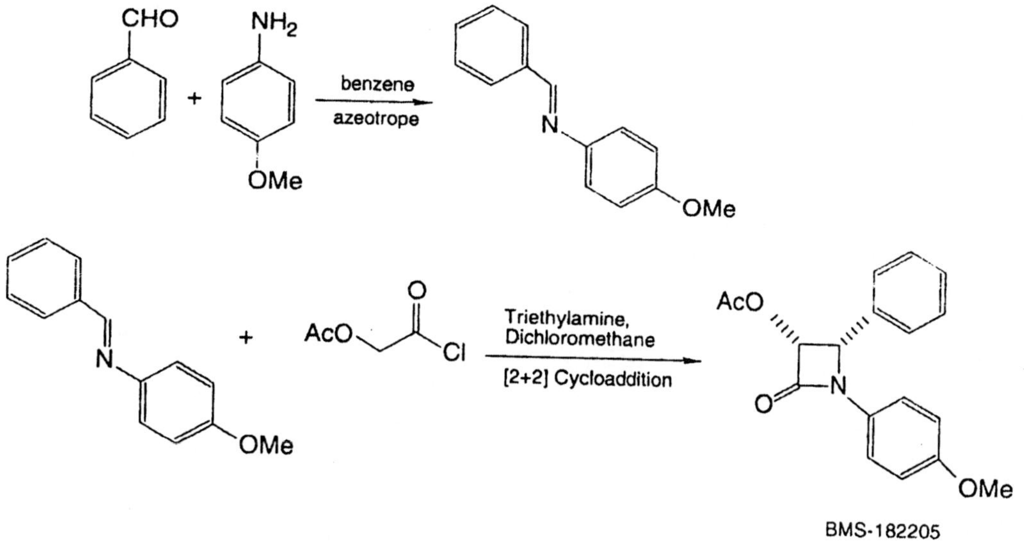

Fig. 3.4. Synthesis of BMS-182205.

Example 1: Process development of BMS-1 82205

Issues: environmental concerns, human safety, waste management, process inefficiency. The first step in the synthesis of the Paclitaxel side chain has been reported in the literature by Holton. The drawbacks of this procedure from a process development standpoint are

1. The use of benzene and dichloromethane (human and environmental concerns).
2. No opportunity for telescoping (since the first reaction is conducted in benzene and the second in dichloromethane)
3. Low yield (68% after crystallization from ethylacetate and hexane), and
4. Brown-black product (color).

Process improvements

Phase I. Benzene was replaced with a safer solvent, toluene, which was also used for the cycloaddition reaction, thus facilitating the telescoping of the two reactions. However, dichloromethane was added during the work-up to prevent product precipitation. The product was crystallized from 2-propanol in 80% yield. The phase I of development eliminated the use of benzene and allowed for telescoping of the two chemical steps. However, a solvent exchange from toluene-dichloromethane to 2-propanol was still needed to crystallize the product. The color of the product after this modification was dark brown.

Phase II. Additional crystallization studies revealed that the product could be crystallized from toluene– heptane and acetone–water. The product also exhibited limited solubility in toluene. With this information at hand, both reactions were conducted in toluene as before; however, during the work-up, dichloromethane was not added. Instead, aqueous hydrochloric acid was added to neutralize excess triethylamine. Heptane was then added to precipitate the product directly from the reaction mixture. The crude wet product was crystallized from acetone–water with an overall yield of 80%. The color of the product was brown. The advantages of this modification are the elimination of several extraction and back-extraction steps and a reduction in processing time and in solvent consumption.

In an attempt to further improve the yield and address the product color issue, the following process variables were studied: the rate of addition of acetoxyacetyl chloride, the reaction temperature, and the effect of other amine bases. The rate of addition of acetoxyacetyl chloride was optimized to be 2–3 h, at 3, 10, and 17°C. Reactions conducted at 3°C afforded the product with the highest quality. Two amines, N-methylmorpholine (NMM) and diisopropylethylamine (DIPEA), were evaluated in addition to triethylamine. In the presence of NMM, the reaction stopped after 65% conversion. In triethylamine the reaction took an additional 3 h for completion, after the addition of acetoxyacetyl chloride. However, in DIPEA, the reaction was instantaneous, the yield was further improved to 87%, and the product was free of brown-colored impurities.

Example 2: Process development of Ifetroban

Issues: environmental concerns, human safety, cost of goods. In the improved synthesis of Ifetroban described previously, environmental concerns due to special handling of copper bromide waste and hazards associated with hexamethylene tetramine (HMT) on manufacturing scale led to further perfection of the synthesis. Mechanistic considerations suggested that an oxidized form of aminoamide B would eliminate the necessity for a late-stage copper-mediated oxidation. This was indeed accomplished. The cyclization–elimination sequence was initiated by a Lewis acid and completed by base-mediated elimination to afford the Ifetroban penultimate. In addition to eliminating the need for copper bromide and HMT, this modification helped to reduce the cost of the product by an additional 15%.

Manufacturing process, route from medicinal chemistry to multi-kilos for clinical study supplies: A highly optimized and concise large-scale synthesis of a purine bronchodilator was developed by the Astra Production Chemical company from Sweden. Supplies for the initial biological studies were generated by the medicinal chemistry route shown in Fig. 3.6. The overall yield was about 14%, which was improved in the environmentally friendly manufacturing process to about 51%.

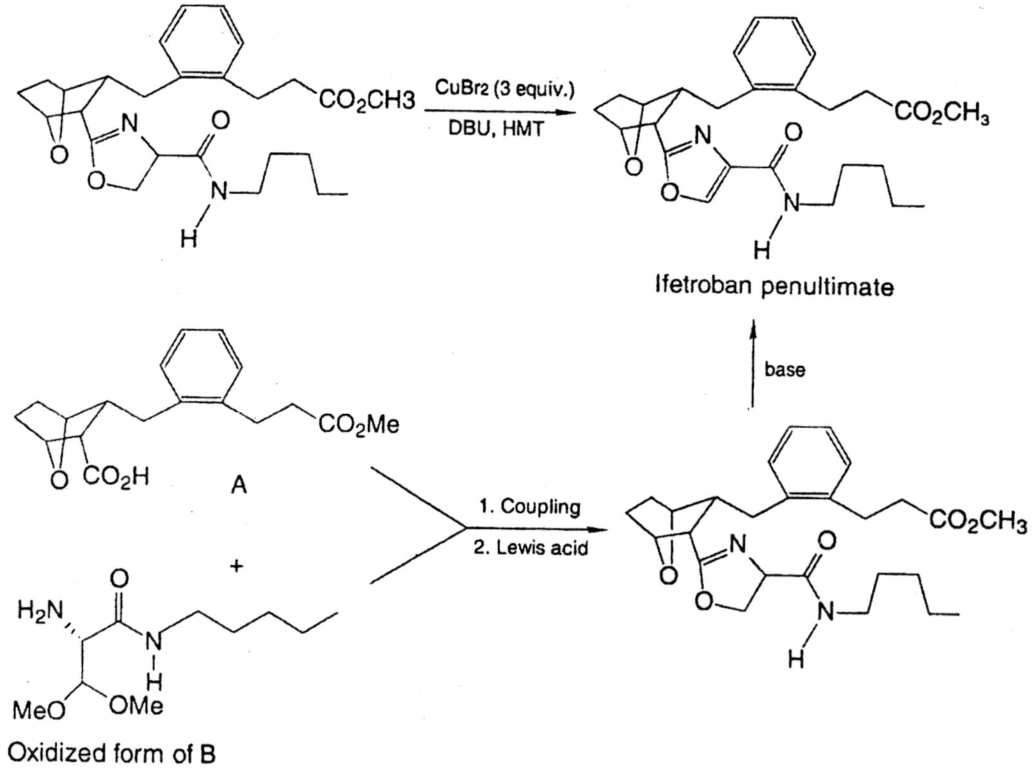

Fig. 3.5. Process development of Ifetroban.

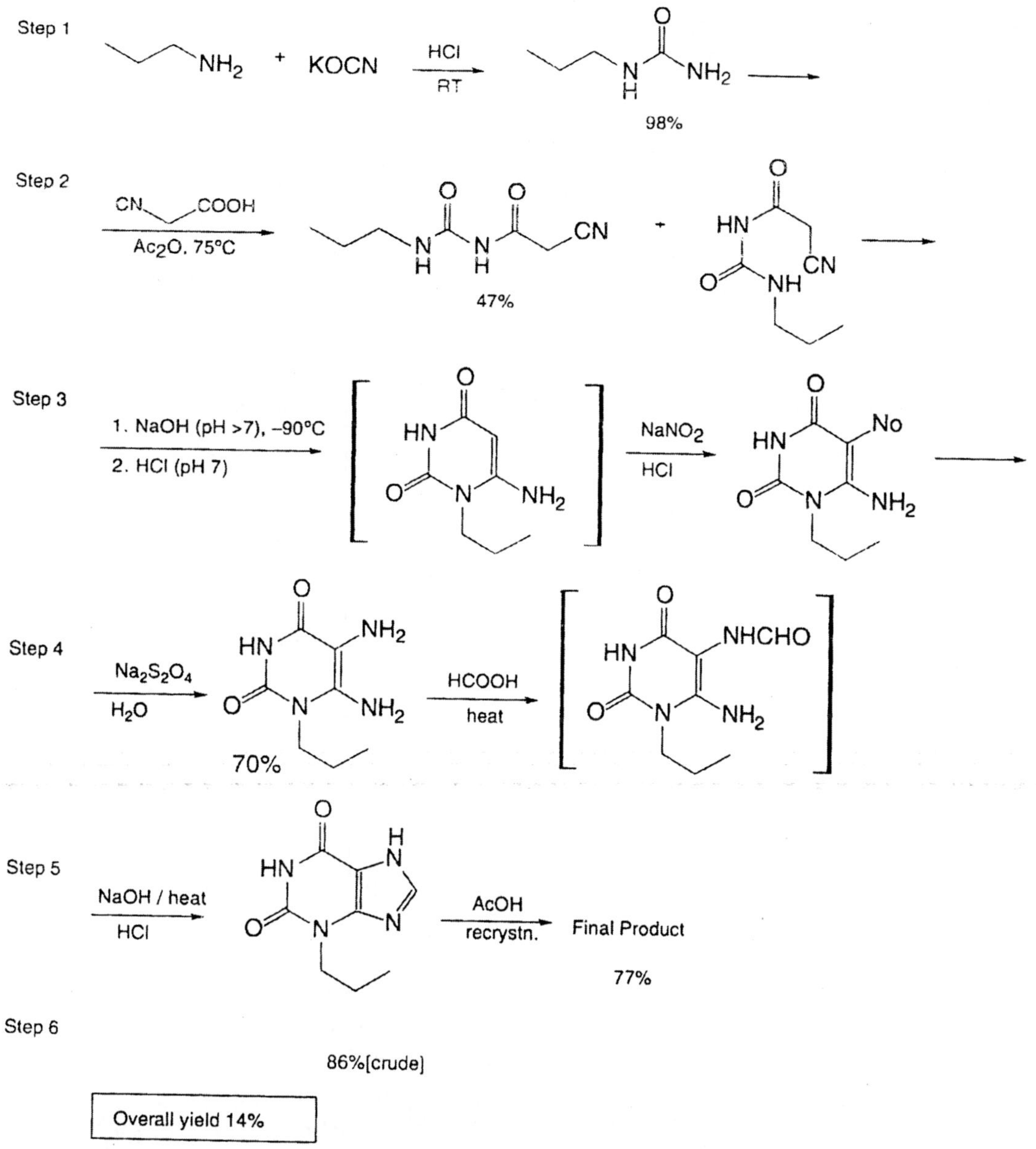

Step 1

Step 2

Step 3

Step 4

Step 5

Step 6

Overall yield 14%

Fig. 3.6. Original synthesis of enprophylline.

Process Hazards and Safety

Process safety has become an integral part of the development of new synthetic routes, and more and more relevant information is gathered in typical process development labs. Many development facilities have now established special process safety departments with state-of-the-art equipment and well-trained personnel. It is important for process chemists considering alternative process routes to know the potential hazards from the main reaction and from the unwanted side reactions in each case so that the hazards of reactivity are included in the factors reviewed in developing and selecting the final process route; three main parameters determine the design of safe chemical processes:

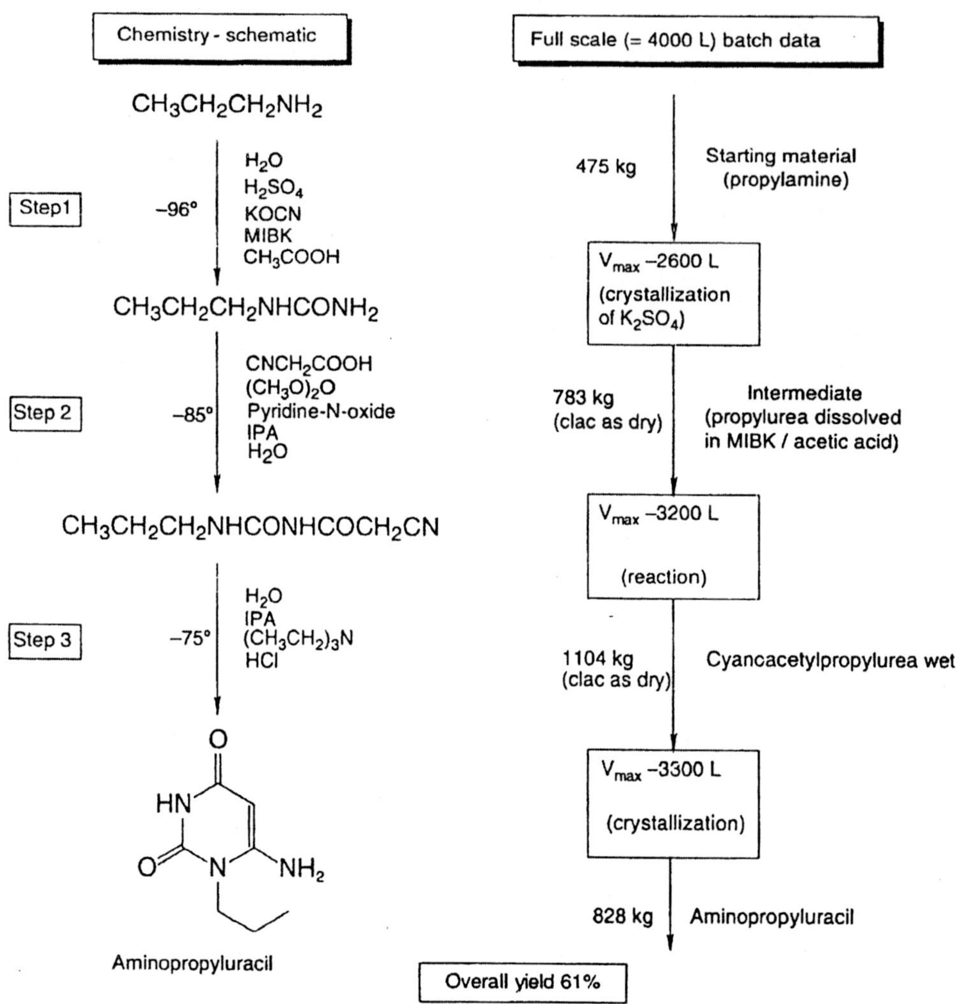

Fig. 3.7. Commercial process of 6-amino-1-propyluracil.

1. The potential energy of the chemicals involved and understanding of the inherent energy (exothermic release or endothermic absorption) during a chemical reaction.
2. The rates of reaction (energy release in the form of heat or pressure) that depend on the temperature, pressure, and concentrations. In any hazard evaluation process, the rates of reaction during normal and abnormal operations (including the worst credible case) must be considered in order to design an inherently safe process.
3. An equipment train must adequately remove any heat or pressure generated in a reaction. The effects and requirements of scale-up must be considered.

In most cases, a team of development chemists, engineers, and safety personnel evaluate and assess hazards associated with each and every step of a process, from performing a reaction to storage of waste streams in drums. The team recommends a set of safety experiments to be conducted, and data are collected for reaction exotherms, powder explosivity, gas evolution, and compatibility of reaction mixtures or reaction waste with pilot-plant equipment and storage drums. Experiments are designed and conducted to determine the potential for initiation of a runaway reaction and the effect of

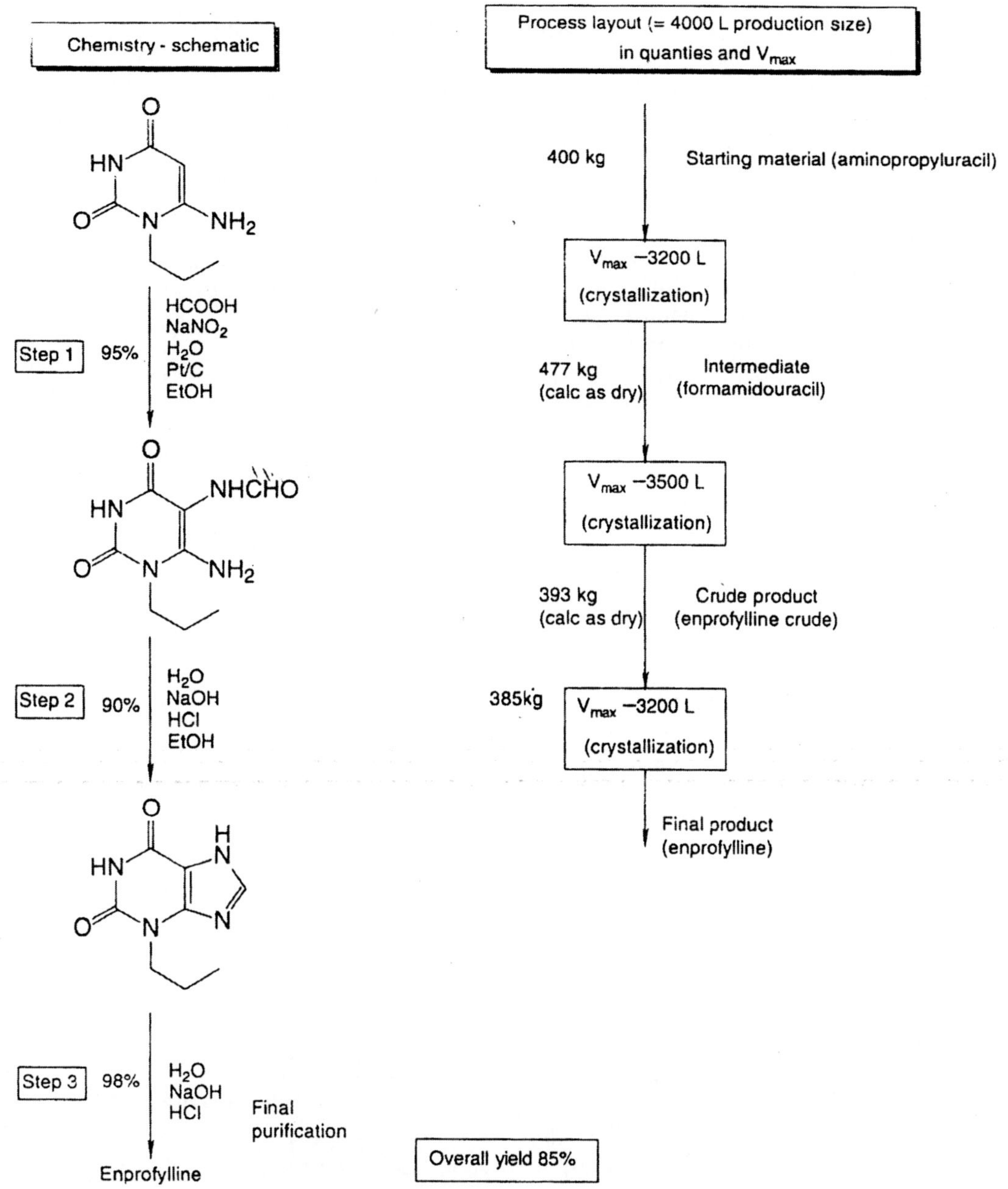

Fig. 3.8. Astra full-scale synthesis of enprofylline from 6-amino-1-propyluracil

decompositions that may occur on runaway. Based on the safety assessment of a process, appropriate measures are taken in the pilot plant to eliminate or minimize any hazard. During the early stages of process research (route scouting), only small amounts of materials are available. In many cases, only theoretical information from the literature or from calculations is readily available. Screening tests can be run to identify the reaction hazards. As the route-scouting efforts enter the process development phase, additional material becomes available so that the reaction hazards can be studied more extensively to test "what-if" scenarios. During full-scale production, the chemical hazards may be reevaluated to address changed production requirements or other process changes such as the use of a different source of raw materials.

Numereous test methods are available using a variety of sample sizes and conditions. The tests provide qualitative or quantitative data on onset of temperature, reaction enthalpy, instantaneous heat production as a function of temperature, maximum temperature, and/or pressure excursions as a consequence of a runaway, and additional data useful for process design and operation.

"Green Chemistry": Environmental Concerns

The research that involves the end-of-process treatments to eliminate pollutants is termed "*green chemistry.*" As Ronald Breslow pointed out, concern for the environment is as old as the biblical injunction, "hurt not the earth, neither the sea, nor the trees." The following example indicates approaches to the environmentally benign chemistry. The process described is high yielding with water as the by-product. Sato et al. have developed an efficient, environmentally friendly method for oxidizing primary and secondary alcohols. The Japanese scientists use hydrogen peroxide as an oxidant, a quaternary ammonium hydrogen sulfate as a phase-transfer agent, and tungsten as catalyst.

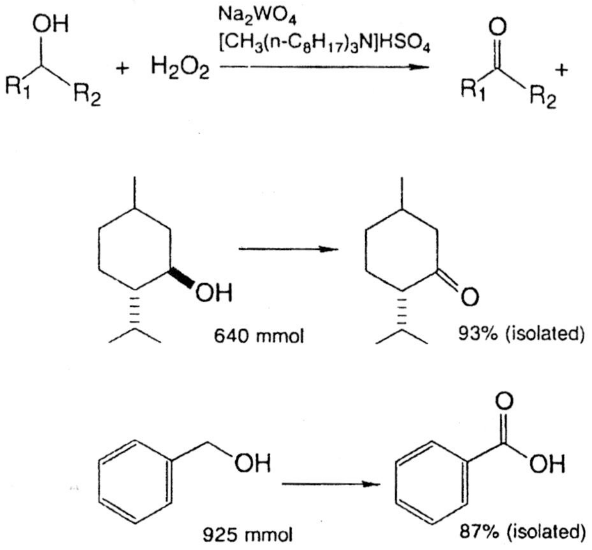

Fig. 3.9. Noyori's oxidation of alcohols.

Enzymatic Intervention

The recent trend in pharmaceutical industries is to incorporate a microbial technology (MT) or enzymatic technology division in the process R&D and manufacturing (need basis) departments. The role of the MT division is usually to provide pharmaceutical drugs (e.g., pravastatin, β-lactam drugs, etc.), and chiral (optically pure) building blocks or synthons for the ongoing synthetic programs.

A number of cholesterol-lowering drugs (Pravachol, Zocor, and Mevacor) are prepared by enzymatic processes. Penicillin antibiotics that have been in the market for decades are produced in large quantities by the enzymatic process.

Enzymatic catalysis

The extensive use of enzymatic catalysts in organic synthesis has been documented. Enzymes represent a broad range of efficient chemical catalysts. They are classified mainly into six categories:

1. Hydrolases (hydrolysis of amides, esters, glycosides, and lactones)
2. Isomerases (C–C bond migration, E/Z isomerization, and racemization)
3. Lyases (addition to *p*-bonds)
4. Oxidoreductases (reversible oxidations and reductions)
5. Synthetase formation and breaking of C–C, C–N, C–O, C–S, and phosphate ester bonds
6. Transferases (transfer of acyl, glycosyl, or phosphoryl groups from one molecule to another)

Design of Experiments (DOE)

An understanding of how various process variables affect the chemistry is necessary for the design of a chemical process that can reliably provide the product in high yield and quality. This understanding can be obtained from experimentally determined rate laws for the main and side reactions that relate

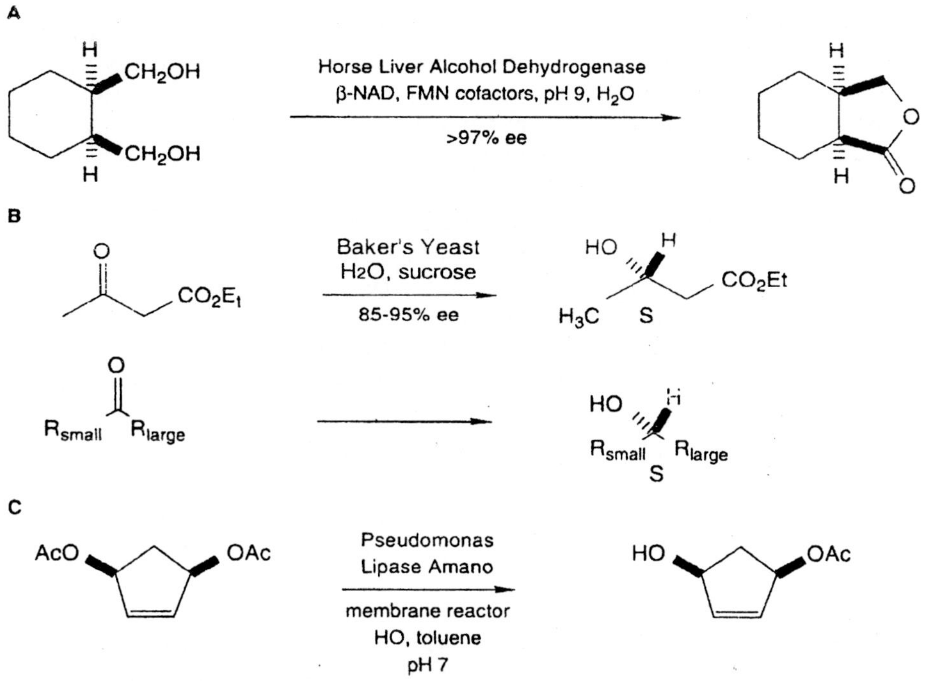

A

B

C

Fig. 3.10. Enzyme-mediated chemical transformations. A-Enatioselective enzymatic oxidation and lactonization; B-enzyme reduction with baker's yeast and enantioselective rule; and C-enzymatic hydrolytic desymmetrization.

temperature, concentration, pressure, solvent effects, and equivalents of each reagent to yield and impurity levels. The process chemist may take the approach of evaluating the importance of process variables by changing one variable at a time. This method can help generate chemical knowledge but is not efficient and does not easily provide the quantitative information needed to rank the importance of process variables. Furthermore, the process chemist is often faced with a task of quickly scaling up the synthesis without the benefit of completely understanding the mechanism of the chemistry involved. With the aid of statistical design approach, a great deal of useful information can be obtained with relatively few experiments. Statistical approaches involving factorial designs are ideal for studying processes where the underlying principles are not well developed or are extremely complicated.

Factorial experiments consists of a systematic variation of two or more process variables at a time. For a two-level experiment, each variable is set to a high or a low value according to a standard pattern. An experimental run is conducted for each possible combination of variable settings. Selection of the low and high levels for each variable is important for obtaining meaningful results. If the levels selected are too close together, the calculated effect could be no larger than the experimental noise. Selecting widely separated levels could result in running the reaction under unrealistic conditions, for example, above the solvent boiling point, or above the decomposition temperature for reagents and reactive intermediates. Data analysis of factorial designs involves a comparison of the experimental responses at the high and low settings of each variable. The results can be plotted in several different ways to develop an understanding of the effect of changing two or more process variables at a time with regard to reaction yield and quality of the product.

Drug Substance Crystal Form

The crystal form of the drug substance is important for pharmaceutical industries, where products are specified not by chemical composition but by their performance. Good crystallinity, good bioavailability, satisfactory aqueous solubility and dissolution rate, and satisfactory physicochemical properties, such as stability, hygroscopicity, and flowability are required. Choosing the appropriate crystal form (final form) often involves crystallizing the drug substance from various solvent systems to search for polymorphism and screening of various salts of the drug substance (if chemically possible).

The chemical, biological, and physical characteristics of the drug substance can be manipulated and hence optimized by conversion to a salt form. Every compound that exhibits acid or base characteristics can participate in salt formation. Various salts of the same compound often behave quite differently because of the physical, chemical, and thermodynamic properties they impart to the parent compound. Only salts of organic compounds have been considered here because most drugs are organic- substances. The relative frequency with which each salt type has been used is calculated as a percentage, based on the total number of anionic or cationic salts in use.

The salt form is known to influence a number of physicochemical properties of the parent compound, such as dissolution rate, solubility, stability, and hygroscopicity. These properties, in turn, influence the absorption, distribution, metabolism, and excretion of the drug. This knowledge is essential for a complete understanding of the onset and duration of action, the relative toxicity, and the possible routes of administration. For example, certain salts of the strong base choline have proved to be considerably less toxic than their parent compound. This observation led to the preparation of choline salicylate as an attempt to reduce the gastrointestinal (GI) disturbances associated with salicylate administration. Clinical studies indicated that choline salicylate elicited a lower incidence of GI distress, was tolerated in higher doses, and was of greater benefit to the patient than was acetylsalicylic acid (aspirin).

The chemical and physical stability of a drug can influence the choice of dosage form, the manufacturing and packaging, and the therapeutic efficacy of the final preparation. Systematic determination of the thermal stability, solution stability (at various pHs), and light sensitivity of a drug and its derivatives, both alone and in the presence of additives (exceptients), provides essential information toward selecting the most suitable salt and dosage forms.

Depending on the mechanism of degradation, different salt forms impart different stability characteristics to the parent drug. Sparingly soluble salts used in the formulation of suspensions reduce the amount of drug in solution and hence its degradation. Differences in hygroscopicity of several salts influence the stability of the drug in the dry state. For example, the stability of penicillin G and its salts has been widely studied because of the drug's therapeutic importance and its characteristic instability.

A solution of penicillin is not stable beyond two weeks even at refrigerator temperatures. However, the use of suspensions of sparingly soluble amine salts (procaine and hydrabamine salts) in aqueous vehicles allowed marketing of a "readymade" penicillin product.

Crystallization of the drug substance and its salt forms

In academia, a synthetic organic chemist rarely thinks about isolating a compound by crystallization, unless a single crystal structure is required. Most of the time, the chemist depends upon column chromatography to purify the compound. In contrast, in the pharmaceutical industry much depends upon crystallization. For example, crystal morphology and particle size have a direct impact on the filtration of a crystal slurry, cake compressibility, bulk stability and dissolution, bulk density, and flow characteristics. Crystallization is the preferred way of isolating the product from a reaction mixture. Knowledge of various crystallization systems from which the drug substance could be crystallized can provide information on polymorphism, thus expediting the selection of final crystal form. In polymorphism, two crystal forms with the same molecular structure are distinguished by the way in which the molecules are packed within the crystal lattice; each form has distinct physical and thermodynamic properties. In 1998, Abbott Laboratories withdrew its HIV drug, Ritonavir, because of the unexpected appearance of a new crystal form that had different dissolution and absorption characteristics than the standard product.

Crystallization is generally preceded by two types of nucleation. The primary nucleation occurs with the formation of clusters of molecules at the submicron level. When the concentration exceeds saturation to afford supersaturation, the clusters become nuclei. The secondary nucleation is caused by particles due to primary nucleation or seeds. There are many strategies to achieve supersaturation to initiate crystallization such as cooling, evaporation, and antisolvent addition.

Early on in the drug development program, only small amounts of material are available for crystallization studies. Parallel crystallization technique in test tubes allows for the identification of many solvent systems using small amounts of material. On a small scale, it is not easy to control the rate of cooling or the rate of evaporation to achieve supersaturation. However, the antisolvent addition strategy to achieve supersaturation in combination with seeding allows rapid identification of several crystallization systems using a minimum amount of compound.

Salts of a substrate having an acid or an amine functionality are prepared by dissolving the substrate and the counter-base (or acid) separately in appropriate solvents, mixing the two solutions in equimolar ratios, and removing the solvents under vacuum to afford a solid. This method has two distinct advantages: First, the composition of the substrate remains the same during various crystallization attempts, and second, this portion of the work can be automated with the use of liquid handling systems.

The next step is to determine the solubility of the substrate (or its salts) in different solvents. This can also be performed by an automated liquid handling system. Depending upon the solubility of the substrate in water-miscible solvents (alcohols, acetone, tetrahydrofuran, etc.) and water-immiscible solvents (ethyl acetate, methyl-tert-butyl ether, heptane, etc.), the process chemist can identify one or many solvent systems from which the substrate (or its salts) could be crystallized using the antisolvent addition strategy.

Another crystallization technique is used when the isolation of a highly water-soluble compound in its salt form is required from aqueous reaction mixtures. This technique takes advantage of the common-ion effect and is based on the le Chatelier's principle, which states that, "if, to a system in equilibrium, a stress is applied, the system will react so as to relieve the stress." Thus, in aqueous solutions, the solubility of the compound in salt form can be reduced by adding large amounts of a common ion that is more soluble than the salt of the compound.

Example: BMS-187745 is a potent inhibitor of squalene synthase and an efficient cholesterol-lowering agent in orally dosed animals. The final step of the synthesis involved oxidation of the penultimate in water with hydrogen peroxide and formic acid. The disodium salt was chosen as the final crystal form. Because of extremely high solubility of the disodium salt in water, it cannot be extracted from water by common organic solvents. However, by employing the concept of the common-ion effect, the disodium salt can be easily crystallized from water. To accomplish this, the pH of the reaction mixture, after quench with hypo-phosphorous acid, is adjusted to the desired range of 6.05–6.25 (pKa of disodium salt of BMS-187745 is 6). In this pH range, sodium salts of formic, hypophosphorous, and phosphoric acids are present in high enough concentration to help lower the solubility of the disodium salt of BMS-187745 and effect crystallization.

Automation in Process Chemistry Laboratories

Since the 1960s, automation has been the major tool for dramatically improving productivity. Automation techniques were introduced on the plant floor to improve quality, increase safety, and streamline the work. Significant savings were realized initially from shorter delivery times, lower unit costs, smaller inventories, and fewer product failures. Due to an escalating cost of bringing a drug to market, companies are under immense pressure to shorten development time. The pharmaceutical industry

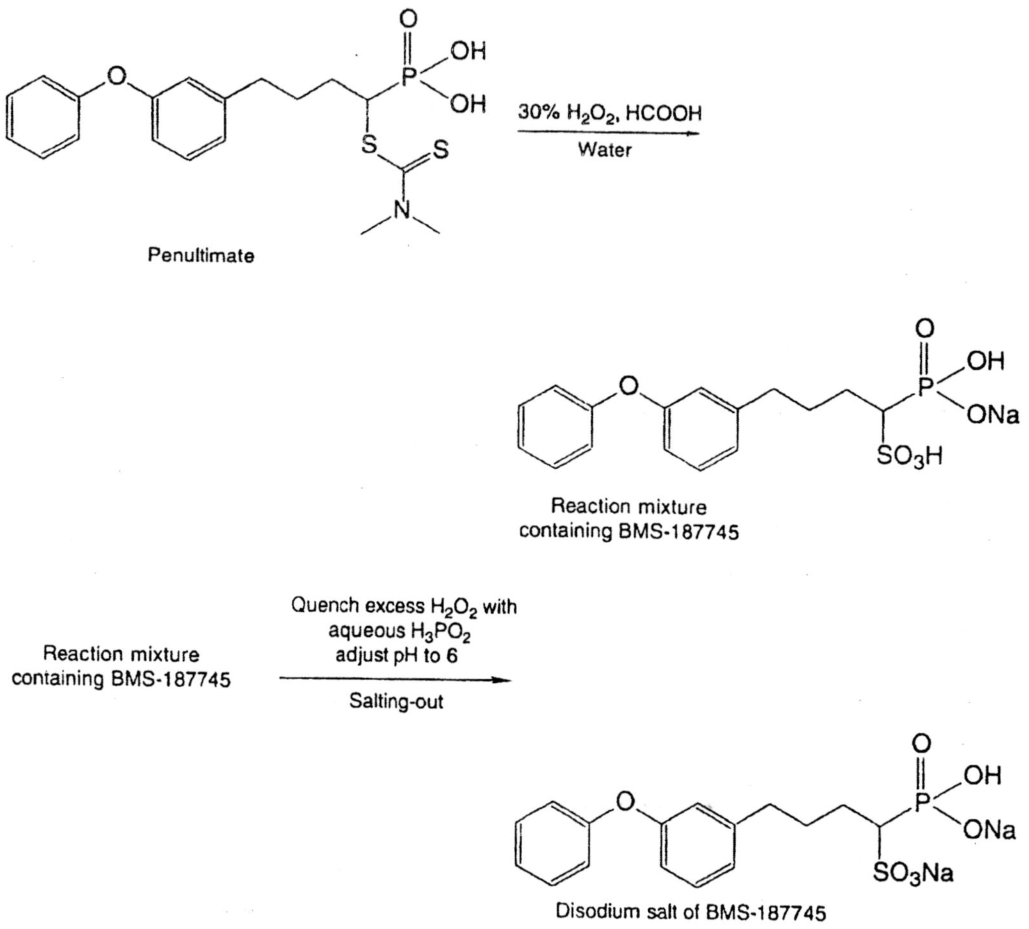

30% H_2O_2, HCOOH
Water

Penultimate

Reaction mixture containing BMS-187745

Reaction mixture containing BMS-187745

Quench excess H_2O_2 with aqueous H_3PO_2 adjust pH to 6
Salting-out

Disodium salt of BMS-187745

Fig. 3.11. BMS-187745 crystallization by salting-out.

has embraced new technologies in its discovery programs to increase throughput, generate precise data, and ensure accuracy.

Drug discovery scientists have already adopted tools such as combinatorial chemistry synthesizers; robotic systems for HTS; and software packages for computational chemistry, molecular modeling, and design of experiments to identify lead compounds ("hits"). As the number of "hits" grows, there is a potential for process R&D to become the "bottleneck." The number of compounds that can enter process development is limited by the number of process chemists available to work on these compounds. Without some type of automated process development machines to increase throughput, it will not be feasible to evaluate all the potential "hits." Created by the results from the HTS, demand for high-throughput development (HTD) tools is growing. Various companies, who in the past may have only addressed the needs of drug discovery scientists, are in the process of inventing and developing instruments that can be used by process chemists to perform many experiments in parallel.

Parallel reactions

Charybdis technologies. In the Calypso Reaction Block, multi-well reaction arrays are designed for both solution and solid-phase synthesis applications. Well volumes range from 2 to 10 ml, pressures up to 207 kPa (30 psi), and temperatures from −80 to +180°C.

Quest synthesis technology. Quest 210 is designed for up to 20 reactions in 5- or 10-ml reaction vessels. Each of the 20 vessels can be efficiently stirred, heated, or cooled, and maintained under an inert atmosphere. Quest 205 is designed for synthesis on a large scale, with two banks of five 100-ml reaction vessels.

Argonaut technologies. Endeavor allows parallel reactions under pressures up to 3.3 MPa (33 atm) and temperatures up to 200°C. Each of the eight vessels (working volume 15 ml) can be independently controlled for temperature, pressure, and gas delivery.

Surveyor: Suitable for parallel process development and optimization with online sampling and integrated HPLC analysis, it employs 10 reaction vessels (working volume 15–45 ml), with individually controlled reaction temperatures from -40° to + 150°C, with the ability to reflux. Reagent addition, reaction parameter control, sampling, and HPLC injection are controlled by built-in software.

Bohdan automation, inc. The process development workstation can run up to 12 independent reactions with working volumes of 25 ml. The following operations are automatically carried out: reagent preparation and addition, individual heating, cooling, and mixing, reaction sampling and quenching, and transfer to optional HPLC or FTIR modules.

Parallel purification

Isco, inc. The CombiFlash Sg 100c System is suitable for purifying 10–35 g of material. It provides time- or peak-based fraction collection with on-line UV detection and a linear and/or step gradient with two solvents at a flow rate of 10–100 ml/min.

The CombiFlash Si 10x System simultaneously purifies up to 10 samples, with a linear and/or step gradient with two solvents with a total flow rate of 10–100 ml.

Automated sample handling and analysis

Bohdan automation, inc. The Balance Automator offers a cost-effective alternative to manual weighing, reduces errors and operator tedium, and processes up to 120 samples per hour. This system can accommodate various container sizes and balances with the help of interchangeable parts.

Gilson. The Gilson 215 Liquid Handler is a versatile, large-capacity, septum-piercing liquid handler for safe and efficient transfer. It helps in transferring samples to other analytical systems or inject samples directly to an on-line HPLC system.

Outsourcing

Outsourcing covers a broad range of services. It can eliminate the need for additional staff, facilities, and/ or equipment. Outsourcing in drug discovery and development is expected to continue its remarkable growth over the next decade as drug synthesis becomes more complex. This dynamic growth is due to a number of factors, including the ongoing consolidation in the pharmaceutical industry and a tight labor market. As larger companies consolidate, they seek synergies resulting in release of R&D personnel. Retrospectively, companies need to get more done with fewer internal resources and this promotes outsourcing. The tight labor market has made it increasingly difficult to recruit and retain staff, and many companies are turning to outsourcing to gain access to highly trained scientists who are available. Pharmaceutical companies are also looking into long-term relationships with outsourcing partners.

Fermentative Production

Streptomyces fradiae produces the 16-membered macrolide antibiotic tylosin, which exhibits antimicrobial activities against Gram-positive bacteria and *Mycoplasma* species. Because of its remarkable effect against infections, tylosin has been widely used as a veterinary antibiotic for livestock for the last several decades. However, as with almost all classes of antibiotics in clinical use, the long-term use of tylosin has eventually induced bacteria and *Mycoplasma* species to become resistant to tylosin.

The mechanisms of resistance are attributed either to diminished uptake of the antibiotic into cells or to the structural alteration of the 70S ribosome, the target site of macrolide antibiotics, which enables the ribosome to escape from tylosin binding. In our studies to investigate tylosin derivatives with increased antimicrobial activities, one of the acyl derivatives of tylosin, 3-*O*-acetyl-4[2]-*O*-isovaleryltylosin (AIV), exhibited excellent activity against such resistant microbes. Tsuchiya et al. have shown that AIV (1) binds more strongly to the altered 70S ribosome, which has only weak affinity to other macrolides, and (2) is taken up rapidly even through cell membranes that have acquired low penetrability to other macrolides. Higher blood levels of AIV after oral administration to rabbits and mice ensure its strong therapeutic effect.

Since tylosin is composed of tylonolide (macrolactone; aglycone ring) and three attached sugars having several chemically reactive hydroxyl groups, it is laborious in terms of industrial production to modify tylosin into AIV by the methods of chemical synthesis. Therefore, an advantageous biotransformation system derived from a streptomycete producing a structurally related macrolide was

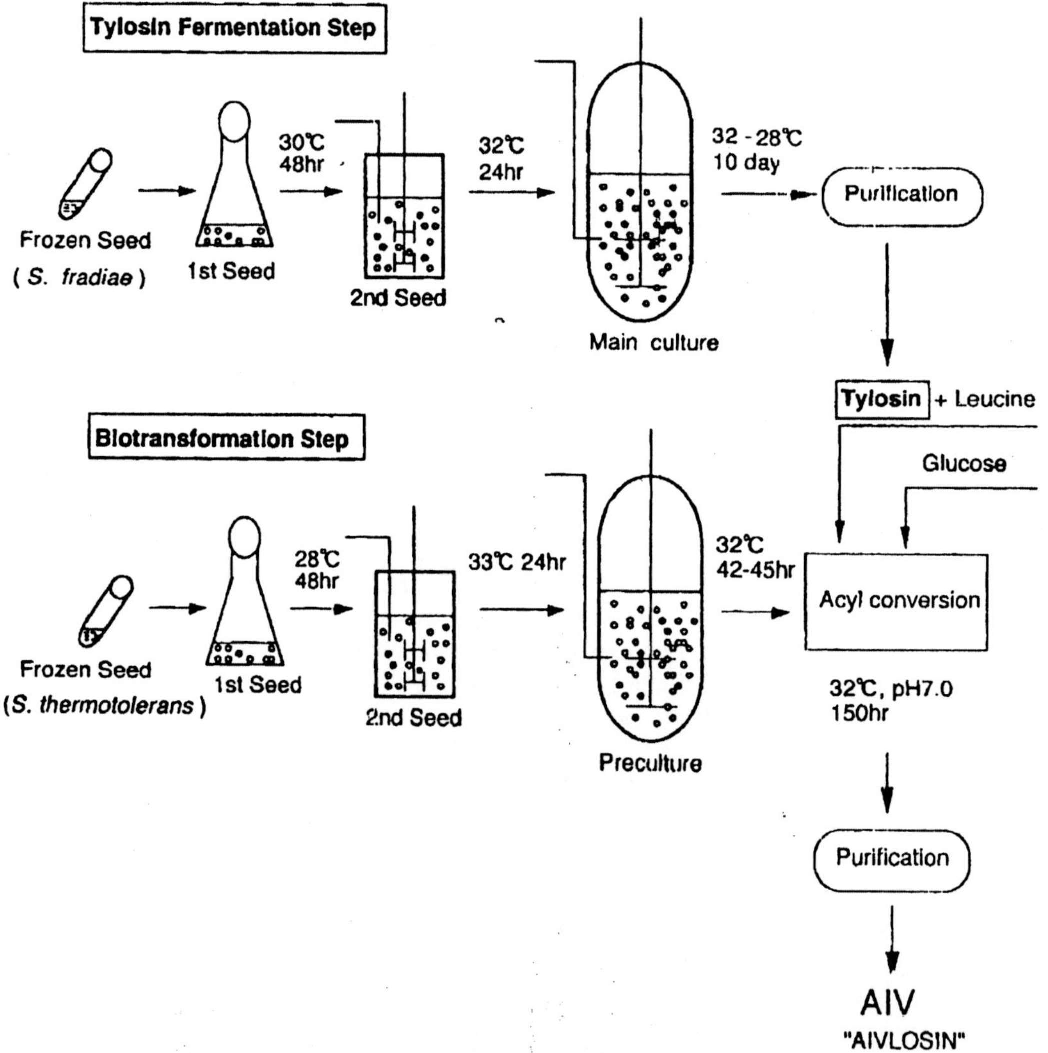

Fig. 3.12. Manufacturing process of AIV.

adopted to produce AIV. In screening for the most suitable converting strain among streptomycetes that have an ability to convert tylosin to AIV, a carbomycin producer, *Streptomyces thermotolerans*, ATCC 11416, was selected. This strain has a 3-*O*-acyltransferase and a 4″-*O*-acyltransferase, both of which are required for the biosynthesis of carbomycin. Tylosin, due to its structural similarity to carbomycin, can serve as a substrate for these acyltransferases. In practice, AIV was produced using a mutant strain of *S. thermotolerans* (strain TH475, a No. 8254 derivative), which lacks the ability to produce the parent antibiotic carbomycin, but which has both acyltransferase activities, by adding the substrate tylosin exogenously to its growing culture. The use of the mutant strain improves recovery of AIV because co-production of carbomycin is eliminated. Utilizing this biotransformation system, industrial manufacturing of AIV was established in 1990 after a number of optimizations of factors influential in large-scale fermentation. AIV is now on the market with the commercial name of Aivlosin and has achieved some market share of antibiotics used for farm animals (particularly, hogs and fowls) in Southeast Asia, South America, and Eastern Europe as well as Japan.

Although some antibiotics are produced in a single fermentation (e.g., erythromycin, leucomycin, streptomycin, kanamycin), the current manufacturing process for AIV includes two distinct fermentations: first, tylosin fermentation by *S. fradiae*; and second, acyl modification of tylosin by *S. thermotolerans*. This two-step process is relatively laborious and time-consuming, and thus it still needs improvement to reduce manufacturing cost. To solve the problem, we started to work on a strain that produces AIV directly, by expressing cloned acyltransferase genes in *S. fradiae*, which would realize a cost-saving single-step fermentation. Around 1990, when we started the project, the basis for gene manipulation technology in streptomycetes had been established, and the features and roles of genes for some antibiotic biosyntheses were beginning to be clarified. These results greatly helped us to move toward the improvement of streptomycetes by DNA recombinant techniques.

Cloning Genes Involved in Acyl Modifications of Macrolides from *S. thermotolerans*

Cloning of 4″-O-Acyltransferase Gene and a Putative Regulatory Gene

Eli Lilly researchers cloned a gene from *S. thermotolerans* for carbomycin 4″-*O*-acyltransferase from the region adjacent to *carB* (carbomycin resistance gene), and designated it *carE*. Independently, we cloned the same gene and designated it *acyB1*. Nucleotide sequence analysis of *acyB1* showed that it encodes a protein comprising 388 amino acids with a calculated molecular weight of 43.5 kDa. Interestingly, when we cloned *acyB1*, the cloned fragment included another gene that was found later to activate *acyB1* expression. This putative regulatory gene, called *acyB2*, seemed to start divergently from two possible start codons about 320 bp upstream of *acyB1*. Each protein comprises 374 or 387 amino acids with a calculated molecular weight of 41.7 or 43.0 kDa, respectively. The function of *acyB2* will be discussed in the next section.

Cloning of 3-*O*-Acyltransferase Gene

We isolated three contiguous cosmids that cover a 120-kb region containing the carbomycin biosynthetic cluster through extensive cloning by chromosome walking. Since it has been known that genes for antibiotic biosynthesis form a cluster on the genome of its producing actinomycete, this strategy facilitated us to clone a gene for 3-*O*-acyltransferase, which is located in a region approximately 60 kb downstream of *acyB1*. The deduced amino acid sequence of *acyA* (389 amino acids with a calculated molecular weight of 42.8 kDa) showed significant homology to the *acyB1* product (45% identity) and greater homology to the *mdmB* product (midecamycin 3-*O*-acetyltransferase from *Streptomyces mycarofaciens*, 66% identity). It is of great interest that comparison of amino acid sequences of those acyltransferases revealed some highly conserved motifs that might provide us with clues to identify domains responsible for regio- and substrate specificity.

A strain of *Streptomyces lividans*, which does not produce macrolide antibiotics, was transformed with plasmids carrying *acyA* and/or *acyB1-acyB2*. The resulting transformants were capable of converting exogenously added tylosin to its expected acyl derivatives (i.e., transformant with *acyA*, 3-*O*-acetyltylosin; *acyB1-acyB2*, 4″-*O*-isovaleryltylosin; both sets of genes, AIV).

Hybridization Studies with Two Acyltransferase Genes

Southern blot hybridization analysis proved that homologes of *acyA* and *acyB1* were almost perfectly conserved in the genomes of streptomycetes producing the 3,4″-di-*O*-acyl group of 16-membered macrolide antibiotics. The only exception was the *acyB1* probe, which weakly hybridized with the genomic DNA of *Streptomyces ambofaciens* that produces spiramycin, whose 4″-hydroxyl group is not acylated, but whose 3-hydroxyl group is acylated. Hybridization conditions were stringent so that the *acyB1* probe was not allowed to cross-hybridize with homologs of *acyA*. The *acyB1* probe hybridized with a 3-kb *Sac* I-digested fragment with which the *acyA* probe did not hybridize, suggesting the presence of an *acyB1* homologous gene that does not function in the *S. ambofaciens* genome. The macrolide *O*-acyltransferase genes are conserved among streptomycetes that produce 16-membered acyl macrolides such as midecamycin, leucomycin, and josamycin, but are not homologous to other types of known *O*-acyltransferases for nonmacrolide compounds (e.g., chloramphenicol acetyltransferase and choline acetyltransferase). These results indicate that the genes for macrolide *O*-acyltransferases have a common ancestry and have evolved specifically in acylation of the 3-hydroxyl group or 4″-hydroxyl group in 16-membered macrolides.

Other Cloned Genes Involved in Carbomycin Biosynthesis

The regions flanking *acyA* were sequenced. Several genes involved in carbomycin biosynthesis have been identified after sequence homology searches or expression experiments.

Regulatory Function of *ACYB2*

Expression assays with deletion plasmids revealed that the *acyB2* gene was essential for expression of the 4″-*O*-acyltransferase gene (*acyB1*). We further characterized the function of *acyB2* in *S. thermotolerans* TH475. When *acyB2* was disrupted by homologous recombination in the strain, the disruptants exhibited quite low activities of both 3-*O*- and 43″-*O*-acyltransferases and failed to convert tylosin to AIV. In contrast, the TH475 transformants in which *acyB2* was overexpressed with a high-copy vector, exhibited elevated activities of both acyltransferases and resulted in a 2.4-fold increased production of AIV. These results suggest that *acyB2* could encode a novel regulatory protein which activates expression of *acyA* and *acyB1* simultaneously.

Bate et al. reported that the deduced product of *tylR* in the biosynthetic gene cluster of tylosin resembled the *acyB2* product (42% identity at amino acid sequence level). They showed that disruption of *tylR* affected tylosin production, thus concluding that *tylR* encodes a global regulator which controls various aspects of tylosin biosynthesis. Similarly, it is very likely that *acyB2* governs not only two acyltransferases but also other genes governing carbomycin formation. We obtained the *acyB2* disruptants from the TH474 strain of *S. thermotolerans*, which fails to produce carbomycin but expresses acyltransferases. Therefore, the regulatory role of *acyB2* for the carbomycin biosynthesis genes other than *acyA* and *acyB1* has not yet been verified.

Production of Acyltylosins including AIV by Genetically Engineered *S. fradiae*

Plasmid Construction and Establishment of Host-Vector System in *S. fradiae*

We screened some strains having an improved productivity of tylosin following a series of conventional mutagenesis on the parent *S. fradiae* ATCC 19609. One of the strains, called MBBF, whose productivity is over 3500 μg/ml, was used as a host for transformation.

Various types of plasmids for producing acyltylosins were designed and constructed. *Streptomyces* high-copy vector pIJ350 and pSK1, a plasmid from *Streptomyces kasugaensis* MB273, were used as vectors. The 1.8-kb *acyA* fragment and/or the 3.4-kb *acyB1-acyB2* fragment were inserted into those vectors and the orientation of the insert(s) was verified. On the other hand, a host-vector system of the MBBF strain was established after rounds of transformation and plasmid curing. The resulting strain, in which the original restriction-modification system seemed to be eliminated or markedly diminished, was designated MBBF-c. Tylosin productivity of MBBF-c remained unchanged, whereas its transformation efficiency remarkably improved as compared with the parent MBBF when pIJ350- and pSK-based plasmids were used. After preliminary fermentation tests, the MBBF-c transformants harboring pMAA25, pMAB3, and pAB11ΔEH were selected for subsequent fermentation studies as strains to produce 3-*O*-acetyltylosin, 4″-*O*-isovaleryltylosin and AIV, respectively. Those transformants showed better productivities of acyltylosins than transformants with other types of plasmids. No morphological changes were observed in the selected transformants. Flask fermentation tests were carried out for each transformant. Acyltylosins extracted from the growing culture were analyzed by high-performance liquid chromatography (HPLC) and evaluated for productivities.

Production of 3-*O*-Acetyltylosin by *acyA*-Expressing *S. fradiae*

The *S. fradiae* transformant harboring pMAA25 (carrying *acyA*) gave a high titer of 3-*O*-acetyltylosin (3690 μg/ml), while a control strain with the pIJ350 vector produced 3250 μg/ml of tylosin. During this fermentation, the 3-*O*-acetylation reaction proceeded completely, since no tylosin was left unacylated. Probably a sufficient pool of substrate acetyl-CoA is present in cells to result in the successful conversion. Reduction in total macrolide productivity was not observed after introducing the plasmid into the host strain. Some 3-*O*-acyltranferases from other macrolide producers are likely to utilize propionyl-CoA as well as acetyl-CoA, based on their products, which include 3-*O*-propionyl components. However, no 3-*O*-propionyltylosin was detected from the fermentative products of the *acyA*-expressing strain in the HPLC analysis. Currently, we have no evidence that the *acyA*-encoded 3-*O*-acyltransferase can utilize propionyl-CoA in the reaction with tylosin.

As discussed in the previous section, *acyA* cannot be expressed efficiently without *acyB2*. In the tested strain with pMAA25 carrying *acyA* alone, however, *acyA* was expressed enough to produce a considerable amount of 3-*O*-acetyltylosin under the condition where *acyB2* was not co-expressed. The mRNA constitutively transcribed from the *tsr* gene (thiostrepton-resistance gene) lying just upstream of *acyA* is likely to run through *acyA*.

Production of 4″-*O*-Acyltylosins by *acyB1*-Expressing *S. fradiae*

After 7 days of flask fermentation in a sucrose-based medium, the MBBF-c strain transformed with pMAB3 (carrying *acyB1* and *acyB2*) produced tylosin and several 4″-*O*-acyltylosins in which the 4″-hydroxyl group had undergone various acylations. In contrast to the *acyA*-encoded 3-*O*-acyltransferase, the *acyB1*-encoded 4″-*O*-acyltransferase seemed to utilize several acyl-CoAs as substrates. The productivity of 4″-*O*-acyltylosins, which was determined by HPLC, is 4″-*O*-butyryltylosin (772 μg/ml), 4″-*O*-acetyltylosin (524 μg/ml), 4″-*O*-propionyltylosin (359 μg/ml), and 4″-*O*-isovaleryltylosin (190 μg/ml), in descending order. In this test, unconverted tylosin was also detected, and its production was 635 μg/ml (25.6% of total macrolide produced). The total macrolide productivity was reduced by 25% as compared with MBBF-c by introducing the plasmid. These results indicated that 74.4% of macrolide produced suffered 4″-*O*-acylation, but that 4″-*O*-isovaleryltylosin was a minor component (7.6% of total macrolide produced). Although 4″-*O*-isovalerylation is the major reaction in *S. thermotolerans* under conditions even without L-leucine, a starting material for isovaleryl-CoA, three other kinds of 4″-*O*-acylation (4″-*O*-acetylation, 4″-*O*-propionylation, and 4″-*O*-butyrylation) are predominant in *S. fradiae*. This finding is well consistent with differences in the macrolide-producing patterns between *Streptomyces kitasatoensis* and *Streptomyces narbonensis* var. *josamyceticus*. *S. kitasatoensis* produces many components of leucomycin (a 16-membered macrolide antibiotic related to carbomycin), which differ in their 4″-*O*- and 3-*O*-acyl groups. In contrast, *S. narbonensis* var. *josamyceticus* selectively produces josamycin (identical to the 3-*O*-acetyl-4″-*O*-isovaleryl component of leucomycin, namely, leucomycin A_3). The production rate of each component of 4″-*O*-acyltylosins is likely to depend on which and how much acyl-CoA is accumulated in the host. The genetic background advantageous for accumulating isovaleryl-CoA in cells will be discussed in the last section.

Production of 3-*O*-Acetyl-4″-*O*-acyltylosins Including AIV by *S. fradiae* Expressing *acyA* and *acyB1*

The *S. fradiae* MBBF-c strain transformed with pAB11ΔEH carrying *acyB1*- *acyB2* and *acyA* produced a variety of 3-*O*-acetyl-4″-*O*-acyltylosins after 7 days of flask cultivation. However, addition of L-leucine in the late period of fermentation increased AIV up to 602 μg/ml. The introduction of pAB11ΔEH decreased the total macrolide production by 77–78%, which was a larger loss than that caused by the introduction of pMAB3 (i.e., 25% loss) in the same host. Since the host *S. fradiae* exhibits high resistance to various acyltylosins as well as to tylosin, the decreased production was not caused by antimicrobial activities of acyltylosins. Probably some aberrant event caused by pAB11ΔEH, for example, overexpression of the acyltransferases and/or the *acyB2*-encoded regulatory factor, might affect the normal secondary metabolism including macrolide biosynthesis. A similar effect of a plasmid on secondary metabolites was previously reported. Such a negative effect of a plasmid on macrolide production was confirmed by the fact that cured strains (strains that lost pAB11ΔEH) were restored to their original productivity of tylosin.

A time course of AIV production together with other acyltylosins was studied by cultivating the transformant of MBBF-c (pAB11ΔEH) in a 3-liter-jar fermenter for 10 days. Macrolide productivity was determined by HPLC on a daily basis from the second day. Production of 3-*O*-acetyltylosin (3-AT) started to rise on day 3 and steadily increased until day 6, when L-leucine was added. Simultaneously, due to acylation at the 4″-hydroxyl group of the intermediate 3-*O*-acetyltylosin, the series of 3-*O*-acetyl-4″-*O*-acyltylosins excluding AIV (3,4″-AAT) began to accumulate and production of AIV followed. The formation of 3,4″-AAT and AIV reached a plateau on day 5, probably because of the shortage of endogenous acyl-CoAs. This assumption is supported by the fact that when exogenous L-leucine was added on day 6, AIV increased exclusively and reached 650 μg/ml on day 9, while the other group of acyltylosins remained unchanged. The AIV productivity was not improved very much in this fermentation experiment using the jar fermenter, even though its control system to keep aeration and pH conditions optimal for macrolide production was expected to ensure better productivity than fermentation in flasks. An unexpected problem appeared upon finding 3-*O*-acetyl-4″-*O*-(3-hydroxyisovaleryl)tylosin (3-HAIV) in the products, which represented a possible further metabolite of AIV that was produced at up to 270 μg/ml. The ratio of 3-HAIV to AIV remained approximately 0.3 throughout the course of the fermentation. Isovaleryl-CoA de-hydrogenase and enoyl-CoA hydratase seem to play key roles in the formation of 3-HAIV. It is likely that a series of reactions by both enzymes may convert isovaleryl-CoA to 3-hydroxyisovaleryl-CoA, which would then be used for 4″-O-acylation of tylosin to form 3-HAIV. Alternatively, the same enzymes may attack AIV directly, to give 3-HAIV.

Other Studies on Cloning Acyltransverase Genes and Heterologous Expression in Macrolide-producing Streptomycetes

In 1989, Epp and her co-workers at Eli Lilly first reported success in production of 4″-*O*-isovalerylspiramycin by expressing *carE* (identical to *acyB1*) in spiramycin-producing *S. ambofaciens*. In the study, the *carE* gene was integrated into the chromosome of *S. ambofaciens*. The resulting

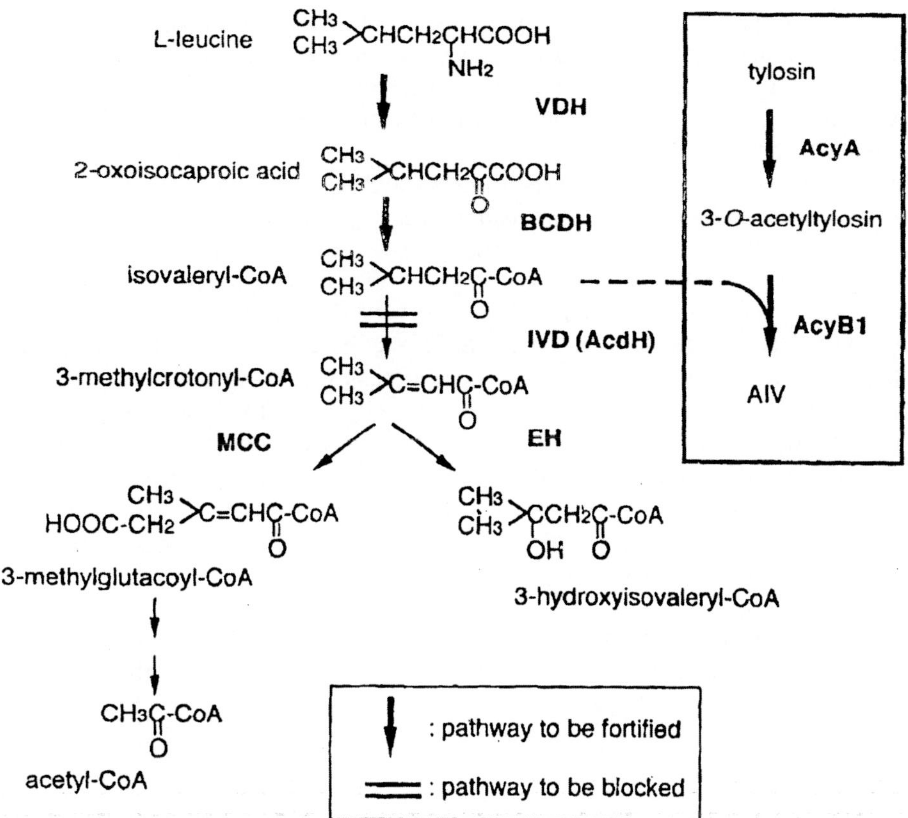

Fig. 3.13. The putative catabolic pathway of L-leucine and implications for strain improvement.

integrant produced 4″-*O*-isovalerylspiramycin II (3-*O*-acetyl-4″-*O*-isovalerylspiramycin I) and 4″-*O*-isovalerylspiramycin III (3-*O*-propionyl-4″-*O*-isovalerylspiramycin I) as the major components, although their productivities were not clarified. A similar study accomplished by Wang et al. expressed the 4″ -*O*-acyltransferase gene from the midecamycin-producer *S. mycarofaciens* in the spiramycin producer *S. ambo-faciens*. They obtained strains that produced 4″-*O*-propionylspiramycin II (3-*O*-acetyl-4″-*O*-propionylspiramycin I) and 4″-*O*-propionylspiramycin III (3,4″-di-*O*-propionylspiramycin I). The midecamycin 3-*O*-acyltransferase gene (*mdmB*) was also cloned and expressed in *S. lividans* by Hara and Hutchinson, although expression of the gene in heterologous macrolide producers was not mentioned. Researchers at Asahi Chemical Industry have looked for strains that acquired an improved productivity of leucomycin by self-cloning a gene for 4″-*O*-acyltransferase from the leucomycin producer *S. kitasatoensis*.

Perspectives for Industrial Manufacture of AIV by Genetically Engineered S. fradiae

Reduction in manufacturing cost has been one of the most general and imporant problems in the fermentation industry. To cope with the problem, strain improvements by both conventional and molecular biology-based strategies have contributed much to increase the productivity of various industrially important bioproducts, including enzymes, chemicals, and pharmaceuticals, especially in the early stage of their development process. Recently, it is becoming acceptable that ge-netic engineering, incorporating applicable aspects of metabolic engineering and directed enzyme evolution, can provide powerful and practical means to improve strains into ones ideal for fermentation with minimum labor and time. In the improvement of AIV-producing strains, as in other cases of antibiotic production, the product must satisfy high qualitative and quantitative demands. In this view, it is more significant to design and alter specific genes in the biosynthetic pathways by genetic engineering than to do random alterations by classical mutagenesis.

The AIV-producing strain that we have constructed and evaluated through the studies mentioned in this chapter is still far from industrial application. As a promising approach to its realization for industrial manufacturing, the use of hosts with highly improved productivity of tylosin is absolutely necessary. Chromosomal integration of *acyA* and *acyB1-acyB2* is thought to be effective to retain the introduced genes stably, and to express enough enzymes for the acyl modifications without a decrease in tylosin productivity during large-scale fermentation. Furthermore, to obtain a host strain which allows accumulation of much endogenous isovaleryl-CoA, we probably need to alter the catabolic path-way of L-leucine. A mutational inactivation of isovaleryl-CoA dehydrogenase gene, together with enhanced expression of valine (branched-chain amino acid) dehydrogenase and branched-chain α-keto acid dehydrogenase, would be most effective. Lately, genes for acyl-CoA dehydrogenase (*acdH*) were cloned from *Streptomyces avermitilis* and *Streptomyces coelicolor*. The gene product oxidized both short straight- and branched-chain acyl-CoAs including isovaleryl-CoA, and a mutant having a disrupted *acdH* was not able to grow on minimal media containing L-leucine as a sole carbon source. These facts show that this gene is substantially the isovaleryl-CoA dehydrogenase (IVD) gene of our interest. Use of the *acdH* gene (or its homolog in *S. fradiae*) will accelerate the work for the IVD mutant. It is hoped that these efforts assisted by genetic engineering and genome technology will lead to the direct and selective fermentation of AIV on an industrial scale.

4

Moisture in Pharmaceutical Products

The earth contains 75% water, some of it in pharmaceutical products. With regard to solid dosage forms, pharmaceutical scientists have struggled for years to answer questions on how much is there, in what form is it, and if, when, and how might it influence a product or manufacturing process. The term moisture, usually defined as wetness conferred by an unidentified liquid, is assumed here to be due to water. Thus, the scope of this article is the characterization of and consequences due to relatively small amounts of water associated with solids of pharmaceutical interest. Chemical stability, crystal structure, powder flow, compaction, lubricity, dissolution rate, and polymer film permeability are some properties of pharmaceutical interest that have been demonstrated to be influenced by the presence of moisture. Wet granulation, extrusion, spheronization, tray drying, freeze drying, spray drying, fluid-bed drying, tableting, and aqueous film coating are some unit operations that obviously depend on the amount and state of water present.

Moisture can and does influence the properties of individual active ingredients and excipients, and it is essential, as a first step, to characterize the effect of moisture on these individual components. Indeed, most of this article examines the sorption behavior of specific chemicals. However, the behavior of a pharmaceutical formulation is a complicated function of the individual component attributes. The following is an example of heterogeneous moisture distribution: A powder blend containing 2% moisture has a 10% content of an hydrophilic binder. If one assumes that all the moisture is associated with the binder, the moisture content of the binder itself would be 20%. Photomicrographic evidence demonstrates dramatically how the presence of a disintegrant, for example, can dramatically alter the environment in which a moisture-sensitive drug may exist at a particular relative humidity. Even though at least one model has been developed that allows the prediction of component moisture contents in a blend, the distribution of water in complicated formulations is largely uncharted territory.

Historical Perspective

In the area of moisture in pharmaceutical products, it is possible to identify three stages in the scientific and regulatory history. The first stage dealt more or less exclusively with the amount of water present in pharmaceuticals, most of which were products of natural origin, with regard to issues of potency and commerce. In the second stage, there was a realization that water could affect the chemical and physical properties of drugs and dosage forms. The fact that water might exist in different states was exemplified by partitioning the water into "bound" or "free" moisture. The implication was that the free, or solvent-like, moisture was responsible for most stability and production problems.

The third stage came with the realization that even small amounts of "bound" moisture could have a dramatic impact on properties and processes of pharmaceutical interest. In the evolution of this scientific pursuit, it is now evident that the state of moisture is as important as the amount present. Although sophisticated thermodynamic characterization of adsorbates has been the subject of research since the pioneering work of Gibbs, this stage has been enhanced by the ability to examine behavior at the molecular level by using powerful new analytical tools. Over the years, only few studies linked a thorough characterization of moisture with physical and chemical stability and production problems. Recent interest indicates that the subject is still important, there are still questions to be answered, and the gap between thermodynamic characterization and technological application will continue to narrow.

Compendial Standards

The methods for moisture determination in USP 24/NF 19 are at best, classical, addressing only the determination of moisture content. The specifications for most official articles are arbitrary and may be excessively restrictive or broad. They are not supported by the type of data referred to previously that relate moisture content to the stability or performance of the article. However, this occurred over 10 years ago and it has not been followed by the inclusion of standard analytical tests that can be used to characterize the state of water. The USP offers two methods for the determination of moisture content in solids: titrimetry and gravimetry (e.g., thermal gravimetric analysis). Applications, advantages, and disadvantages of these methods are addressed later. Most articles listed in the official compendia contain specifications on "water" or "loss on Drying (LOD)." As volatile components other than water may be present, loss on drying is not a de facto moisture content determination. Inclusion of a "water" specification is an indication that the only volatile component present is water.

The nature of moisture content determinations is perhaps best exemplified by the fact that the Handbook of Pharmaceutical Excipients lists 31 separate versions of laboratory tests to determine moisture content and one to determine equilibrium moisture content. These methods were used to assess the moisture content in the compilation of 148 monographs, many of which do not deal with solids.

Background

Conventions, Definitions, and Terminology

The subjects of moisture and solids have not been distinguished by clear definitions and consistent usage. Several conventions will be followed in this article. Moisture contents are expressed on a dry weight basis. When necessary, the subscript 1 is used for water, and the subscript 2 for the other component in the adsorbent; in the absence of a subscript, the property is to be attributed to water. Results of many routine tests conducted in my laboratory have been included here. Although the specific equipment used and all the experimental details are not provided, an effort has been made to include information that can substantially influence the results of the test (e.g., heating rate in thermal gravimetric analysis). These data should be taken as being representative of the substance tested and not necessarily as the results to be expected for a given lot of the substance examined with different instrumentation under different experimental conditions.

The sorption isotherm is the most widely used expression to quantify a substance's affinity for water. It is, as the term implies, a relationship at a constant temperature.

$$n = f(x) \qquad \ldots(1)$$

where n, the number of moles of water sorbed, is a function of x, the partial pressure of water in the atmosphere at that temperature. The correspondence of n to moisture content and x to relative humidity, suggests that this functional relationship may be stated in numerous ways. Often, the graphical presentation of sorption isotherms is a plot of the dependent variable moisture content versus relative humidity, with both expressed on a percentage basis.

Idealized moisture isotherms are presented in this article for substances that sorb moisture in discrete stages (e.g., crystalline materials capable of forming a hydrates) and for substances that do not interact with water in discrete stages. These idealized isotherms form a basis for the discussion of deviations and unexpected effects of moisture sorption that can influence the physical or chemical properties of the solid. Fig. 4.1 is a sorption isotherm constructed for a hypothetical solid with a molecular weight of 180, which is capable of forming a monohydrate. In this case, the solubility of the substance in water is assumed to be 50 wt% and the critical humidity for the transition from anhydrous to monohydrate is assumed to be 60% RH. It is also assumed that a solution of the solid in water behaves ideally.

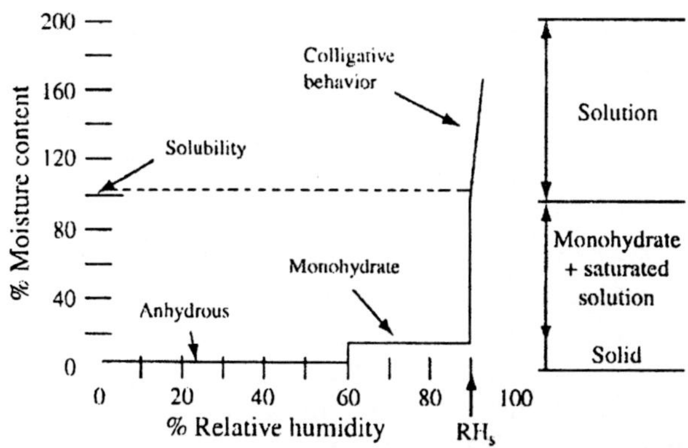

Fig. 4.1. Stepwise sorption isotherm for a hypothetical substance.

The stepwise character demonstrated in this profile is characteristic of a substance capable of forming a hydrate. At humidities below 60% RH, the moisture content of the solid remains virtually unchanged. When the activity of water reaches a critical relative humidity of 60%, water is sorbed by the solid as the anhydrous form converts to the monohydrate. For this example, the moisture content associated with the complete transition to the monohydrate is 10% (e.g., 1 mole of water = 18g; 1 mole of the substance = 180 g).

Further increase of humidity has no appreciable effect on moisture content until a water activity is reached equal to that associated with a saturated solution of the substance in water at the temperature of the analysis. The relative humidity associated with this activity will be referred to as RH_s. In this case, RH_s = 91% relative humidity, as the solubility of 50 wt% is $x_2 = 0.09$. On a mole fraction basis, and, assuming ideal solution behavior, $x_1 = 1 - x_2 = P_1/P_1^o$. In this hypothetical case, the moisture content of the saturated solution when all the solid is dissolved is 100%; therefore, at 91% RH the monohydrate sorbs water from the atmosphere until dissolution is complete. The fact that constant humidity is produced by a saturated solution of a substance has been used as a basis for establishing controlled-humidity chambers.

At relative humidities above 91%, the colligative behavior of the solution results in absorption of water until the solution is in equilibrium with water vapor in the atmosphere. Although some specific examples are given, several aspects of the sorption of water by crystalline substances deserve attention at this point. First, it is important to recognize that the large quantity of water that associates with these systems actually obscures small changes in moisture content that occur between hydrate transitions. It has been stated that lactose monohydrate, for example, "contains 5% water of crystallization and approximately 0.1% adsorbed water", indicating that adsorption takes place on the hydrate.

Furthermore, this sorption isotherm is a thermodynamic relationship. Although it represents the equilibrium position, it does not provide any information about the rate at which the transitions take place. For example, the desiccant calcium sulfate goes through two stages of hydration, as shown in Eq. (2)

Stage 1:

$$CuSO_4 + \frac{1}{2}H_2O \rightarrow CuSO_4 + \frac{1}{2}H_2O$$

Stage 2:

$$CuSO_4 + \frac{1}{2}H_2O + 1\frac{1}{2}H_2O \rightarrow CuSO_4 + 2H_2O \qquad \ldots(2)$$

The first stage where the hemihydrate is formed takes place instantaneously in the presence of water vapor, whereas the second stage requires a matter of weeks or months to reach completion, depending on the humidity at which the hemihydrate is stored. Finally, the critical relative humidities are dependent on the nature of the solid. For example, the spontaneous dissolution process has been observed for many water-soluble substances at relative humidities significantly below that associated with a saturated solution of the substance in water. Van Campen, Amidon, and Zograf have examined the moisture sorption kinetics of deliquescent solids at relative humidities above what they term the "*critical relative humidity*" (RH_0), where adsorbed water takes on the character of condensed water and serves as a solvent. It is important to recognize that a highly undesirable process such as deliquescence can occur when it may not be expected (e.g., when $RH_0 < RH < RH_s$).

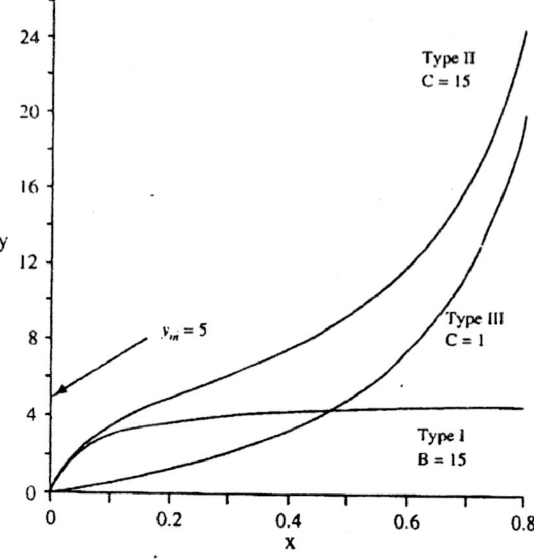

Fig. 4.2. Hypothetical type I, II, and III sorption isotherms with a monolayer capacity of y_m = 5.

In all the previous examples, the process was absorption, and water ultimately had access to the entire solid; variations in particle size, and consequently, surface area, would not effect the profile. In many of the subsequent examples, not only is surface area a determinant of moisture content, but perturbation of the solid can occur during sorption to produce unexpected and dramatic effects. Brunauer organized the experimental isotherms observed for vapor sorption into the now classical five groups, Types I to V. Brunauer, Emmett, and Teller presented a unified theory of multilayer physical adsorption that was purported to describe all types of isotherms. Numerous texts present detailed discussion of the basis for this theory. In the context of this discussion, capillary condensation will not be considered and the focus will be Types I, II, and III behavior.

Type I isotherms, where sorption occurs on strong sorption sites, are characterized by a monotonic increase in the amount of vapor adsorbed, up to a maximum value assumed to represent a completed unimolecular layer. The Langmuir equation is generally a suitable functional relationship for $n = f(x)$, as given by

$$\frac{y = y_m Bx}{1 + Bx} \quad \ldots(3)$$

where y is the amount of water adsorbed at $x = P/P_0$, y_m is the monolayer capacity, and B is a constant, often referred to as the adsorption coefficient. Using the generally assumed value of 1250 nm^2 for the area occupied by a molecule of water on the adsorbent surface, the surface area can be estimated from y_m.

The characteristic inflection in Type II behavior occurs when multilayer sorption starts. The Brunauer, Emmett, Teller (BET) equation, shown as Eq. (4), can describe isotherms where multilayer sorption is evident:

$$\frac{y = y_m Cx}{(1-x)(1+(C-1)x)} \quad \ldots(4)$$

Based on the assumptions in the kinetic derivation of the BET equation, the constant C is related to the average heat of adsorption in the first layer. Type III isotherms occur when this value is low.

Application of the BET equation to experimental data has become the standard method for surface area determinations. The constants are determined from data at low humidities (5–30% RH). Based on these parameters, the BET equation almost always over-estimates the amount of water associated with the solid at high humidity.

As 100% RH is approached, the BET theory predicts that the amount of water adsorbed will be infinite. As the influence of the solid surface does not extend indefinitely, it should be expected that a finite number of molecular layers would be adsorbed (presuming that the solid is not soluble.) Many authors attribute the "*infinity catastrophe*" of the BET theory to the lack of consideration of lateral adsorbate interactions.

Ostensibly the constant C relates to the state of water associated with the solid; however, the simplistic assumptions (all molecules in the second and higher layers are assumed to have the same character as bulk water and horizontal interactions between molecules are ignored for all layers) used in the derivation preclude really useful thermodynamic information.

Eq. (5), a modification of the BET equation which assumes a third thermodynamic state for the adsorbate, was developed independently by Guggenheim et al.

$$\frac{y = y_m CKx}{(1 - Kx)(1 + (C - 1)Kx)} \qquad \ldots(5)$$

where K is a constant that accounts for the intermediate state between tightly bound water in the first layer and bulk liquid. This model is also simplistic but it does fits data at high relative humidities better than the BET equation. Eq. (5) is termed the GAB equation.

All of the equations presented thus far are single-valued relationships between the amount adsorbed and the pressure of water in the atmosphere. However, hysteresis is frequently observed. When a sample that has reached a specific equilibrium moisture content is exposed to lower relative humidity, desorption occurs. In many cases, adsorption and desorption isotherms are not superimposable. Fig. 4.3 is an example of a Type II sorption isotherm with hysteresis. Although the etiology of hysteresis has been the subject of many discussions, the phenomena usually can be attributed to

1. Irreversible perturbation of the solid, that is, sorption can increase (swelling) or decrease (collapse of a freeze-dried cake) the surface area;
2. Kinetic origin, that is, the new equilibrium position has actually not yet been reached; and
3. An actual change in state of the adsorbate.

Most individuals recognize hysteresis in terms of a substance having different moisture contents at a specified relative humidity. The implications of this situation are obvious: the moisture content of a material depends on its history of exposure to different relative humidity conditions. Controlling relative humidity can only insure that the moisture content lies within the range specified by the isotherm. The other aspect of hysteresis is that substances with equal moisture contents can have adsorbed water with different chemical activity.

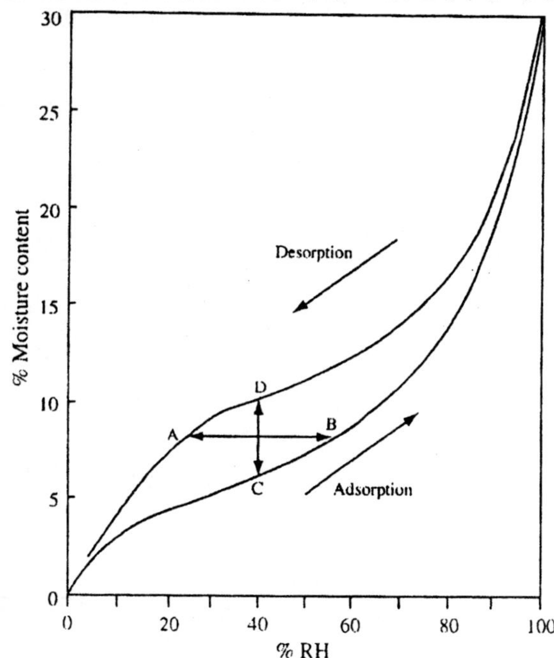

Fig. 4.3. Type II isotherm with hysteresis.

Although the sorption isotherm is fundamental to the characterization of moisture interaction with water, it is generally not possible to make any judgments about the effect of water on the substrate from the isotherm alone. For example, it is not possible to determine if an increase in moisture content is due to multilayer adsorption, swelling of the substrate, or some combination of the two. Compressible sugar NF is an example of a material that very slowly sorbs relatively small amounts of water, with a resulting isotherm that is not smooth. The adsorption isotherm was generated from a sample that had been carefully preconditioned to remove moisture. The dramatic difference between the desorption and adsorption branches of the isotherm indicates that water forms a hydrate-like phase. Zografi and Kontny have demonstrated that almost all of the water taken up by compressible sugar is associated with the maltodextrin.

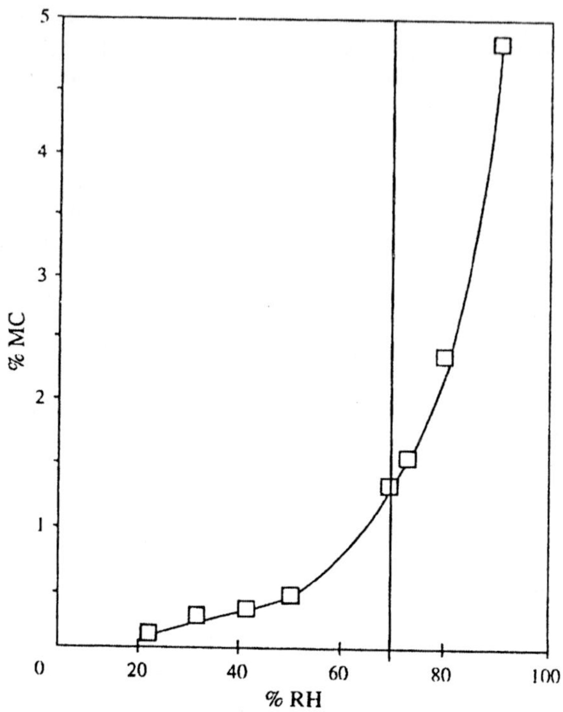

Fig. 4.4. Moisture sorption isotherm for lactose.

Moisture sorption of microcrystalline cellulose has been studied extensively. The inserts are plots of moisture content versus time, which approximately represent the kinetics of sorption and desorption at each humidity. The equilibrium adsorption isotherm (Type II) has been fit to the BET equation (C = 16.48, y_m = 0.033g/g solid) and this curve is presented along with a curve described by the GAB equation by using the same monolayer capacity.

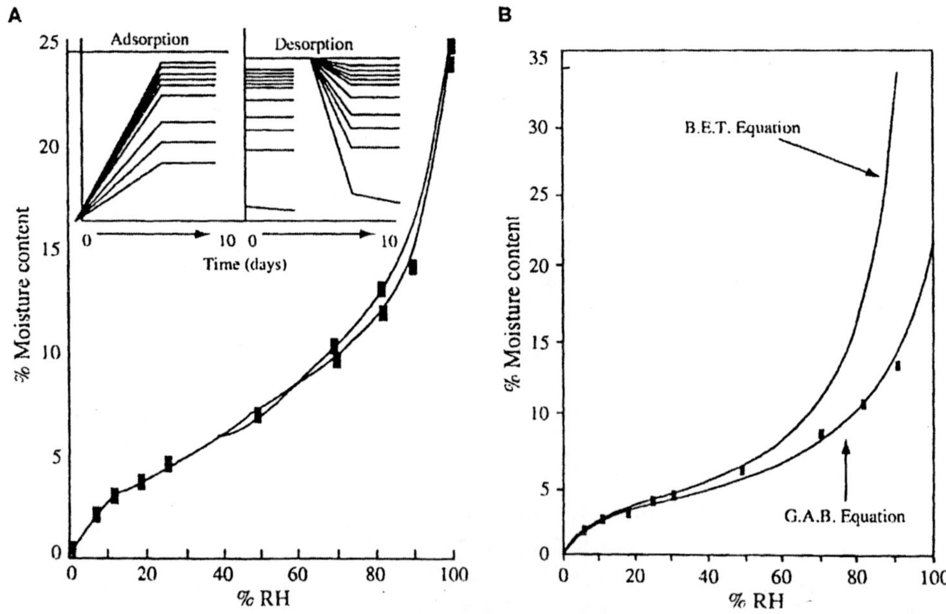

Fig. 4.5. A–Moisture sorption isotherm for microcrystalline cellulose: adsorption and desorption. B–BET and GAB equations describing the adsorption branch.

The isotherm for aspirin would be classified as Type III, indicating a low affinity for water followed by multilayer sorption. These four isotherms cover a broad range of moisture interaction with solids of pharmaceutical interest.

Analytical Methods

There is no single analytical method that suffices in the characterization of moisture associated with solids. The best approach is a judicious combination of the following techniques. In this era of automatic titrators, microprocessor- controlled thermal analysis, and definitive spectral techniques, one of the most powerful techniques, that is, optical microscopy, is frequently overlooked. The value of direct sample observation, preferably while it is exposed to different relative humidities, cannot be overstated. In the author's laboratory, a plexiglass chamber was constructed that can be placed on the stage of the microscope, through which air of known humidity can be circulated. This simple technique has been very useful in examining the swelling (or lack) of disintegrants and the influence of very hydrophilic excipients in combination with a moisture sensitive drug.

In a moisture determination by the physical separation of water from the solid, it is important to recognize that free and bound moisture must be dissociated from the solid by an applied stress, using

$$\text{Solid} \cdot xH_2O \rightarrow \text{Solid} \cdot yH_2O + (x - y)H_2O \quad \ldots(6)$$

where x is the moles of water initially associated with the solid, y the moles of water still associated with the solid, and $(x - y)$ the amount of water released as a consequence of the stress. The stresses used differ according to the conditions (e.g., high temperature, low vapor pressure, anhydrous solvent systems). Hence, the moisture contents determined by different methods may very well be different. There is no guarantee that $y = 0$, and no reason to expect that y has the same value for different methods. An equally important consideration is the fact that these stresses are different than those that may be responsible for moisture release during manufacturing or within the product after manufacture. One should approach the determination of moisture content with the disconcerting realization that different methods can produce different results and that none of these results may be relevant.

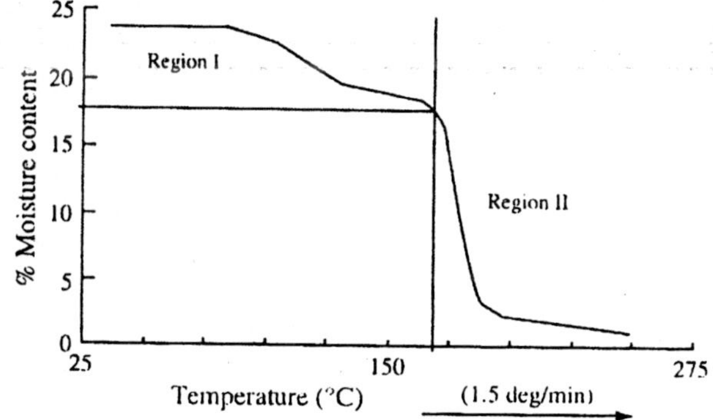

Fig. 4.6. Thermal gravimetric analysis of dicalcium phosphate dihydrate.

Thermal Methods

Thermal gravimetric analysis (TGA) is undoubtedly the most widely used method of moisture content determination. The sensitivity and sophistication of TGA instruments ranges from the classical moisture balance (LOD) to specially designed microbalances enclosed in chambers that may be evacuated. Microprocessor control of the temperature increase has led to more reproducible and discriminating information. The profile represents the weight loss with increasing temperature (1.5°C/min) in an environment containing a desiccant. The total weight loss is the difference between the initial weight and the final constant weight of the dry solid. There are two regions in the profile, the first beginning at about 90°C and the second at about 170°C. Assuming that the only volatile component is water, calculations indicate $W_D = 0.228$ (22.8% MC), with WD values of about 0.042 and 0.186 associated with Regions I and II, respectively.

The profile is characteristic of a crystal hydrate, showing discrete regions of moisture loss occurring at relatively high temperature. This particular profile is consistent with the dehydration scheme shown in Eq. (7).

Reaction 1 :

$$CaHPO_2 \cdot 2H_2O \rightarrow CaHPO_4 \cdot 1\frac{1}{2}H_2O + \frac{1}{2}H_2O$$

Reaction 2 :

$$CaHPO_2 \cdot 1\frac{1}{2}H_2O \rightarrow CaHPO_4 + 1\frac{1}{2}H_2O \qquad \ldots(7)$$

Differential scanning calorimetry (DSC) is a thermal method that measures the energy change accompanying a non-adiabatic process. A small sample of the moist solid contained in a metal sample container is exposed to a controlled increase in temperature. Water dissociated from the sample is swept out of the heating chamber by a nitrogen stream and the dynamic energy consumption (mcal/sec) required to keep the sample at the same temperature as an empty sample container is recorded. When the temperature is increased at a constant rate, the area under the DSC curve reflects the energy, in the form of heat, associated with the phase change. The DSC profile for dicalcium phosphate dihydrate includes two endotherms consistent with the dehydration scheme shown in Eq. (7). (In all DSC plots reported here, endotherms are positive deflections from the base line.) It should also be noted that the energy change measured is not specific for water; it includes, for example, energy consumed or released because of changes in crystal structure. Thus, it is generally not appropriate to estimate moisture content from the enthalpy change for dehydration and the specific heat of vaporization of water.

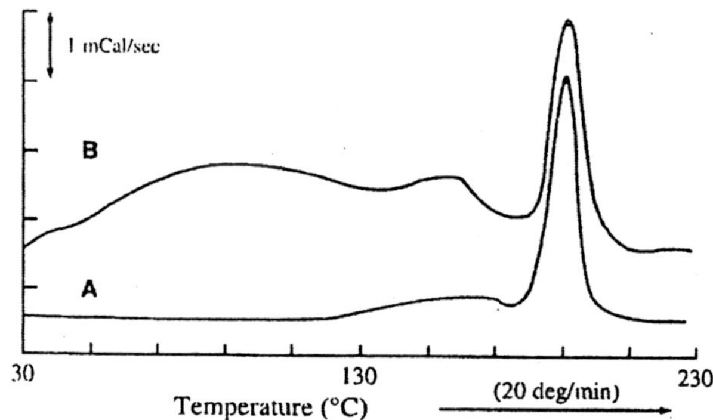

Fig. 4.7. Differential scanning calorimetry of dicalcium phosphate samples. A-dicalcium phosphate dihydrate; B-anhydrous dicalcium phosphate with adsorbed moisture.

A common error is to look at temperature profiles (TGA or DSC) and conclude, for example, that no water is released from dicalcium phosphate dihydrate at 50°C. It is important to recognize that this is a dynamic test with a large temperature increase examined over a relatively short time periods. Exposure of dicalcium phosphate dihydrate at 50°C may indeed drive off water of hydration; the system is not held at any particular temperature and the relative rate of moisture loss is slow. Curve B in Fig. 4.7 is the result of an interesting test on a sample of anhydrous dicalcium phosphate that had been exposed to 100% RH for three months. Clearly, some of the moisture acquired by the solid was converted into water of hydration. However, the broad endotherm from about 50 to 130°C represents the energy consumed in the dissociation of water that is not part of the crystal structure. The existence of two states of water in the same solid raises a number of questions pertaining to the wisdom of using anhydrous dicalcium phosphate as an excipient for moisture-sensitive drugs.

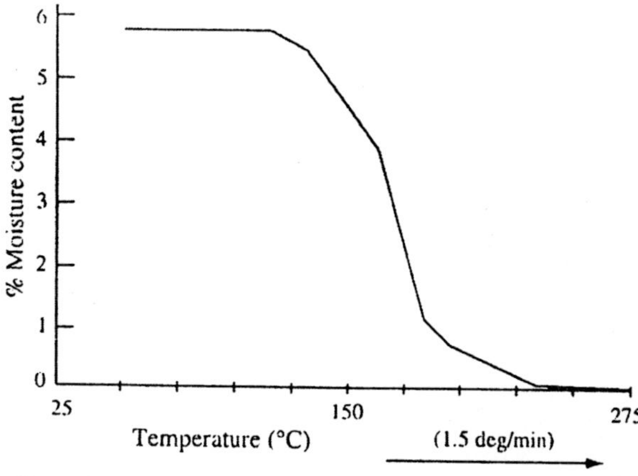

Fig. 4.8. Thermal gravimetric analysis of lactose monohydrate.

The TGA profile for lactose is shown in Fig. 4.8. This profile is consistent with a monohydrate that loses its water of hydration in one step. DSC data for lactose are shown in Fig. 4.9. Scan A for anhydrous lactose is rather uneventful, although comparison with the other scans seems to indicate the presence of a small quantity of water. Scan B is for lactose monohydrate; the single water of hydration is lost at approximately 135°C, with decomposition occurring at about 200°C. Scan C is for an anhydrous lactose sample that had been exposed to 100% RH for three days. Clearly, the water sorbed by anhydrous lactose was quickly and completely converted to water of hydration.

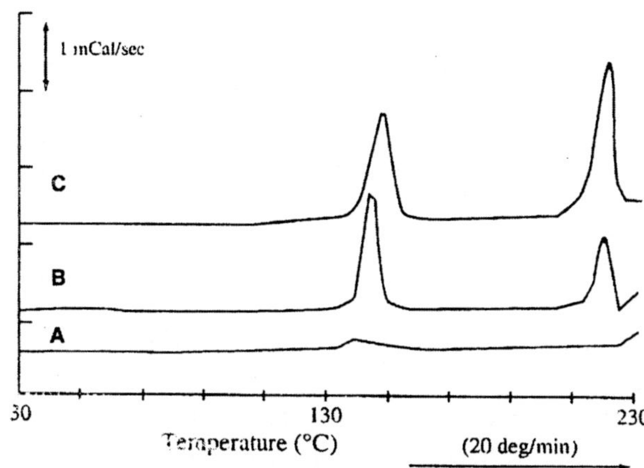

Fig. 4.9. Differential scanning calorimetry of lactose samples. A–anhydrous lactose; B–lactose monohydrate; C–anhydrous lactose with adsorbed moisture.

Thermal analyses of microcrystalline cellulose reveal distinctly different results. The TGA shows a loss of moisture at low temperature and a reasonably monotonic decrease that does not indicate discrete stages of hydration. The DSC shows a broad region of moisture loss at temperatures well below the boiling point of water. The principal advantage of the thermal methods is convenience; however, these analyses are not specific for water, and exposure to high temperature may be an unrealistic stress or alter the sample. An acceptable determination of moisture content using a thermal method provides a result with minimal residual moisture and only minor alteration of the solid. Thermal methods can be combined with a specific titration of water by bubbling the evolved gas from TGA or DSC through the titration medium.

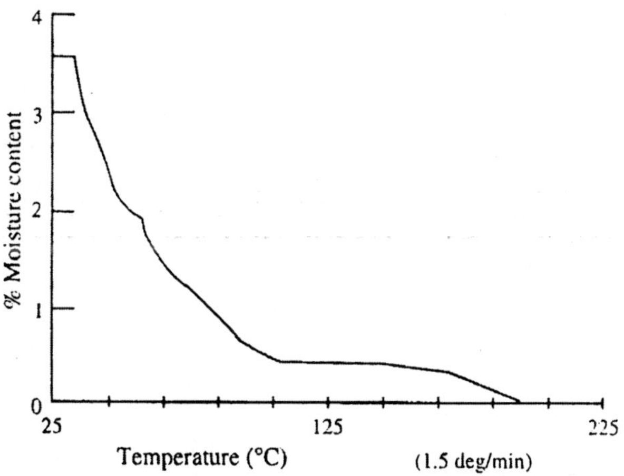

Fig. 4.10. Thermal gravimetric analysis of microcrystalline cellulose.

Karl Fisher Titration

For over 60 years, the specific titration of water has used a reagent developed by Karl Fisher, which consists of iodine, sulfur dioxide, and pyridine in methanol. The Karl Fisher titration of water is addressed in most analytical chemistry texts and is not presented here. However, the advantages and disadvantages of this method for the characterization of water associated with solids are discussed later.

In its simplest form, the Karl Fisher titration is a one-point determination of moisture content. The principal advantage is specificity for water. It is also a non-thermal method, which is very sensitive and can be easily automated. The main disadvantage is that the solid must dissolve in the titration medium to be sure that the total amount of moisture is released. If the analysis is carefully designed in such a way that moisture is "extracted" from the solid to the same degree each time, accurate and reproducible results can be obtained for solids that do not dissolve.

With automation, the Karl Fisher titration provides a titration kinetics profile (e.g., milliliters of titrant vs. time). If the rate of water release from the solid is the rate-limiting step, the kinetics of the Karl Fisher titration profile can provide indirect information about the state of water associated with the solid. Fig. 4.11 shows the titrations of two different samples of dicalcium phosphate dihydrate.

Here, and in the titration profiles in Fig. 4.12, the data have been normalized in such a way that each titration ultimately consumes 25 mL of reagent. This normalization is analagous to increasing the sample size in such a way that it contains an amount of available water which would require 25 mL of reagent to neutralize. Also, the direct titration of water can be finished in less than 90s.

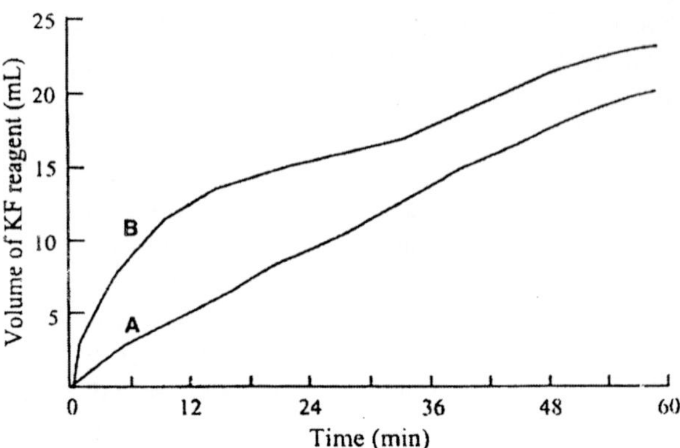

Fig. 4.11. Normalized Karl Fisher titrations of dicalcium phosphate dihydrate; A-unmilled form; B-milled form.

The titration profiles for dicalcium phosphate are not monotonic, but exhibit stages of dehydration consistent with the scheme shown in Eq. (7). It is also evident that the release of moisture is faster from the milled form of the excipient. This is consistent with the increased total surface area and shorter diffusional path expected with smaller particle size. In Fig. 4.12, Karl Fisher titration of anhydrous dicalcium phosphate, which had been exposed to 100% RH for 3 months, is compared to with that of milled dicalcium phosphate dihydrate. The adsorbed water, which was not incorporated into the crystal lattice, was released from the solid very rapidly. Results of normalized Karl Fisher titrations for lactose monohydrate and microcrystalline cellulose both present profiles not significantly different from water, indicating a very rapid release of moisture.

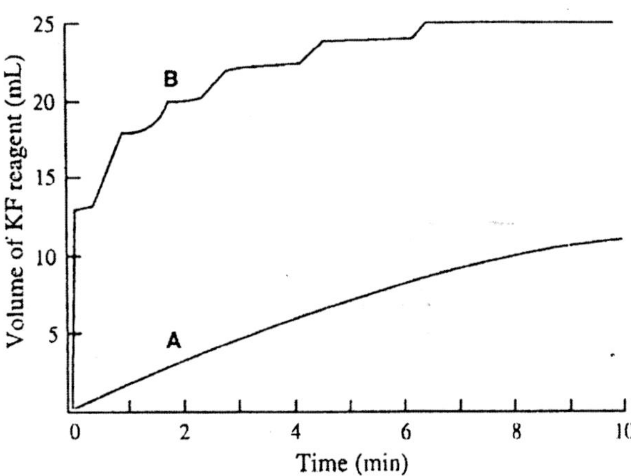

Fig. 4.12. Normalized Karl Fisher titration for dicalcium phosphate; A-milled sample; B-anhydrous sample with adsorbed moisture.

Spectroscopic Methods

The most useful spectral methods for the characterization of water in solids are Fourier transform infrared spectroscopy (FTIR), nuclear magnetic resonance (NMR), and powder X-ray diffraction (XRD). A thorough treatment of these methods is not given here; instead the example of ampicillin presented by Brittan, et al. is summarized. Hydrates normally form crystal structures (pseudopolymorphs) that differ from the anhydrous form. Although moisture contents often present values that are close to being stoichiometric, X-ray confirmation of the differing crystal structure should be a requisite for designation as a hydrate.

The X-ray method is not just useful from the qualitative perspective. In samples that contain both anhydrous and hydrate forms, diagnostic regions of the pattern can be identified, and the relative areas of peaks in these regions may be used to establish the relative amounts of each phase. Infrared analysis of water associated with a solid centers on an assessment of the degree to which the environment influences the stretching frequency associated with the -OH group. The -OH stretching mode for free water in the gaseous state has a characteristic energy of 3655 cm^{-1}. The frequency of this stretching is lowered when water is condensed and/or bound. Ice has a characteristic -OH stretching frequency of 3400 cm^{-1}. By comparison of the FTIR spectra for the anhydrous form with those of the sample with water, the -OH bands for water can be identified. The distinctive, sharp peak for crystalline water is shown in Fig. 4.13; when water is present in several states, multiple bands may be seen in the spectrum.

Solid-state NMR is a method that promises to increase the understanding of the state of water in solids and its specific influence on the chemicals of interest. For example, it is clear that the solid-state ^{13}C NMR spectra of ampicillin trihydrate is a very different form than that for the anhydrous form. Although three carbonyl resonances present in the anhydrous form (169.7, 172.7, and 174.6 ppm), it is interesting that only two (170.4 and 172.6 ppm) are fully resolved in the hydrate form. Thus, in the latter, two of the three carbonyls are equivalent. Evidence also exists for differences in carbons in the aromatic ring based on the presence of water of hydration.

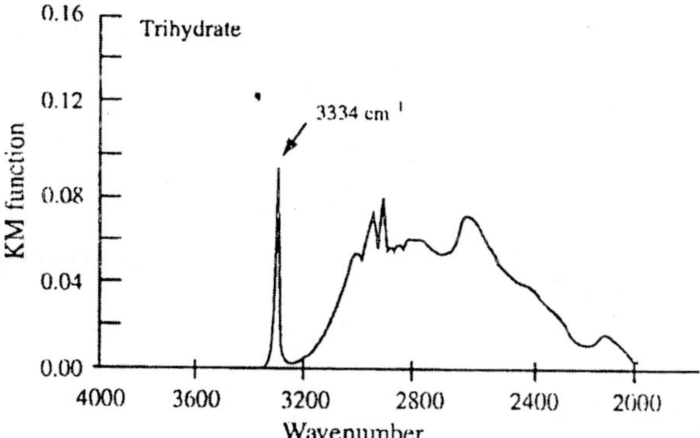

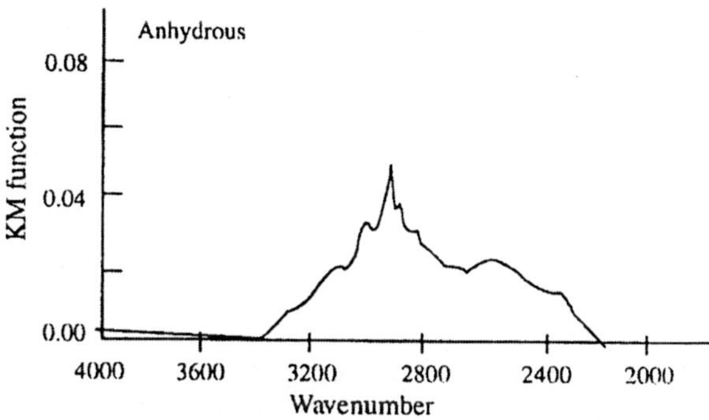

Fig. 4.13. Partial FTIR spectra of ampicillin.

Influence of Moisture on Product and/or Process Attributes

No attempt will be made to provide a comprehensive summary of the numerous studies that have been conducted and which show how water influences the processing and stability of pharmaceutical solids and dosage forms. For more information, the reader is referred to some classical texts, recent general articles on the subject, and those with specific emphasis on the role of water on stability or compaction properties. In an earlier section, the potential for a water-soluble substance to deliquesce was discussed. The emphasis here is on less obvious effects of moisture on solid dosage forms, and three associated areas that link to information presented earlier in this article are discussed: (1) moisture-induced changes in the state of the solid; (2) the effect of moisture on the performance of excipients in the manufacture of compressed tablets; and (3) the chemical stability of bioactive agents alone and in combination with excipients.

Moisture-Induced Changes

That moisture can have a dramatic effect on the physical character of a substance has been demonstrated recently by Carstensen and Van Scoik. Amorphous sucrose spheres were prepared by lyophilization and placed in an environment at 33% RH. Lyophilization characteristically produces a highly porous, amorphous solid cake. Its moisture content increases considerably in the first few days of the study. However, the moisture absorbed by the porous amorphous sucrose phase eventually caused a collapse of the structure and a commensurate reduction in moisture content because of the dramatic decrease in available "surface." Not only did the physical structure change from a loose to a more dense amorphous structure, but also the amorphous sucrose was shown to convert to the crystalline form at a rate that was dependent on relative humidity. This example is consistent with the increased emphasis being placed on changes in state of the solid as a result of sorption. One of the difficulties associated with a thermodynamic treatment of solids is the problem of dealing with changes in surface area as a continuous variable. An early thermodynamic treatment to address this problem was presented by Copeland and Young in 1961. These authors considered a change in the number of moles of adsorbent as an addition or removal of particles with the same specific surface area, and, therefore, presented a basis for treating thermodynamic properties of powder systems as continuous functions. Wu and Copeland used this approach in the characterization of barium sulfate. They found clear evidence to discount the "inert" adsorbent theory and stressed that even though thermodynamic variables of adsorbents are generally smaller than these for adsorbates, this can be misleading. Adsorbent properties are average properties of the respective component. When the adsorbed moisture is homogeneously distributed within the solid, this estimate is reasonable. However, if the process is adsorption and only the first few layers of the adsorbent are affected, the thermodynamic changes would be dramatically increased. Very few pharmaceutical studies involve the determination of thermodynamic properties of the adsorbent which is a promising area for further research.

The need to address changes in adsorbent is discussed by Zografi. He observes that water absorbed into the bulk structure of a solid can act as a plasticizer and depress the glass transition temperature. At temperatures above the glass transition point, the mobility of molecules or segments of molecules in the system increases. The change from the "*glassy state*" to the "*rubbery state*" can account for a number of physical chemical processes of pharmaceutical interest, including the collapse and subsequent crystallization of lyophilized cakes, direct compaction properties, powder caking, permeability of coatings and packaging materials, and solid-state chemical stability. Recognition of this fact has been the single greatest recent advance in establishing a framework for understanding and predicting the impact of moisture. Zografi and Kontny corrected the experimentally determined monolayer capacities of microcrystalline cellulose for degree of crystallinity and found reasonably consistent values. This result supported the conclusion that water in microcrystalline cellulose is confined to the non-crystalline regions.

Effect of Moisture on Excipients and Tablet Manufacture

The bulk properties of celluloses are generally influenced by adsorbed moisture. The effect of the change in bulk solid properties for microcrystalline cellulose has been demonstrated by a tableting operation in a very simplistic manner. Dry microcrystalline cellulose (%MC = 0.07) was compared with material with a moisture content above that associated with completion of the monolayer (%MC = 5.1). A thermodynamic picture of the character of water in these samples can be based on the adsorbate thermodynamic properties: $\Delta H > 3.5$ kcal/mole (14.65 kJ/mole), $\Delta G > 2.3$ kcal/mole (9.6 kJ/mole), $\Delta S < 4.12$ entropy units (e.u.) per mole with the dry solid, and $\Delta H = 1.5$ kcal/mole (6.27 kJ/mole, $\Delta G = 0.53$ kcal/mole (2.21 kJ/mole), $\Delta S = 3.35$ e.u./mole for moisture at the 5.1% level, or 1.5 times monolayer capacity. (The differential entropy goes through a maximum near the level where a monolayer is completed, and the large difference in free energy between the two states can be accounted for primarily in terms of the bonding of the water to the solid.)

In each case, preconditioned material was placed in the hopper of an instrumented tablet machine and the performance of these two materials was compared at constant machine settings. The sample with 5.1% MC produced tablets that weighed slightly less (an effect on flow and bulk density), and as a result were exposed to lower compression force. However, the moist micro- crystalline cellulose resulted in harder tablets, even though it had been exposed to lower compression force. The loci of points on the compression force versus hardness profile for the tablets indicate a different fundamental behavior for the two materials. In a similar, yet more extensive study, the compaction of compressible sugar was examined for materials preconditioned at different relative humidities. The hardness versus compression profiles for these samples show a group of lines whose slope appears to be a function of moisture content. This index is a linear function of moisture content; samples with "desorbed" moisture did not differ from those with adsorbed moisture.

Chemical Stability of Bioactive Agents

Despite recent advances in understanding the influence of moisture on the physical state of the solid, it is perhaps the effect of sorbed moisture on the chemical stability of moisture-sensitive drugs that is most important, particularly because many new bioactive agents are expensive moisture-sensitive proteins. The literature related to the study of the influence of moisture on the properties and stability of proteins is extensive and growing rapidly. The examination of water associated with proteins and polymers is relevant to the pharmaceutical scientist dealing with the formulation and processing of small drug molecules as well because many excipients used belong in this large- molecule category. A review of protein stability from the pharmaceutical perspective has been presented by Hageman. He ascribes the effect of water content and activity on the solid-state stability of proteins to

1. Changes in dynamic activity;
2. Changes in conformational stability;
3. Participation of water as a reactant or inhibitor; and
4. Participation of water as a medium for mobilization of reactants.

Using an analysis of the hydration data of lysozyme and other proteins, Hageman describes critical ranges of hydration based on certain properties of bound water (carboxylate absorbance at 1580 cm^{-1}, amide-1 shift at 1660 cm^{-1}, OD stretching frequency at 2570 cm^{-1}, specific heat capacity, diamagnetic susceptibility). Below monolayer capacity, these physical properties of water do not change significantly, and this water has very little mobility. Between 6% and 25% water, the properties of bound water change dramatically, above 25% water, the properties of bound water are similar to bulk water.

The role of moisture in bimolecular reactions is classified by Hageman into three cases. The increases in reaction rate are attributed to a change in state of the water associated with the solid as reflected by a lower effective viscosity. In Case I, there is a continual increase in reaction rate with increasing water content above the monolayer. When all the reactant has been solubilized and further water dilutes the medium, Case II results. If the dilution is extensive, or if water is a product inhibitor of decomposition, a rate reduction can be observed (Case III). Case III behavior is an example of the effect of moisture on the progress of the Malliard reaction for the glucose-containing formulations of α-N-acetyl-L-lysine, poly-L-lysine, insulin, casein, and plasma proteins. The fact that there can be a maximum degradation rate at a humidity other than 100% RH is observed in other situations as well.

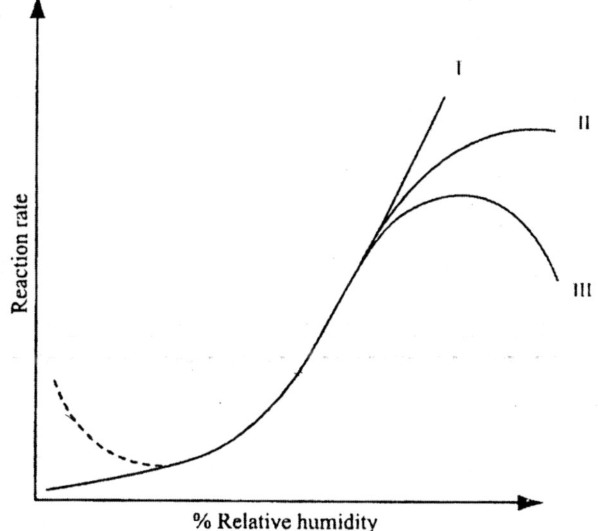

Fig. 4.14. Effect of sorbed water on the reaction rates of bimolecular reactions in the solid state.

The presence of excipients in a formulation can influence product stability. The conceptually appealing strategy of including a "*moisture scavenger*" in a formulation is based on this. In glucose-containing systems, it was demonstrated that liquid and solid humectants can influence the mobility of water in the system. The location of the maximum rate of reaction was found to vary from 40% to 80% RH, depending on the additives. The addition of liquids such as glycerol or propylene glycol lowered the mobilization point and facilitated the reaction at lower humidities. The addition of the solid humectant sorbitol reduced the reaction rate dramatically by decreasing free water for mobilization of reactants. Carstensen has presented a summary of the effects of moisture on the stability of smaller molecules by addressing three cases: decomposition with non-depleting moisture, simultaneous decomposition in the solid and dissolved states, and decomposition with limited amounts of water. In the context of this discussion, emphasis here is placed on hydrolytic degradation processes.

The first case with abundant moisture was initially modeled by Leeson and Mattocks by assuming that the solid particle was surrounded by a layer of moisture sufficiently mobile to permit dissolution of the drug substance. If the layer remains saturated with drug, this approach yields an apparent zero-order degradation process given

$$-\frac{dM}{dt} = kS[H_2O] \qquad \ldots(8)$$

where $-dM/dt$ is the rate of drug loss, k is a rate constant appropriate for the order of the reaction, S is the saturation concentration of the drug in the layer, and $[H_2O]$ is the concentration of water. Although this simple approach often suffices in form to describe data observed in a stability study, it should not be expected to account for the effects of moisture present in the different states described previously.

The degradation of aspirin powder after 120 days at 100% RH and 25°C, for example, was found to be more than ten times greater than what would be expected based on suspension data. In addition, the actual rate of aspirin degradation has been found to increase with time. Carstensen presented a theory to describe this non-linear behavior based on the fact that the formation of salicylic acid actually exposes moisture adsorption sites of higher energy on aspirin, thereby leading to the acquisition of more water.

This explanation accounts for an increase in rate with time, but does not explain why the rate is higher for the powder than a suspension where the supply of water is in huge excess. This increased rate could be due to specific acid catalysis in a film of relatively small volume where the pH is dramatically affected by the hydrolysis itself. Finally, the complicated situation faced when a moisture sensitive drug is combined with an hydrophilic excipient. In this study, aspirin was combined with 4% of the disintegrant and stored for 120 days at 25°C at the respective humidity. The moisture contents stabilized within the first few days, and the degradation results are presented as moles of the degradation product salicylic acid per mole of water. Point A is the result for aspirin powder alone at 100% RH.

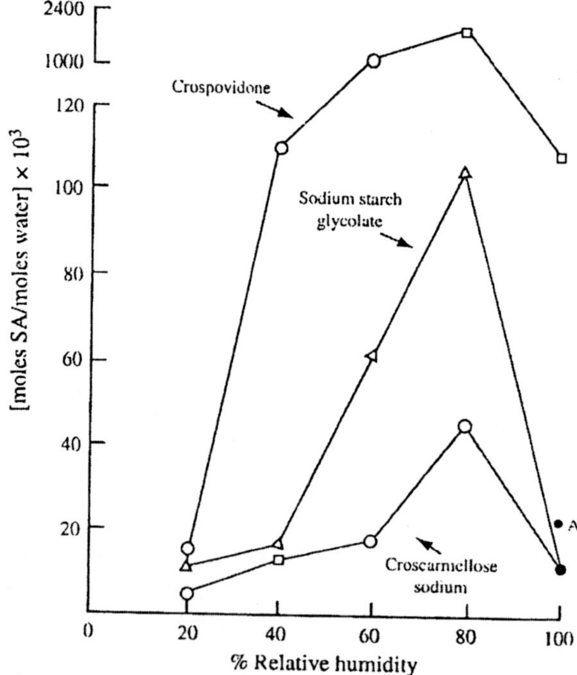

Fig. 4.15. Effect of humidity on the salicyclic acid content in aspirin-disintegrant mixtures at 120 days and 25°C (A, aspirin powder).

These results demonstrate many of the points presented here. At 100% RH, the reaction rate is lower than that expected for croscarmellose and sodium starch glycolate, because the disintegrants swelled and in doing so diminished the available moisture (crospovidone does not swell). Normalizing based on the total moisture present overstates the amount of water available to react and underestimates the actual reaction rate. At the other extreme (20% RH), the analysis is also biased by overstating the amount of water available, but for a different reason. The water associated with the system here is tightly bound to the disintegrant and not available. At intermediate humidities, depending on the excipient, the observed rate for degradation of the solid is higher than expected. This behavior may be a consequence of the activated sorption process and a specific acid catalysis described by Carstensen. Nevertheless, results of this sort are disconcerting for the product development pharmacist interested in making a stable tablet that disintegrates quickly. Real progress has been made in the last 10 years, providing pharmaceutical scientists with a solid basis for understanding the interaction of water with solids of pharmaceutical interest. Much of this progress has been the consequence of a paradigm shift: the model of the solid as an inert substrate is almost never valid. Further characterization of the state of water in solid–water systems may ultimately provide a basis for the design of stable formulations and permit the establishment of performance-based specifications for pharmaceutical excipients.

5

ANTIBODIES, VACCINES AND ADJUVANTS

Few substances have had a greater positive impact upon human healthcare management than antibodies, vaccines and adjuvants. For most of this century, these immunological agents have enjoyed widespread medical application, predominantly for the treatment/prevention of infectious diseases. As a group, they are often referred to as 'biologics'. Polyclonal antibody preparations have been used to induce passive immunity against a range of foreign (harmful) agents, and vaccines are used efficiently, and safely, to promote active immunization. Adjuvants are usually co-administered with the vaccine preparation, in order to enhance the immune response against the vaccine. The development of modern biotechnological methodology has had a significant impact upon the therapeutic application of immunological agents. Monoclonal/engineered antibodies find a range of therapeutic uses, and many of the newer vaccine preparations are now produced by recombinant DNA technology.

TRADITIONAL POLYCLONAL ANTIBODY PREPARATIONS

Polyclonal antibody preparations have been used for several decades to induce passive immunization against infectious diseases and other harmful agents, particularly toxins. The antibody preparations are usually administered by direct i.v. injection. While this affords immediate immunological protection, its effect is transitory, usually persisting for only 2–3 weeks (i.e. until the antibodies are excreted). Passive immunization can be used prophylactically (i.e. to prevent a future medical episode) or therapeutically (i.e. to treat a medical condition that is already established). An example of the former would be prior administration of a specific anti-snake toxin antibody preparation to an individual before they travel to a world region in which these snakes are commonly found. An example of the latter would be administration of the anti-venom antibody immediately after the individual has experienced a snake bite.

Antibody preparations used to induce passive immunity may be obtained from either animal or human sources. Preparations of animal origin are generally termed '*antisera*', and those sourced from humans are called '*immunoglobulin preparations*'. In both cases, the predominant antibody type present is IgG. Antisera are generally produced by immunizing healthy animals (e.g. horses) with appropriate antigen. Small samples of blood are subsequently withdrawn from the animal on a regular basis and quantitatively analysed for the presence of the desired antibodies (often using ELISA-based immunoassays). This facilitates harvesting of the blood at the most appropriate time points. Large animals, such as horses, can withstand withdrawal of 1 or 2 l of blood every 10–14 days, and antibody levels are usually maintained by administration of repeat antigen booster injections.

The blood is collected using an aseptic technique into sterile containers. It can then be allowed to clot with subsequent recovery of the antibody-containing antisera by centrifugation. Alternatively, the blood may be collected in the presence of heparin, or another suitable anticoagulant, with subsequent removal of the suspended cellular elements, again by centrifugation. In this case, the resultant antibody-containing solution is termed 'plasma'.

The antibody fraction is then purified from the serum (or plasma). Traditionally, this entailed precipitation steps, usually using ethanol and/or ammonium sulfate as precipitants. The precipitated antibody preparations, however, are only partially purified and modern preparations are generally subjected to additional high-resolution chromatographic fractionation. Ion-exchange chromatography is often employed, as is protein A affinity chromatography. (IgG from many species binds fairly selectively to protein A.)

Following high resolution purification, the antibody titre is determined, usually using an appropriate bioassay, or an immunoassay. Stabilizing agents, such as NaCl (0.9 per cent w/v) or glycine (2–3 per cent w/v) are often added, as are antimicrobial preservatives. Addition of preservative is particularly important if the product is subsequently filled into multi-dose containers. Phenol, at concentrations less than 0.25 per cent, is often used. After adjustment of the potency to fall within specification, the product is sterile filtered and aseptically filled into sterile containers. These are sealed immediately if the product is to be marketed in liquid form. Such antibody solutions are often filled under an oxygen-

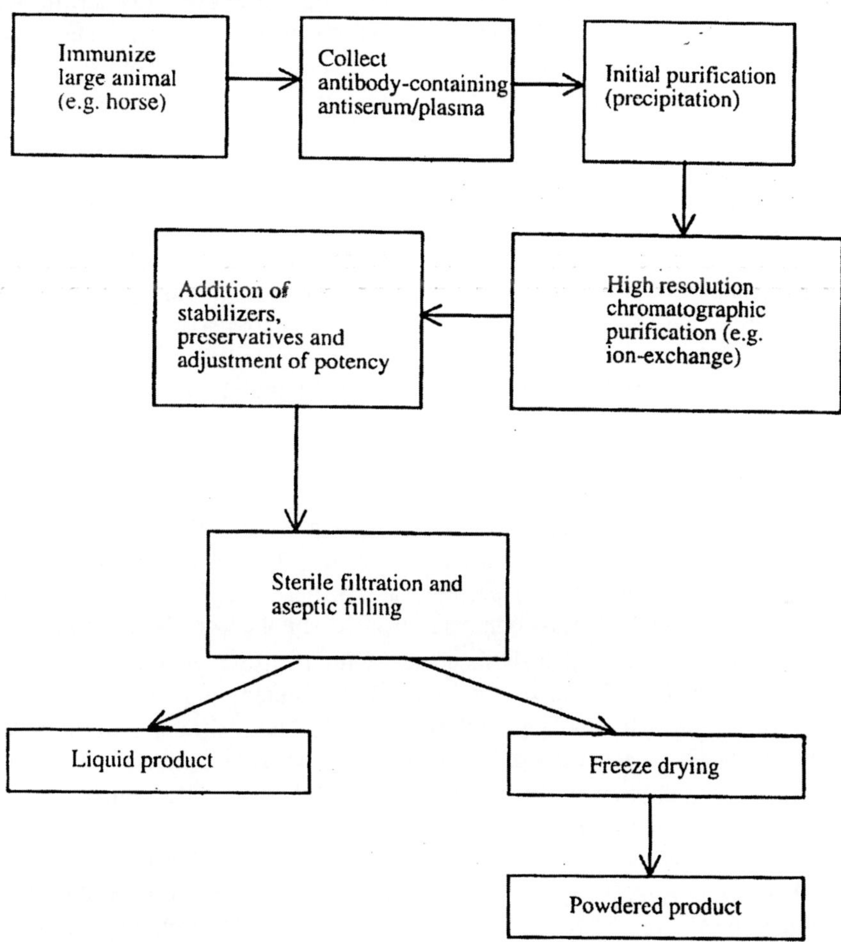

Fig. 5.1. Overview of the production of antisera for therapeutic use to induce passive immunization.

free nitrogen atmosphere in order to prevent oxidative degradation during subsequent storage. Such a product, if stored between 2 and 8°C, should exhibit a shelf life of up to 5 years.

Although specific antisera have proven invaluable in the treatment of a variety of medical conditions, they can also induce unwanted side effects. Particularly noteworthy is their ability to induce hypersensitivity reactions; some such sensitivity reactions (e.g. 'serum sickness') are often not acute, whereas others (e.g. anaphylaxis) can be life threatening. Because of such risks, antibody preparations derived from human donors (i.e. immunoglobulins) are usually preferred as passive immunizing agents.

Immunoglobulins are purified from the serum (or plasma) of human donors by methods similar to those used to purify animal-derived antibodies. In most instances, the immunoglobulin preparations are enriched in antibodies capable of binding to a specific antigen (usually an infectious microorganism/ virus). These may be purified from donated blood of individuals who have recently:

1. Been immunized against the antigen of interest;
2. Recovered from an infection caused by the antigen of interest.

Although hypersensitivity reactions can occur upon administration of immunoglobulin preparations, the incidence of such events is far less frequent than is the case upon administration of antibody preparations of animal origin. As with all blood-derived products, the serum from which the immunoglobulins are due to be purified is first assayed for the presence of infectious agents before its use. These may generally be categorized into one of several groups upon the basis of their target specificities. These groups include antibodies raised against:

1. Specific microbial or viral pathogens;
2. Microbial toxins;
3. Snake/spider venoms (anti-venins).

Monoclonal Antibodies

In the last 20 years or so, antibody-based therapeutics have mainly focused upon the medical application of monoclonal antibodies. Monoclonal antibody technology was first developed in the mid 1970s, when Kohler and Milstein successfully fused immortal myeloma cells with antibody-producing B-lymphocytes. A proportion of the resultant hybrids were found to be stable, cancerous, antibody-producing cells. These '*hybridoma*' cells represented an inexhaustible source of monospecific (monoclonal) antibody. Hybridoma technology facilitates the relatively straightforward production of monospecific antibodies against virtually any desired antigen.

The production process entails initial immunization of a mouse with the antigen of interest. The mouse is subsequently sacrificed and its spleen removed. (The spleen is an organ enriched in B-lymphocytes. Because of the immunization process, a significant proportion of these lymphocytes are likely capable of producing antibodies recognizing specific epitopes on the antigen.)

Spleen-derived B-lymphocytes are then incubated with mouse myeloma cells in the presence of propylene glycol. This promotes fusion of the cells. The resultant immortalized antibody- producing hybridomas are subsequently selected from unfused cells by culture in a specific selection medium. Individual hybridomas can be separated from each other by simple dilution and subsequently grown in culture, producing a clone. Individual clones can be screened to identify which ones produce murine (monoclonal) antibody that binds the antigen of interest. Appropriate clones are then selected and grown on a larger scale in order to produce biotechnologically useful quantities of antibody. Whereas many of the monoclonal antibodies approved in the 1980s and early 1990s were produced by such means, the majority of more recent approvals are engineered products produced by recombinant means, as described later.

Antibody Screening: Phage Display Technology

Phage display technology provides an extremely powerful modern way to generate a library of (protein) ligands and, subsequently, screen these ligands for their ability to bind a selected target molecule. The technique, as the name implies, employs filamentous phage (bacteriophage) that replicate in *E. coli*. These genes are inserted (batch cloned) into a phage library fused to a gene encoding one of the phage coat proteins (pIII, pIV or pVIII). The phage are then incubated with *E. coli*, which facilitates phage replication. Expression of the fusion gene product during replication and the subsequent incorporation of the fusion product into the mature phage coat results in the gene product being 'presented' on the phage surface. The entire phage library can then be screened in order to identify the one(s) coding for the protein of interest. This is usually achieved by affinity selection (biopanning). Biopanning entails passing the library over immobilized target molecules, usually in immobilized column format. Only the phage expressing the protein of desired specificity should be retained in the immobilized column. The bound phage can subsequently be eluted, e.g. by reducing the pH of the elution buffer or inclusion of a competitive ligand (usually free target molecules) in the buffer. Eluted phage can then be repassed over the affinity column in order to isolate those binding the immobilized ligand with the highest specificity/affinity. Once this is achieved, the gene coding for the protein of interest can be excised from the phage genome by standard techniques of molecular biology. It can then be incorporated into an appropriate microbial/animal cell/transgenic expression system, facilitating large-scale production of the gene product. Variations of the phage display approach have been developed, some of which

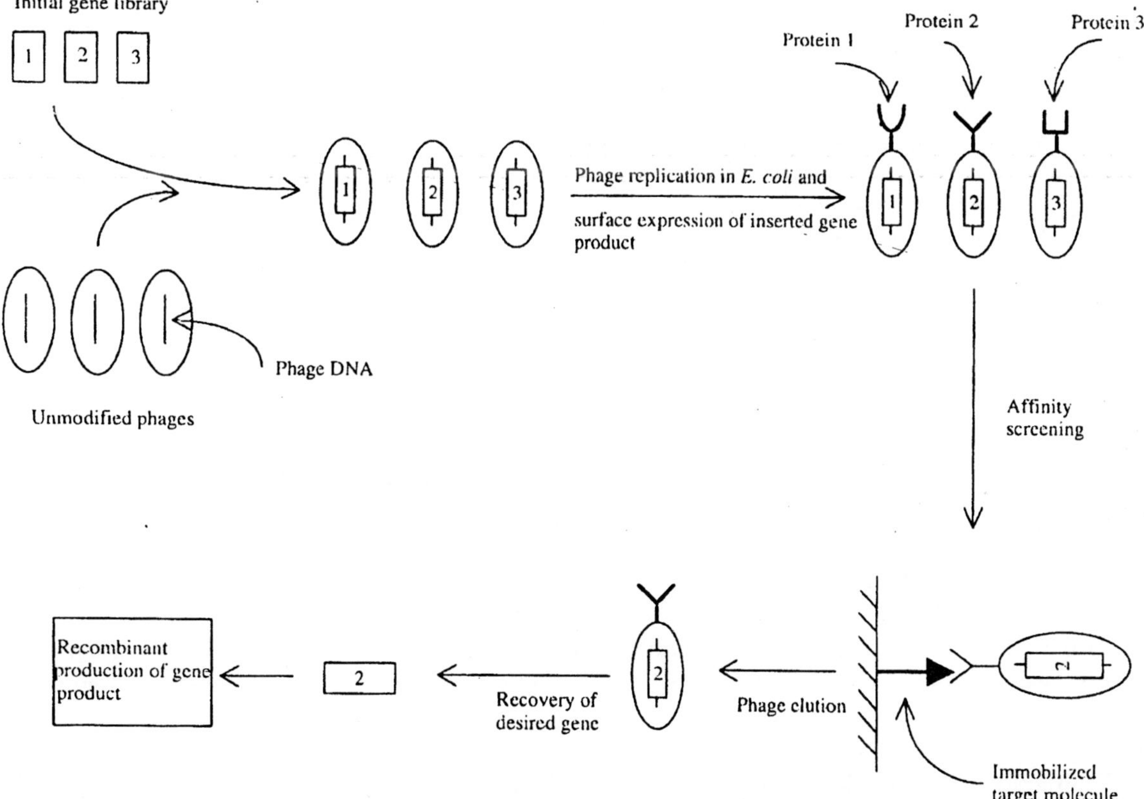

Fig. 5.2. Phage display technology and the screening of a library for a protein capable of binding to a desired target molecule. In this simplified example an initial library of three genes is inserted into three phages.

utilize engineered phage (phagemids), whereas others achieve library expression not on the surface of phage but on the surface of bacteria. Amongst the first and still most prominent application of phage display technology is the production and screening of antibody libraries in order to isolate/identify an antibody capable of binding to a desired target molecule. As such, this technology has now come to the fore in identifying antibodies suited to clinical application.

Genes/cDNA libraries coding for antibodies/antigen-binding antibody fragments have been obtained from human and animal (e.g. mice, rabbit and chicken) sources. Two types of library can be generated. '*Immune libraries*' are obtained by cloning antibody/antibody fragment coding sequences derived from B-lymphocytes (usually from spleens) of donors previously immunized with the target antigen. A high number of hits (positive clones) should be obtained from such libraries. Non-immune libraries are produced in a similar fashion, but using B-lymphocytes from non-immunized donors as a source of antibody genes. This approach becomes necessary if initial immunization with the antigen of interest is not possible (e.g. due to ethical considerations). Although such libraries will generate a lower number of positive clones, they can be screened against multiple antigens. Such native non-immune libraries can also be the starting point for the generation of so-called synthetic immune libraries. Their generation entails initial *in vitro* engineering of the non-immune library of antibody genes in order to increase still further the level of antibody diversity generated.

Therapeutic Application of Monoclonal Antibodies

The unrivalled specificity of monoclonal antibodies, coupled to their relatively straightforward production and their continuity of supply, renders them attractive biochemical tools. Therapeutically, they represent by far the single largest category of biopharmaceutical substances under investigation. Several hundred such preparations are currently undergoing preclinical and clinical trials. Throughout the 1980s the focus of attention rested upon their use either as *in vivo* imaging (i.e. diagnostic) agents or as direct therapeutic agents. Initial studies centred mainly around cancer, but monoclonal antibody preparations are now used in a variety of other medical circumstances:

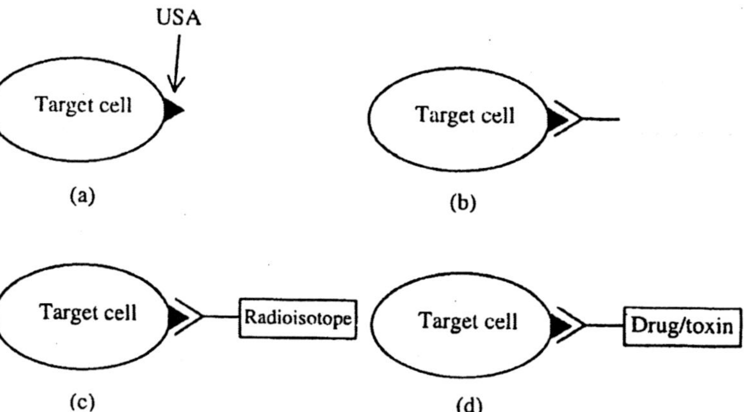

Fig. 5.3. Underlying principle/approaches taken during the development and use of antibody-mediated target cell detection/destruction.

1. Induction of passive immunity;
2. Diagnostic imagining;
3. Therapeutically (e.g. treatment of cancer, transplantation and cardiovascular disease).

All *in vivo* diagnostic/therapeutic applications are dependent upon the selective interaction of a monoclonal antibody with a specific target cell type in the body (e.g. a cancer cell). Therefore, a prerequisite to application of monoclonal antibody-based products in this way is the identification of a cell surface antigen unique to the target cell type. Once identified and characterized, monoclonal antibodies may be raised against that unique surface antigen (USA or USAg). The specificity of antibody-antigen binding should ensure that, once injected into the body, the antibody will selectively congregate on the surface of only the target cells. Depending upon the specific intended therapeutic/diagnostic application, antibodies employed may have nothing attached to them or may be conjugated to a radioisotope, drug or toxin. With the latter approaches, the antibody is used as a 'magic bullet', delivering a radioactive/drug load to specific cells in the body.

In the context of antibody-mediated cell targeting, it is also important to appreciate that binding of an antibody to a USA can, by itself, trigger a number of responses. In some instances, the antibody–antigen (Ab–USA) complex is quickly internalized. In other instances, the Ab–USA complex is shed from the cell surface, whereas in yet other cases binding induces neither response. The specific response triggered is generally only determined by direct experimentation. The induction of Ab–USA shedding renders an anti-type-specific antigen (TSA) antibody clinically useless.

By 2006, a total of 29 such antibody-based products had gained marketing approval in some world regions at least. Over half of these aim to detect/treat various cancers, and cancer represents the single most significant indication for antibody-based products currently in clinical trials. The application of antibodies in the context of cancer is overviewed in the next section. A minority of the products approved/in trials are intact antibodies produced by classical hybridoma technology. The majority are engineered antibodies ('*chimaeric*' or '*humanized*') or antibody fragments.

Tumour Immunology

The transformation of a cell to the cancerous state is normally associated with increased surface expression of antigens recognized as foreign by the host immune system. These surface antigens, often termed tumour antigens or tumour surface antigens, are either not expressed at all by the untransformed cell or are expressed at such low levels that they fail to induce immunological tolerance.

The presence of tumour-specific antigens implies that the immune system should be capable of recognizing and destroying transformed cells. This concept, known as immunosurveillance, probably does function to some extent in the body. The immune system does respond to the presence of some tumours, causing their partial or complete regression. The major anti-tumour immune elements include:

1. T-lymphocytes, which are capable of recognizing and lysing malignant cells.
2. NK cells, which, like some T-cells, can induce lysis of tumour cells. The tumouricidal activity of NK cells is potentiated by various cytokines (e.g. IL-2 and TNF).
3. Macrophages can destroy tumour cells, largely by releasing damaging lysosomal enzymes and reactive oxygen metabolites at the tumour cell surface. Macrophages also produce TNF, which can kill tumour cells by (a) binding to high-affinity TNF cell surface receptors (which is directly toxic to the cells) and (b) promoting synthesis of additional cytokines (which can, indirectly, lead to tumour destruction via activation of other elements of immunity).
4. Antibodies that, by binding to the cell surface antigen, mark the tumour cell for destruction. NK cells and macrophages express cell surface receptors that bind to the antibody F_c region. Thus, antibody bound to tumour antigens directs these immune elements directly to tumour surface. Antibodies also activate complement, which is capable of directly lysing tumour cells.

Antibody-based strategies for tumour detection/destruction

Clear identification of tumour-associated antigens would facilitate the production of monoclonal antibodies capable of selectively binding to tumour tissue. Such antibodies could be employed to detect and/or destroy the tumour cells. The antibody preparations could be administered unaltered or (more commonly) after their conjugation to radioisotopes or toxins. Binding of unaltered monoclonal antibodies to a tumour surface alone should facilitate increased destruction of tumour cells. This approach, however, has yielded disappointing results, as the monoclonal antibody preparations used to date have been murine in origin. The F_c region of such mouse antibodies is a very poor activator of human immune function. Technical advances, allowing the production of human/humanized monoclonals may render this therapeutic approach more attractive in the future.

Several clinical trials have evaluated (or continue to evaluate) monoclonal antibodies to which a radioactive tag has been conjugated. These are usually employed as potential anti-cancer agents. The rationale is selective delivery of the radioactivity directly to the tumour site. Most of the radioisotopes being evaluated are β-emitters. These include istopes of iodine (^{125}I, ^{131}I), rhenium (^{186}Re, ^{188}Re) and yttrium (^{90}Y). The medium-energy radioactivity these emit is capable of penetrating a thickness of several cells. Congregation of radioactivity at the tumour surface could thus promote irradiation of several layers of tumour cells, as well as nearby healthy cells. Higher energy á-emitters are also being evaluated. Although their effective path length is only about one cell deep, each emission has a greater likelihood of killing all cells in its path.

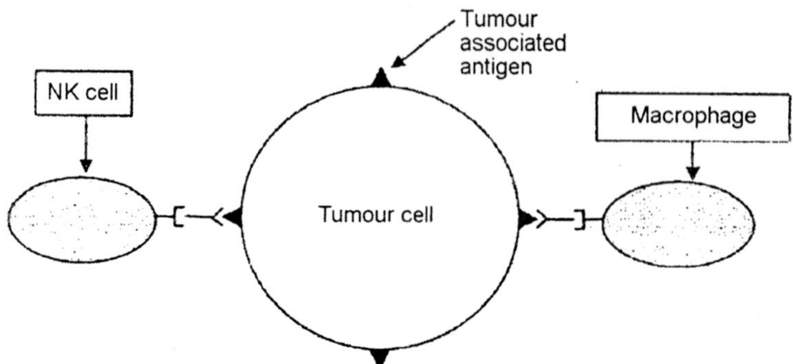

Fig. 5.4. Binding of appropriate antibody to tumour-associated antigens marks the tumour cell for destruction.

An allied application of radiolabelled anti-tumour monoclonal antibodies is that of diagnostic imaging (immunoscintigraphy). In this case, the radioisotope employed must be a γ-emitter (such that the radioactivity can penetrate outward through the body for detection purposes). Although various radioisotopes of iodine have been evaluated, technetium (^{99m}Tc) is the one most commonly employed. It has a γ-ray emission energy that is sufficient, but a relatively short half life of 6 h (this minimizes long-term exposure of patient to high-energy γ-rays). It can also be generated at nuclear installations relatively easily and is inexpensive. Equally important, chemical methodologies exist which facilitate its (stable) coupling to antibody molecules. Direct labelling with ^{99m}Tc generally entails initial reduction of antibody disulfide residues, forming free sulfahydryl (—SH) groups. This is achieved by incubation with a suitable reducing agent, such as ascorbic acid or sodium dithionite. A source of ^{99m}Tc (e.g. $Na^{99m}TcO_4$) is then reduced separately. Subsequent mixing under nitrogen gas (to maintain reducing conditions) results in direct linkage of the radioisotope to the antibody.

Upon administration, the anti-tumour ^{99m}Tc conjugate will congregate at the tumour site. The tumour can then be visualized using suitable γ-ray detection equipment, such as a planar gamma camera.

A number of radiolabelled monoclonal antibodies have been approved as tumour diagnostic imaging agents. Carcinoembryonic antigen (CEA)-SCAN, for example, is an antigen- binding fragment (Fab) of a specific murine monoclonal raised against human CEA. CEA is expressed at high levels by some tumours. This is particularly true of tumours of the gastrointestinal tract, such as carcinomas of the colon or rectum. CEA-SCAN (non-proprietary name: Arcitumomab) is used to detect these carcinomas. However, CEA is expressed naturally (all be it at much lower levels) by some non-transformed cells. Therefore, this antibody fragment is used mostly to image recurrence and/or metastases of histologically demonstrated carcinoma of the colon or rectum. It is used as an adjunct to standard imaging techniques, such as a computed tomography scan or ultrasonography. The product is administered by i.v. injection, and only relatively mild side effects are usually noted. These can include nausea, fever, rash and headaches. Anti-tumour monoclonal antibodies can also be used to deliver toxins to tumour sites. Toxins conjugated to therapeutic antibodies include ricin, pokeweed toxin, *Pseudomonas* toxin and diphtheria toxin. After binding to the cell surface, the antibody–toxin conjugate is often internalized via endocytosis. It is presumed that, rather than being destroyed, the toxin is subsequently made available inside the

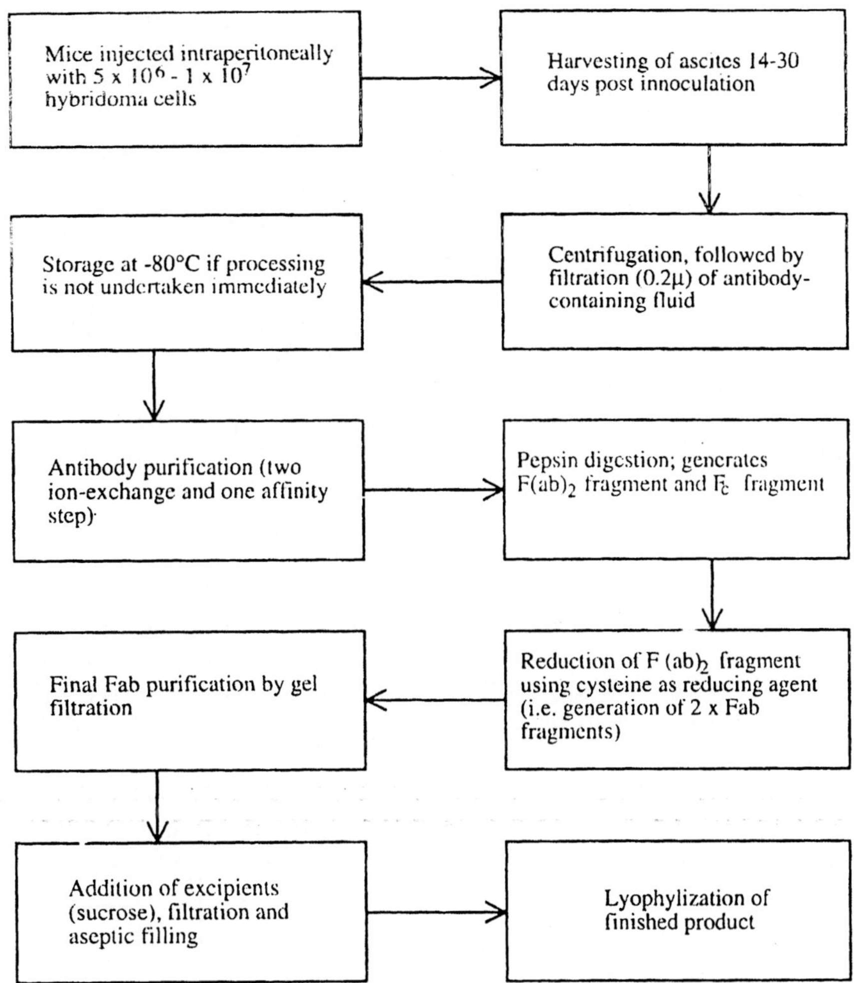

Fig. 5.5. Outline of the production strategy of CEA-SCAN.

cell, such that it can induce its toxic effects. One such antibody-based product now approved for general medical use is Mylotarg. The product consists of an engineered antibody (a 'humanized' antibody, as described later), conjugated to a cytotoxic anti-tumour antibiotic, calicheamicin. The antibody binds specifically to a cell surface antigen, CD33. This is a sialic-acid-dependent adhesion protein found on the surface of leukaemic cells in more than 80 per cent of patients suffering from acute myeloid leukaemia. The product production process entails initial culture of the antibody-producing mammalian cell line with subsequent purification of the antibody by a series of chromatographic steps. Downstream processing also incorporates ultrafiltration and low-pH incubation steps designed to remove/inactivate any virus potentially present. The cytotoxic antibiotic is obtained separately via fermentation of its producer microrganism, *Micromonospora echinospora* sp. *calichensis*. Direct chemical linkage of antibiotic to antibody is achieved using a bifunctional linker.

Mylotarg administration results in congregation of the antibody–toxin conjugate on the surface of (CD33 positive) leukaemic cells. Binding triggers internalization of the conjugate. Lysosomal degradation ensues, but a significant proportion of the intact antibiotic escapes and induces its cytotoxic affect by binding DNA in its minor groove. This, in turn, induces double-strand breakage.

Fig. 5.6. Schematic diagram of the antibody based product mylotarg, with emphasis upon the toxin's chemical structure.

Mylotarg (like most other drugs) does induce some side effects, the most significant of which is immunosuppression. This is induced because certain additional (non-cancerous) white blood cell precursors also display the CD33 antigen on their surface. The immunosuppressive effect is reversed upon termination of treatment, as pluripotent haematopoietic stem cells are unaffected by the product.

Drug-based tumour immunotherapy

In addition to tumour-selective delivery of toxins and radioisotopes, antibodies may also be used to mediate tumour-targeted drug delivery. At its simplest, this involves conjugation of a chemotherapeutic drug to a tumour-specific antibody. Therapeutic drugs used include adriamycin, aminopterin, methotrexate and vinca alkaloids. This direct approach to tumour drug delivery has met with some success, mainly in animal studies. However, a limited number of drug molecules can be conjugated to each antibody molecule, thus somewhat limiting the drug delivery load.

An alternative approach is the use of a tumour-specific antibody to which a prodrug activating enzyme has been attached. Therapeutically inactive prodrugs could be administered by, for example, i.v. injection. This would subsequently be activated only at the tumour surface. This approach has been termed ADEPT or antibody-directed catalysis.

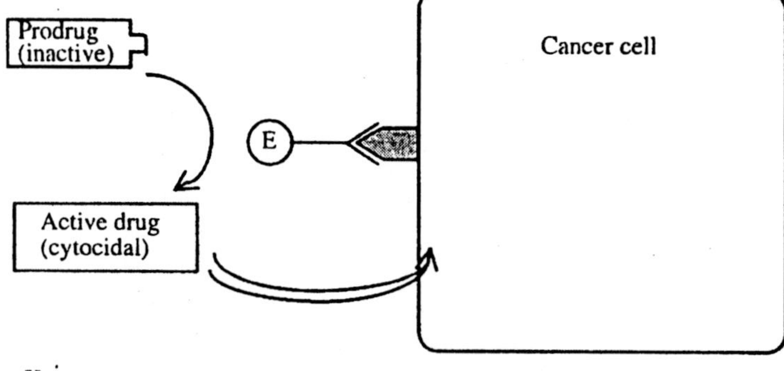

Key:

= (Prodrug activating) enzyme-antibody conjugate

= Tumor-associated antigen

Fig. 5.7. Outline of antibody-directed enzyme prodrug therapy (ADEPT). Subsequent to its enzymatic activation, the active drug is taken up by the cell, upon which it exhibits a cytocidal effect.

Because of its catalytic nature, a single antibody–enzyme conjugate would activate many molecules of the prodrug in question. Much of the active cytocidal agent released at the tumour surface would be taken up by the tumour cells via simple diffusion or carrier-mediated active transport.

Administration of etoposide in prodrug form exemplifies this approach. Etoposide ($C_{29}H_{32}O_{13}$; molecular mass 588.6) is a semi-synthetic derivative of podophyllotoxin, produced naturally by the North American plant *Podophyllum peltatum*. It is used as an anti-cancer agent. Its cellular uptake is diffusion dependent, and once inside the cell it exerts its cytocidal effect. Phosphorylated etoposide is non-diffusable and, hence, represents an inactive prodrug form of etoposide. (Attachment of a charged group to most diffusion-dependent drugs prevents their cellular uptake.) Alkaline phosphatase, however, can cleave the phosphate group, releasing free cytocidal agent. Administration of a tumour-detecting antibody–alkaline phosphatase conjugate thus effectively targets the enzyme to the tumour surface.

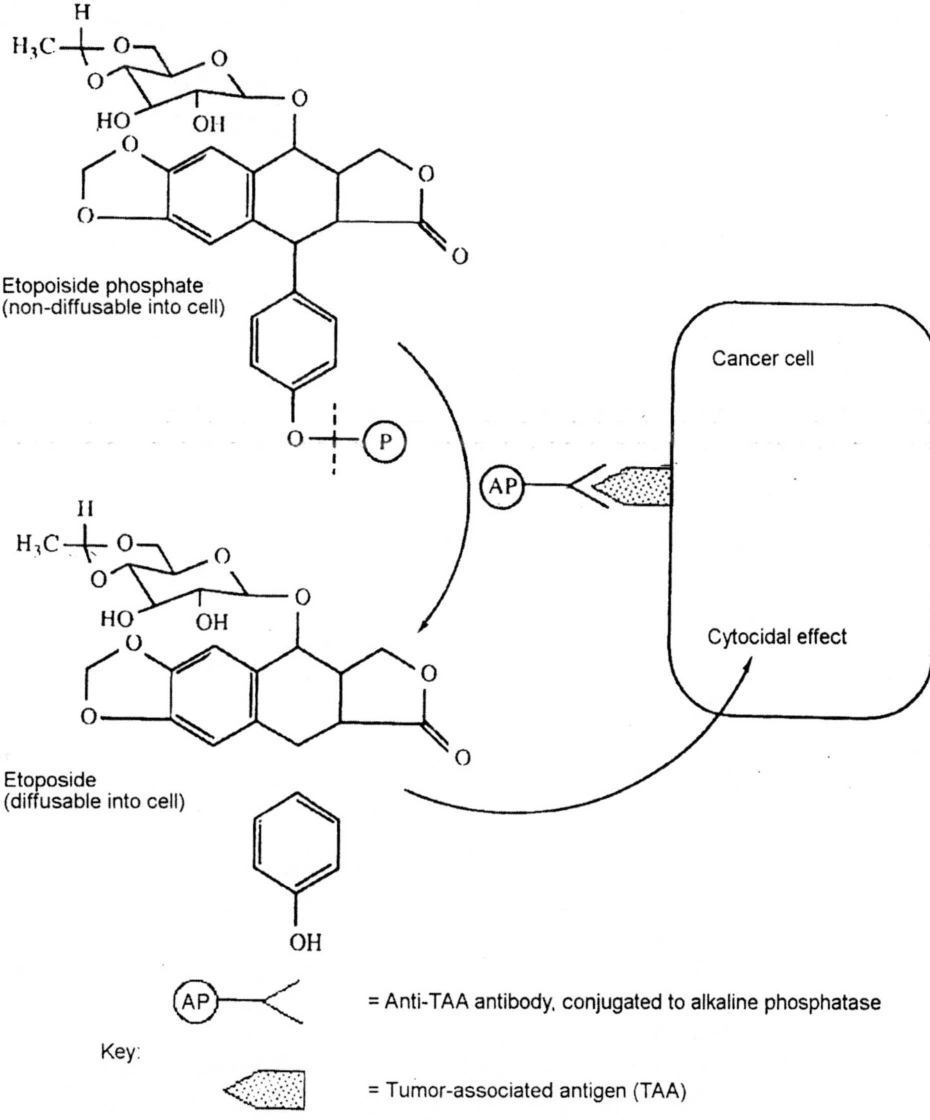

Fig. 5.8. The etoposide-alkaline phosphatase ADEPT system.

Subsequent administration of phosphorylated etoposide results in etoposide liberation at the tumour surface, which can then enter tumour cells by diffusion. Various other prodrug–enzyme combinations have now been developed, including phenoxyacetamide derivatives of doxorubicin (activated by penicillin amidase) and 5-fluorocytosine (activated by cytosine deaminase).

The prodrugs used should be inexpensive, readily available and should be stable to chemical/ enzymatic degradation *in vivo*. Enzymes used should also be stable under physiological conditions, display a reasonable turn over number *in vivo* and not be dependent upon a co-factor for activity. Mammalian enzymes would be likely less immunogenic than microbial enzymes. However, the use of a prodrug capable of being activated by a mammalian enzyme can lead to complications if that enzyme's (human) endogenous counterpart is capable of activating the drug at sites distant from the tumour.

First-generation anti-tumour antibodies: clinical disappointment

Despite the scientific elegance of the antibody-mediated approach to tumour detection/destruction, initial clinical trials proved disappointing. A number of factors contributed to their poor therapeutic performance, particularly against solid tumours. Most such factors relate directly/ indirectly to the fact that the first generation of such drugs utilized whole monoclonal antibody preparations of murine origin. These factors include:

1. Insufficient information exists regarding tumour antigens;
2. Murine monoclonals prompt an immune response when administered to humans;
3. Poor penetration of tumour mass by antibody;
4. Murine monoclonals display a relatively short half-life when administered to humans;
5. Poor recognition of murine antibody F_c domain by human effector mechanisms.

Tumour-associated Antigens

In this text, the term '*tumour-associated antigen*' represents any antigen associated with any cancer cell, no matter what factor(s) originally prompted cellular transformation. (In some circles, the term 'tumour-associated antigen' is often applied more specifically: to antigens associated with virally transformed cells.) Identification of tumour-associated antigens forms a core requirement for effective tumour immunotherapy. Identification of such tumour-associated antigens remains a very active area of biomedical research. From the limited data generated to date, tumour-associated antigens can generally be categorized into one of three groups.

Many tumour types are induced by chemical and/or physical carcinogens we encounter in our living/working environments. Most of these tumours are initiated when the carcinogen induces a point mutation in a nucleotide sequence, thus perhaps altering expression levels of the gene product or altering its functional characteristics. Because such mutations are random, it is not surprising that each resulting tumour displays its own unique tumour-associated antigen(s). This renders an immunological approach to detection/therapy impractical in such instances, as the specific tumour-associated antigens unique to that case would first have to be identified.

In contrast to the above situation, cancers induced by viruses generally exhibit immunological cross-reactivity. Any specific virus will often induce expression of the same tumour antigen no matter what cell type it transforms. Moreover, in some cases, different transforming viruses can induce production of the same tumour antigen(s). Immunodetection/immunotherapy of such cancers is thus rendered attractive. Once a tumour antigen is identified, antibodies raised against it will likely cross-react with several other tumour types.

DNA viruses, such as adenoviruses and papovaviruses (e.g. polyoma and SV40), induce cellular transformation in rodents. Other viruses have been implicated in human cancers. Epstein–Barr virus, for example, has been implicated with nasopharyngeal carcinoma, β-cell lymphomas and Hodgkin's lymphoma. Human papilloma virus is linked to most cervical cancers. Certain RNA viruses, particularly retroviruses, have also proven capable of inducing cancer. Retroviruses known to induce cancer in animals include Rous sarcoma virus, Kirsten murine sarcoma virus, avian myelocytomatosis virus, and various murine leukaemia viruses. Thus far, the only well-characterized human RNA transforming virus is that of human T-cell lymphotropic virus-1 (HTLV-1), which can induce adult T-cell leukaemia/ lymphoma. The identification of antigens uniquely associated with various tumour types and the identification of additional cancer-causing viruses remain areas of very active research.

Another group of antigens associated with some tumour types are oncofoetal antigens. These antigens are proteins that are normally expressed during certain stages of foetal development. Subsequent repression of their structural genes, however, prevents their expression at later stages of development and/or into adulthood. Characteristic of some cancers is the re-expression of oncofoetal antigens. Some such antigens remain attached to the cancer cell surface, whereas others are secreted in soluble form. Although these oncofoetal proteins are not recognized as foreign by the host's own immune system, they do represent important potential diagnostic markers. Although some such markers have been identified, efforts continue to identify additional members of this family.

CEA and α-fetoprotein (AFP) represent the most extensively characterized oncofoetal antigens thus far. We have already encountered CEA in the guise of its use as a marker for cancers of the colon and rectum. CEA is a 180 kDa integral membrane glycoprotein. It also may be secreted into the blood in soluble form. It is expressed mainly in the gut, liver and pancreas, during the first 6 months of foetal development. However, it is now known to be expressed (although at greatly reduced levels) by adult colonic mucosal cells and in the lactating breast. Elevated levels of either soluble (serum) or cell-bound CEA are normally indicative of cancers of the gastrointestinal tract.

AFP is a 70 kDa glycoprotein found in the circulatory system of the developing foetus. It is synthesized primarily by the yolk sac and (foetal) liver. AFP is present only in vanishing low quantities in the serum of adults (where it is replaced by serum albumin). Elevated adult serum levels of this marker are often associated with various cancers of the liver, as well as germ cell tumours. It is also sometimes expressed by gastric and pancreatic cancer cells. Although a useful tumour marker, increased serum AFP levels also often accompany cirrhosis and some other noncancerous liver diseases.

CA125 represents an oncofoetal protein that is expressed by up to 90 per cent of ovarian adenocarcinomas. Some of the protein is released from the tumour site into the general circulation. Elevated serum CA125 levels, therefore, have some diagnostic value. Imaging of actual tumour sites can also be undertaken using radiolabelled antibody coupled to immunoscintigraphy. Indimacis-125 is the trade name given to such a product approved in 1996 for use in the EU. The product is an ^{111}In-labelled $F(ab)_2$ fragment derived from a murine hybridoma cell line. Although some of the product is likely absorbed by the circulatory form of the oncofoetal protein, the product has proven effective in imaging relapsing ovarian adenocarcinoma.

In summary, TSA-based complications in the context of developing antibody-based cancer therapies include:

1. Limited numbers of TSAs currently characterized.
2. Some cancer types, depending upon their cause, may display unique TSAs in different patients.
3. TSAs are often expressed, albeit at lower levels, by one or more additional (non-transformed) body cell types.
4. In some instances, binding of antibody results in immediate shedding of Ab–TSA from the cell surface.
5. TSA expression can be transitory. For many tumours, only a proportion (albeit a large one) of the tumour cells express TSAs at any given time.

Antigenicity of Murine Monoclonals

Antibody immunogenicity remains one of the inherent therapeutic limitations associated with administration of murine monoclonals to human subjects. In most instances, a single injection of the murine monoclonal will elicit an immune response in 50–80 per cent of patients. Human anti-mouse antibodies (HAMA) will generally be detected within 14 days of antibody administration. Repeated administration of the monoclonal (usually required if the monoclonal is used for therapeutic purposes) will increase the HAMA response significantly. It will also induce an HAMA response in the majority of individuals who display no such response after the initial injection. The HAMA response will effectively and immediately destroy subsequent doses of monoclonal administered. In practice, therefore, therapeutic efficacy of murine monoclonals is limited to the first and, at most, the second dose administered.

An obvious strategy for overcoming the immunogenicity problem would be the generation and use of monoclonal antibodies of human origin. This is possible but difficult. Human antibody- producing lymphocytes can potentially be rendered immortal by:

1. Transformation by Epstein–Barr virus infection;
2. Fusion with murine monoclonals;
3. Fusion with human lymphoblastoid cell lines.

However, a number of technical hurdles remain that prevent routine production of human monoclonal preparations. These include:

1. Source of antibody-producing cell;
2. Reliable methods for lymphocyte immortalization;
3. Stability and antibody-producing capacity of resulting immortalized cells.

Initial stages in the production of murine monoclonals entail administration of the antigen of interest to a mouse. This is followed by sacrifice and recovery of activated B-lymphocytes from the spleen. A similar approach to the production of human monoclonals would be unethical. Administration of some antigens to humans could endanger their health. Although B-lymphocytes could be obtained from the peripheral circulation, the majority of these are unstimulated, and recovery of (stimulated) B-lymphocytes from the spleen is impractical.

Although Epstein–Barr virus is capable of inducing cellular transformation, few antibody- producing B-lymphocytes display the viral cell surface receptor. Most, therefore, are immune to Epstein–Barr virus infection. Even upon successful transformation, most produce low-affinity IgM antibodies, and the cells are often unstable. Having said that, one monoclonal antibody approved for medical use is produced by a human lymphoblastoid cell line originally transformed by Epstein–Barr virus.

Fusion of human lymphocytes with human lymphoblastoid cell lines is a very inefficient process. Fusion of human lymphocytes with murine myeloma cells lead to very unstable hybrids. Upon fusion, preferential loss of human genetic elements is often observed. Unfortunately, particularly common is the loss of chromosomes 2, 14 and 22, which encode antibody light and heavy chain loci. The production yields of human monoclonals upon immortalization of the human B-lymphocyte (by whatever means) are also low.

Chimaeric and Humanized Antibodies

Recombinant DNA technology has provided an alternative (and successful) route of reducing the innate immunity of murine monoclonals. The genes for all human immunoglobulin sub-types have been cloned, and this has allowed generation of various hybrid antibody structures of reduced immunogenicity.

The first strategy entails production of '*chimaeric*' antibodies, consisting of mouse variable regions and human constant regions. The chimaeric antibody would display the specificity of the original murine antibody, but would largely be human in sequence.

It was hoped that such chimaeric antibodies, when compared with murine antibodies, would be:

1. Significantly less immunogenic;
2. Display a prolonged serum half-life;
3. Allow activation of various F_c-mediated functions.

Reduced immunogenicity was expected, as only a minor part of the chimaeric antibodies is murine in origin. Furthermore, the HAMA response is normally directed largely at epitopes on the antibody's F_c domains. The variable region appears inherently less immunogenic. In practice, the expected reduced immunogenicity was observed. Early clinical trials with chimaerics have shown them to be generally safe and non-toxic. The rate of immune responses observed after single dose administration dropped from almost 80 per cent (murine) to in the region of 5 per cent (chimaeric). However, repeated administration of chimaerics did eventually raise an immune response in most recipients.

When compared with human monoclonals (half-life 14–21 days), murine monoclonals administered to humans display a relatively short half-life (30–40 h). Chimaerization increased serum half-life by fivefold, with typical values of 230 h being recorded. A prolonged half-life is desirable if the antibody is to be used therapeutically, as it decreases the required frequency of product administration. Chimaeric antibodies also allow activation of F_c-mediated functions (e.g. activation of complement, etc.), as this domain displays human sequence. Although chimaeric antibodies contain an entire murine-derived variable region, it is only the CDRs within this variable domain that actually dictate antigen specificity. A method of reducing still further the antigenicity of murine antibodies is to '*humanize*' them. This entails transferring the nucleotide sequences coding for the six CDR regions of the murine antibody of the desired specificity into a human antibody gene. The resulting hybrid antibody will, obviously, be entirely human in nature except for the CDRs.

Transfer of murine-derived CDR sequences into human antibody framework regions, sometimes generates an antibody with greatly reduced antigen binding affinity. Selected murine framework sequences are often also included in the humanized antibody. This process (known as reshaping the human antibody) facilitates folding of the CDRs into their true native conformations. This, in turn, normally restores antibody–antigen-binding affinity. Over 95 per cent of antibodies are human in sequence. Clinical trials indicate that such proteins do indeed behave similarly to native human antibodies. Humanization has overcome many of the major factors that limited the therapeutic effectiveness of first-generation (murine) monoclonals as therapeutic agents.

Antibody Fragments

One limitation to antibody-mediated treatment of solid tumours relates to their poor penetration of tumour mass. Antibody-based tumour therapy (e.g. using radiolabelled murine monoclonals) has proved more effective in treating disseminated cancers (e.g. leukaemias and lymphomas) as opposed to solid tumours. The physical size of the intact antibody likely hinders tumour penetration. As a result, recent interest has focused upon using antibody fragments that retain their antigen-binding capabilities. Fragments, such as F(ab), $F(ab)_2$ and F_v, can be easily generated, mainly via recombinant DNA technology. These have been labelled with, for example, radioactive tags with the intention of using them as diagnostic and therapeutic agents. Although their lower molecular mass may aid more effective tumour penetration, whole chimaeric/humanized antibodies may be more effective, particularly if used for therapeutic purposes. Fragments generally display greatly reduced serum half-lives and cannot initiate effector functions. Radiolabelled fragments may be better suited to diagnostic imaging purposes.

Additional Therapeutic Applications of Monoclonal Antibodies

Thus far, the discussion relating to the medical uses of monoclonals has focused exclusively upon cancer. Monoclonal antibodies (and their derivatives), however, have a far broader potential therapeutic application. Actual/potential additional uses include detection and treatment of cardiovascular disease, infectious agents, and various additional medical conditions. Various antibody preparations have been developed that facilitate imaging of vascular-related conditions, including myocardial infarction, deep vein thrombosis and atherosclerosis. Anti-myosin monoclonal antibody fragments (Fab) labelled with ^{111}In, for example, have been used for imaging purposes in conjunction with a planar gamma camera. The antibody displays specificity for intracellular cardiac myosin, which is exposed only upon death of heart muscle tissue induced by a myocardial infarction (heart attack).

Imaging monoclonals could be of use in visualizing the sites/extent of focused bacterial infections. This could be achieved by using radiolabelled antibodies displaying binding affinity for specific bacterial surface antigens. A related, but indirect, approach may entail use of imaging antibodies capable of detecting granulocytes and various other leukocytes that congregate at the sites of infection. It has been estimated that 1–2 per cent of the US population suffer from autoimmune conditions, including rheumatoid arthritis, MS and some forms of diabetes. In many instances, an autoimmune response results from the inappropriate activation of a specific subset of B- and/or T-lymphocytes. The most common immunotherapeutic approach to potentially treat such diseases is to induce depletion of the individual's T- and B-cell populations. This could be achieved by administration of an antibody raised against a surface antigen present on such cells. Initial trials, for example, have shown that injection of an (unconjugated) anti-CD4 antibody (cell surface glycoprotein present on many T-lymphocytes) over 7 days significantly reduced the clinical symptoms of rheumatoid arthritis for several months.

Antibodies have and likely will find additional use in transplantation-related medicine. In general, cell-mediated immunological mechanisms are responsible for mediating rejection of transplanted organs. In many instances, transplant patients must be maintained on immunosuppressive drugs (e.g. some steroids and, often, the fungal metabolite cyclosporine). However, complications may arise if a rejection episode is encountered that proves unresponsive to standard immunosuppressive therapy. Orthoclone OKT-3 was the first monoclonal antibody-based product to find application in this regard. This antibody is raised against the protein-based CD3 antigen, present on the cell surface of most T-lymphocytes. I.v. administration of (unconjugated) antibody appears to block normal functioning of such T-cells and promote their clearance from the blood. However, upon cessation of antibody administration, CD3 positive cell numbers rapidly revert to normal values. Therefore, maintenance immunosuppressives (e.g. with cyclosporine) must subsequently be restored. A number of additional antibody-based products aimed at preventing transplant rejection have now gained general marketing authorization. Simulect (chimaeric antibody) and Zenapax (humanized antibody) were approved in the late 1990s. Their engineered nature has greatly reduced the HAMA response upon their administration to humans. Both products target the IL-2 receptor and, hence, bind fairly selectively to activated immune system cells, especially activated T-lymphocytes, monocytes and macrophages. Binding prevents further cellular proliferation and, hence, dampens the immune system's attempts to destroy the transplanted tissue.

Vaccine Technology

The application of vaccine technology forms a core element of modern medicinal endeavour. It plays a central role in both human and veterinary medicine and represents the only commonly employed prophylactic (i.e. preventative) approach undertaken to control many infectious diseases. The current (annual) global vaccine market stands at in excess of US$3 billion. Immunization programmes, particularly those undertaken on a multinational scale, have served to reduce dramatically the incidence of many killer/disabling diseases, such as smallpox, polio and tuberculosis.

Continued/increased emphasis upon the implementation of such immunization programmes is likely. This is true not only of poorer world regions, but also amongst the most affluent nations. An estimated 500 000 adults die annually in the USA from conditions that could have been prevented by vaccination. These include pneumococcal pneumonia, influenza and hepatitis B.

Vaccination seeks to exploit the natural defence mechanisms conferred upon us by our immune system. A vaccine contains a preparation of antigenic components consisting of, derived from or related to a pathogen. In most instances upon vaccine administration, both the humoral and cell-mediated arms of the immune system are activated. The long-term immunological protection induced will normally prevent subsequent establishment of an infection by the same or antigenically related pathogens. Although some vaccines are active when administered orally, more are administered parenterally. Normally, an initial dose administration is followed by subsequent administration of one or more repeat doses over an appropriate time-scale. Such booster doses serve to maximize the immunological response.

Traditional vaccine preparations have largely been targeted against viral and bacterial pathogens, as well as some bacterial toxins and, to a lesser extent, parasitic agents, such as malaria. However, an increased understanding of the molecular mechanisms underlying additional human diseases suggests several novel applications of vaccines to treat/prevent autoimmune conditions and cancer (discussed later). Despite such potentially exciting future applications, recent scientific surveys indicate that the most urgently required vaccines are those that protect against more mundane pathogens. Although the needs of the developing world are somewhat different to those of developed regions, an effective AIDS vaccine is equally important to both. Approaches to development of such AIDS vaccines are discussed later in this chapter. Of particular consequence to developing world regions is the current lack of a truly effective malaria vaccine. With an estimated annual incidence of 300–500 million clinical cases (with up to 2.7 million resulting deaths), development of an effective vaccine in this instance is a priority.

Traditional Vaccine Preparations

For the purposes of this discussion, the term 'traditional' refers to those vaccines whose development predated the advent of recombinant DNA technology. Approximately 30 such vaccines remain in medical use. These can largely be categorized into one of several groups, including:

1. Live, attenuated bacteria (e.g. bacillus Calmette–Guerin (BCG), used to immunize against tuberculosis);
2. Dead or inactivated bacteria (e.g. cholera and pertussis vaccines);
3. Live attenuated viruses (e.g. measles, mumps and yellow fever viral vaccines);
4. Inactivated viruses (hepatitis A and polio (Salk) viral vaccines);
5. Toxoids (e.g. diphtheria and tetanus vaccines);
6. Pathogen-derived antigens (e.g. hepatitis B, meningococcal, pneumococcal and *Haemophilus influenzae* vaccines).

Attenuated, dead or inactivated bacteria

Attenuation (bacterial or viral) represents the process of elimination or greatly reducing the virulence of a pathogen. This is traditionally achieved by, for example, chemical treatment or heat, growing under adverse conditions or propagation in an unnatural host. The attenuated product should still immunologically cross-react with the wild-type pathogen. Although rarely occurring in practice, a theoretical danger exists in some cases that the attenuated pathogen might revert to its pathogenic state. An attenuated bacterial vaccine is represented by BCG. BCG is a strain of tuberculae bacillus that fails to cause tuberculosis, but retains much of the antigenicity of the pathogen. Killing or inactivation of pathogenic bacteria usually renders them suitable as vaccines. This is usually achieved by:

1. Heat treatment;
2. Treatment with formaldehyde or acetone;
3. Treatment with phenol or phenol and heat;
4. Treatment with propiolactone.

Attenuated and inactivated viral vaccines

Viral particles destined for use as vaccines are generally propagated in a suitable animal cell culture system. Although true cell culture systems are sometimes employed, many viral particles are grown in fertilized eggs or cultures of chick embryo tissue. Many of the more prominent vaccine preparations in current medical use consist of attenuated viral particles. Mumps vaccines consist of live attenuated strains of *Paramyxovirus parotitidis*. In many world regions, it is used routinely to vaccinate children, often a part of a combined measles, mumps and rubella vaccine.

Several attenuated strains have been developed for use in vaccine preparations. The most commonly used is the Jeryl Linn strain, which is propagated in chick embryo cell culture. This vaccine has been administered to well over 50 million people worldwide and, typically, results in seroconversion rates of over 97 per cent. The Sabin (oral poliomyelitis) vaccine consists of an aqueous suspension of poliomyelitis virus, usually grown in cultures of monkey kidney tissue. It contains approximately 1 million particles of poliomyelitis strains 1, 2 or 3 or a combination of all three strains. Hepatitis A vaccine exemplifies vaccine preparations containing inactivated viral particles. It consists of a formaldehyde-inactivated preparation of the HM 175 strain of hepatitis A virus. Viral particles are normally propagated initially in human fibroblasts.

Toxoids and antigen-based vaccines

Diphtheria and tetanus vaccines are two commonly used toxoid-based vaccine preparations. The initial stages of diphtheria vaccine production entail the growth of *Corynebacterium diphtheriae*. The toxoid is then prepared by treating the active toxin produced with formaldehyde. The product is normally sold as a sterile aqueous preparation. Tetanus vaccine production follows a similar approach. *Clostridium tetani* is cultured in appropriate media. The toxin is recovered and inactivated by formaldehyde treatment. Again, it is usually marketed as a sterile aqueous-based product.

Traditional antigen-based vaccine preparations consist of appropriate antigenic portions of the pathogen (usually surface-derived antigens). In most cases, the antigenic substances are surface polysaccharides. Many carbohydrate-based substances are inherently less immunogenic than protein-based material. Poor immunological responses are thus often associated with administration of carbohydrate polymers to humans, particularly to infants. The antigenicity of these substances can be improved by chemically coupling (conjugating) them to a protein- based antigen. Several conjugated *H. influenzae* vaccine variants are available. In these cases, the *Haemophilus* capsular polysaccharide is conjugated variously to diphtheria toxoid, tetanus toxoid or an outer membrane protein of *Neisseria meningitidis* (group B).

Impact of Genetic Engineering on Vaccine Technology

The advent of recombinant DNA technology has rendered possible the large-scale production of polypeptides normally present on the surface of virtually any pathogen. These polypeptides, when purified from the producer organism (e.g. *E. coli*, *Saccharomyces cerevisiae*) can then be used as 'subunit' vaccines. This method of vaccine production exhibits several advantages over conventional vaccine production methodologies. These include:

1. Production of a clinically safe product; the pathogen-derived polypeptide now being expressed in a non-pathogenic recombinant host. This all but precludes the possibility that the final product could harbour undetected pathogen.

2. Production of subunit vaccine in an unlimited supply. Previously, production of some vaccines was limited by supply of raw material (e.g. hepatitis B surface antigen).
3. Consistent production of a defined product that would thus be less likely to cause unexpected side effects.

A number of such recombinant (subunit) vaccines have now been approved for general medical use. The first such product was that of hepatitis B surface antigen (rHBsAg), which gained marketing approval from the FDA in 1986. Two billion people are infected with hepatitis B worldwide, 350 million individuals suffer from life-long chronic infection, and more than 1 million infected patients die each year from the associated complications of liver cirrhosis and/or liver cancer. Prior to its approval, hepatitis B vaccines consisted of HBsAg purified directly from the blood of hepatitis B sufferers. When present in blood, HBsAg exists not in monomeric form, but in characteristic polymeric structures that display a diameter of 22 μm. Production of hepatitis B vaccine by direct extraction from blood suffered from two major disadvantages:

1. The supply of finished vaccine was restricted by the availability of infected human plasma.
2. The starting material will likely be contaminated by intact, viable hepatitis B viral particles (and perhaps additional viruses, such as HIV). This necessitates introduction of stringent purification procedures to ensure complete removal of any intact viral particles from the product stream. A final product QC test to confirm this entails a 6-month safety test on chimpanzees.

The HBsAg gene has been cloned and expressed in a variety of expression systems, including *E. coli*, *S. cerevisiae* and a number of mammalian cell lines. The product used commercially is produced in *S. cerevisiae*. The yeast cells are not only capable of expressing the gene, but also assembling the resultant polypeptide product into particles quite similar to those found in the blood of infected individuals. This product proved safe and effective when administered to both animals and humans.

Various other companies have also produced recombinant HBsAg-based vaccines. SmithKline Beecham secured FDA approval for such a product in 1989. Subsequently, SmithKline Beecham have also generated various combination vaccines in which recombinant HBsAg is a component. Twinrix (tradename), for example, contains a mixture of inactivated hepatitis A virus and recombinant HBsAg. Tritanrix, on the other hand, contains diphtheria and tetanus toxoids (produced by traditional means), along with recombinant HBsAg. Dukoral is the tradename given to an additional recombinant protein-containing vaccine now on the market. Indicated for active immunization against disease caused by *Vibrio cholerae* (serogroup 01), the product contains recombinant cholera toxin subunit B and four whole (heat- or formalin-inactivated) *V. cholerae* strains.

It seems likely that many such (recombinant) subunit vaccines will gain future regulatory approval. One such example is that of *Bordetella pertussis* subunit vaccine. *B. pertussis* is a Gram-negative coccobacillus. It is transmitted by droplet infection and is the causative agent of the upper respiratory tract infection commonly termed 'whooping cough'.

Peptide Vaccines

An alternative approach to the production of subunit vaccines entails their direct chemical synthesis. Peptides identical in sequence to short stretches of pathogen-derived polypeptide antigens can be easily and economically synthesized. The feasibility of this approach was first verified in the 1960s, when a hexapeptide purified from the enzymatic digest of tobacco mosaic virus was found to confer limited immunological protection against subsequent administration of the intact virus. (The hexapeptide hapten was initially coupled to bovine serum albumin, used as a carrier to ensure an immunological response.)

Similar synthetic vaccines have also been constructed that confer immunological protection against bacterial toxins, including diphtheria and cholera toxins. Although coupling to a carrier is generally

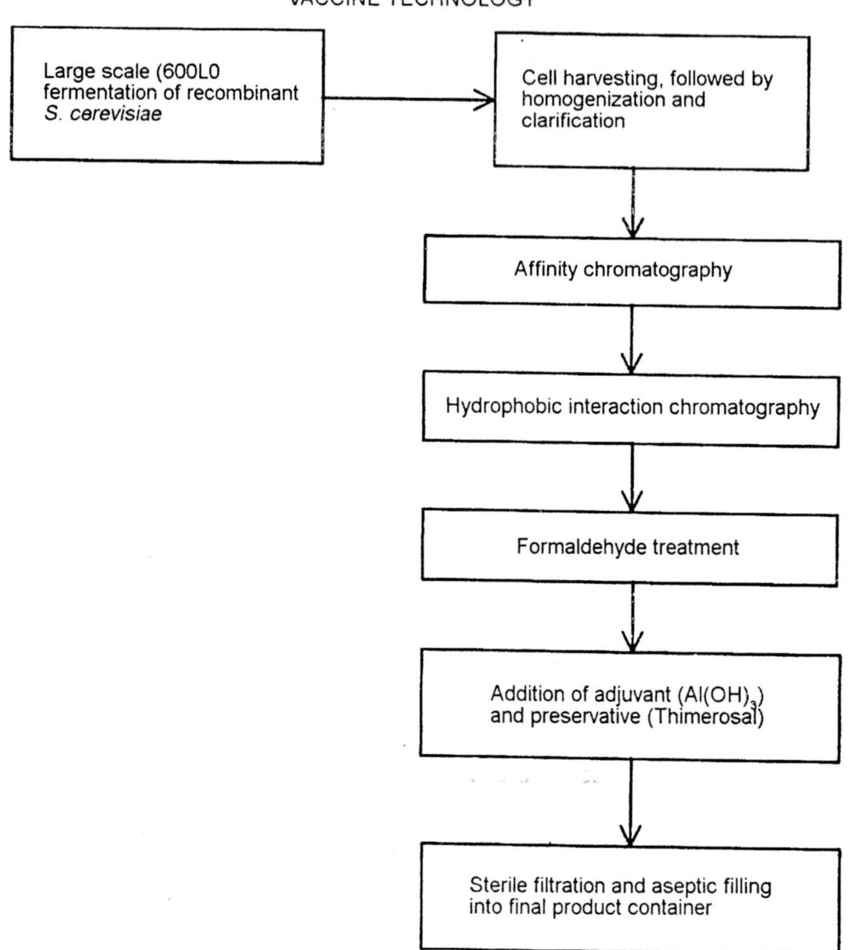

Fig. 5.9. Overview of the production of recombinant HBsAg vaccine.

required to elicit and immunological response, some carriers are inappropriate due to their ability to elicit a hypersensitive reaction, particularly when repeat injections are undertaken. Such difficulties can be avoided by judicious choice of carrier. Often, a carrier normally used for vaccination itself is used. For example, tetanus toxoid has been used as a carrier for peptides derived from influenza haemaglutanin and *Plasmodium falciparum*.

Vaccine Vectors

An alternative approach to the development of novel vaccine products entails the use of live vaccine vectors. The strategy followed involves incorporation of a gene/cDNA coding for a pathogen-derived antigen into a non-pathogenic species. If the resultant recombinant vector expresses the gene product on its surface, then it may be used to immunize against the pathogen of interest. Most vaccine vectors developed to date are viral based, with poxviruses (as well as picorna viruses and adenoviruses) being used most. In general, such recombinant viral vectors elicit both strong humoral and, in particular, cell-mediated immunity. The immunological response (especially the cell-mediated response) to subunit vaccines is usually less pronounced. Poxviruses and, more specifically, the vaccinia virus remain the most thoroughly characterized vector systems developed. These are large, enveloped double-stranded

DNA viruses. They are the only DNA-containing viruses that replicate in the cytoplasm of infected cells. The most studied members of this family are variola and vaccinia. The former represents the causative agent of smallpox, and the latter (being antigenically related to variola but non-pathogenic) was used to immunize against smallpox. Vaccinia-based vaccination programmes led to the global eradication of smallpox, finally achieved by the early 1980s.

A number of factors render vaccinia virus a particularly attractive vector system. These include:

1. Capacity to assimilate large quantities of DNA in its genome successfully;
2. Prior history of widespread and successful use as a vaccination agent;
3. Ability to elicit long-lasting immunity;
4. Ease of production and low production costs;
5. Stability of freeze-dried finished vaccine product.

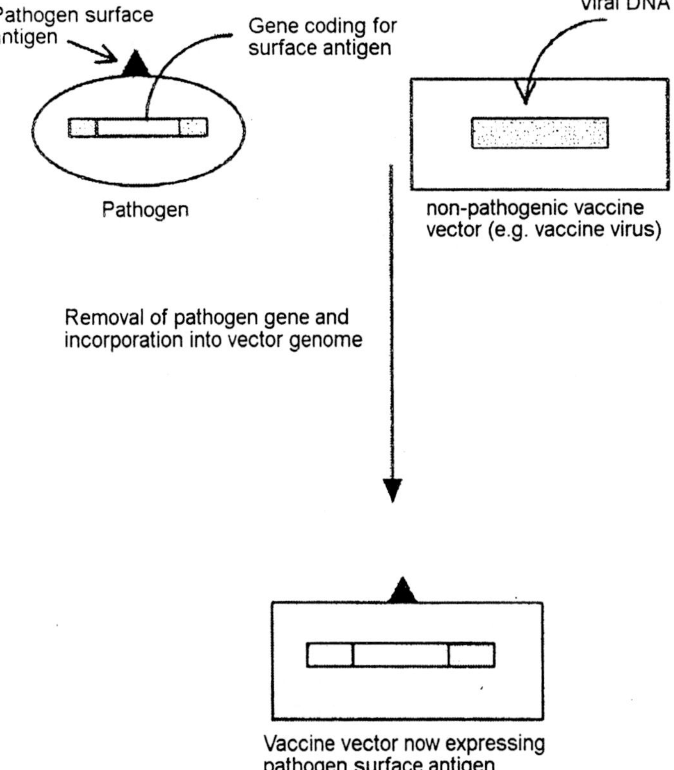

Fig. 5.10. Strategy adopted for the development of an engineered vaccine vector.

Adenoviruses also display potential as vaccine vectors. These double-stranded DNA viruses display a genome consisting of in the region of 36 000 bp, encoding approximately 50 viral genes. Several antigenically distinct human adenovirus serotypes have been characterized, and these viral species are endemic throughout the world. They can prompt respiratory tract infections and, to a lesser extent, gastrointestinal and genitourinary tract infections.

Live adenovirus strains that cause asymptomatic infection and which have proven to be very safe and effective adenovirus vaccines have been isolated. Unlike vaccinia, few sites exist in the adenoviral genome into which foreign DNA can be integrated without comprising viral function. Furthermore, packing limitations curb the quantity of foreign DNA that can be accommodated in the viral genome. However, an approximately 3000 bp region can be removed from a section of the genome termed the E3 region. This facilitates incorporation of pathogen-derived or other DNA at this point.

Recombinant adenoviruses containing the hepatitis B surface antigen gene, the HIV P160 gene, the respiratory syncytial virus F gene, and the herpes simplex virus glycoprotein B gene have all been generated using this approach. Many have been tested in animal models and have been found to elicit humoral and cell-mediated immunity against the pathogen of interest.

The use of recombinant viral vectors as vaccination tools displays considerable clinical promise. One potential complicating factor, however, centres around the possibility that previous recipient exposure to the virus being used as a vector would negate the therapeutic efficacy of the product. Such prior exposure would likely indicate the presence of circulating immune memory cells that could initiate an immediate immunological response upon re-entry of the virus into the host. Studies involving repeat administration of vaccinia virus have, to some extent, confirmed this possibility. However, the degree to which such an effect limits the applicability of this approach in a clinical setting remains to be elucidated.

Development of an AIDS Vaccine

AIDS was initially described in the U.S. in 1981, although sporadic cases probably occurred for at least two decades prior to this. By 1983, the causative agent, now termed HIV, was identified. HIV is a member of the lentivirus subfamily of retroviruses. It is a spherical, enveloped particle, 100–150 nm in diameter, and contains RNA as its genetic material.

The viral surface protein, gp 120, is capable of binding to a specific site on the CD4 molecule, found on the surface of susceptible cells. Some CD4 negative cells may (rarely) also become infected, indicating the existence of an entry mechanism independent of CD4.

Infection of $CD4^+$ cells commences via interaction between gp 120 and the CD4 glycoprotein, which effectively acts as the viral receptor. Entry of the virus into the cell, which appears to require some additional cellular components, occurs via endocytosis and/or fusion of the viral and cellular membranes. The gp 41 transmembrane protein plays an essential role in this process. Once released into the cell, the viral RNA is transcribed (by the associated viral reverse transcriptase) into double-stranded DNA. The retroviral DNA can then integrate into the host cell genome (or, in some instances, remain unintegrated). In resting cells, transcription of viral genes usually does not occur to any significant extent. However, commencement of active cellular growth/differentiation usually also triggers expression of proviral genes and, hence, synthesis of new viral particles. Aggressive expression of viral genes usually leads to cell death. Some cells, however (particularly macrophages), often permit chronic low-level viral synthesis and release without cell death.

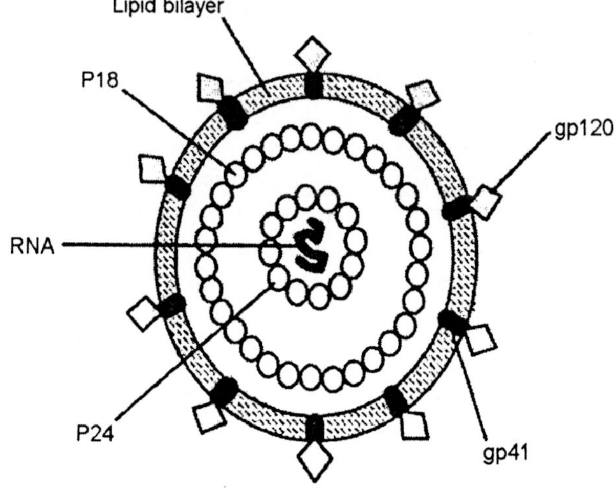

Fig. 5.11. Simplified schematic representation of a cross-section of HIV.

Entry of the virus into the human subject is generally accompanied by initial viral replication, lasting a few weeks. High-level viraemia (presence of viral particles in the blood) is noted and p24 antigen can be detected in the blood. Clinical symptoms associated with the initial infection include an influenza-like illness, joint pains and general enlargement of the lymph nodes. This primary viraemia is brought under control within 3–4 weeks. This appears to be mediated largely by HIV-specific cytotoxic T-lymphocytes, indicating the likely importance of cell-mediated immunity in bringing the initial infection under control. Although HIV-specific antibodies are also produced at this stage, effective neutralizing antibodies are detected mainly after this initial stage of infection. After this initial phase of infection subsides, the free viral load in the blood declines, often to almost undetectable levels. This latent phase may last for anything up to 10 years or more. During this phase, however, there does seem to be continuous synthesis and destruction of viral particles. This is accompanied by a high turnover rate of ($CD4^+$) T-helper lymphocytes. The levels of these T-lymphocytes decline with time, as does antibody levels specific for viral proteins. The circulating viral load often increases as a result, and the depletion of T-helper cells compromises general immune function. As the immune system fails, classical symptoms of AIDS-related complex (ARC) and, finally, full-blown AIDS begin to develop.

In excess of 40 million individuals are now thought to be infected by HIV. In 2001 alone, it was estimated that 3 million people died from AIDS and a further 5 million became infected with the virus. Over 20 million people in total are now thought to have died from AIDS. The worst affected geographical region is the southern half of Africa. Some 90 per cent of sufferers live in poorer world regions. So far, no effective therapy has been discovered, and the main hope of eradicating this disease lies with the development of safe, effective vaccines. The first such putative vaccine entered clinical trials in 1987; but, thus far, no effective vaccine has been developed.

Difficulties Associated with Vaccine Development

A number of attributes of HIV and its mode of infection conspire to render development of an effective vaccine less than straightforward. These factors include:

1. HIV displays extensive genetic variation even within a single individual. Such genetic variation is particularly prominent in the viral *env* gene whose product, gp160, is subsequently proteolytically processed to yield gp120 and gp41.
2. HIV infects and destroys T-helper lymphocytes, i.e. it directly attacks an essential component of the immune system itself.
3. Although infected individuals display a wide range of antiviral immunological responses, these ultimately fail to destroy the virus. A greater understanding of what elements of immunity are most effective in combating HIV infection is required.
4. After initial virulence subsides, large numbers of cells harbour unexpressed proviral DNA. The immune system has no way of identifying such cells. An effective vaccine must thus induce the immune system to (a) bring the viral infection under control before cellular infection occurs or (b) destroy cells once they begin to produce viral particles and destroy the viral particles released.
5. The infection may often be spread not via transmission of free viral particles, but via direct transmission of infected cells harbouring the proviral DNA.

AIDS Vaccines in Clinical Trials

A number of approaches are being assessed with regard to developing an effective AIDS vaccine. No safe attenuated form of the virus has been recognized to date, nor is one likely to be developed in the foreseeable future. The high level of mutation associated with HIV would, in any case, heighten fears that spontaneous reversion of any such product to virulence would be possible. The potential of inactivated viral particles as effective vaccines has gained some attention, but again fears of accidental transmission of disease if inactivation methods are not consistently 100 per cent effective have dampened enthusiasm for such an approach. In addition, the stringent containment conditions required to produce large quantities of the virus render such production processes expensive. Not withstanding the possible value of such inactivated viral vaccines, the bulk of products assessed to date are subunit vaccines. Live vector vaccines expressing HIV genes have also been developed and are now coming to the fore.

Much of the preclinical data generated with regard to these vaccines entailed the use of one of two animal model systems: simian immunodeficiency virus infection of macaque monkeys and HIV infection of chimpanzees. Most of the positive results observed in such systems have been in association with the chimp–HIV model. However, no such system can replace actual testing in humans.

Most of the recombinant subunit vaccines tested in the first half of this decade employed gp 120 or gp 160 expressed in yeast, insect or mammalian (mainly CHO) cell lines. Eukaryotic systems facilitate glycosylation of the protein products. Like all subunit vaccines, these stimulate a humoral-based immune response but fail to elicit a strong T-cell response. The failure to elicit a cell-based response, in particular a cytotoxic T-cell response (now seen as critical to mounting an effective immune response), explains at least in part why subunit vaccines were a clinical disappointment.

Several HIV vaccine systems based upon live vectors have also been developed in an attempt to stimulate a significant T-cell, as well as B-cell, immune response. Both envelope and core antigens have been expressed in a number of recombinant viral systems. The clinical efficacy of these remains to be established. Expression in engineered vaccinia has been undertaken, but its use as an HIV vaccine is likely precluded by the fact that the virus can apparently disseminate and cause fatal encephalitis in immunosuppressed infected individuals. Modified vaccinia Ankara, canarypox and fowlpox viruses have come to the fore as vectors. These likely can produce sufficient protein to initiate both a humoral and cellular immune response during an abortive replication cycle in humans. A vaccination schedule variation of potential interest entails the use of a vector-based primary dose (to induce a cellular response in particular) followed by a subunit-based booster (to induce mainly a humoral response). Whatever the schedule however, the induction of effective (i.e. broadly neutralizing) antibodies remains a challenge, as the regions of HIV envelope proteins that are most highly conserved seem to be shielded from antibody access by loop structures and sugar side-chains on these surface proteins.

Large-scale clinical trials are likely to be the only way by which any HIV vaccine may be properly assessed. In addition, a greater understanding of the molecular interplay between the virus and immune system may provide clues as to the development of novel vaccine and/or therapeutic products. For example, a small proportion of infected individuals remain clinically asymptomatic for periods considerably greater than the average 10–15 years. An understanding of the immunological or other factors that delay onset of ARC/full-blown AIDS in these individuals may aid in the design of more effective vaccines.

Cancer Vaccines

The identification of tumour-associated antigens could pave the way for the development of a range of cancer vaccines. A number of tumour-associated antigens have already been characterized, as described previously. Theoretically, administration of tumour-associated antigens may effectively immunize an individual against any cancer type characterized by expression of the tumour-associated antigen in question. Co-administration of a strong adjuvant would be advantageous, as it would stimulate an enhanced immune response. This is important, as many tumour-associated antigens appear to be weak immunogens. Administration of subunit- based tumour-associated antigen vaccines would primarily stimulate a humoral immune response.

The use of viral vectors may ultimately prove more effective, as a T-cell response appears to be central to the immunological destruction of cancer cells.

The latter approach has been adopted in experimental studies involving malignant melanoma. These transformed cells express significantly elevated levels of a surface glycoprotein, p97. p97 is also expressed (but at far lower levels) on the surface of many normal cell types. Initial animal studies have indicated that administration of a recombinant vaccinia vector expressing p97 has a protective effect against challenge with melanoma cells. However, protracted safety studies would be required in this, or similar, instances to prove that such vaccines would not, for example, induce an autoimmune response if the antigen was not wholly tumour specific. The development of truly effective cancer vaccines probably requires a more comprehensive understanding of the transformed phenotype and how these cells normally evade immune surveillance in the first place. Not withstanding this, limited clinical studies in this field have already begun.

Recombinant Veterinary Vaccines

Amongst the limited number of biopharmaceuticals approved for animal use, recombinant vaccines represent the single largest subgroup. Several such products target pigs, including 'Porcilis pesti' and 'Bayovac CSF E2'. Porcilis pesti, for example, contains a recombinant form of the classical swine fever virus E2 antigen, the immunodominant surface antigen associated with this viral pathogen. It is used to immunize young pigs. The process is initiated by growth of *Spodoptera frugiperda* cells, typically in a 500 l fermenter. The cells are then infected with the recombinant baculovirus vector, resulting in high-level expression of the recombinant E2 antigen. The antigen is harvested from the production medium by low-speed centrifugation and membrane filtration steps, which serve to remove intact cells/cellular debris. The antigen-containing supernatant is then treated with β-propiolacetone in order to inactivate viral particles present. The antigen is not subjected to subsequent high-resolution chromatographic purification steps, and hence is not purified to homogeneity. The product is then formulated as an oil-in-water emulsion.

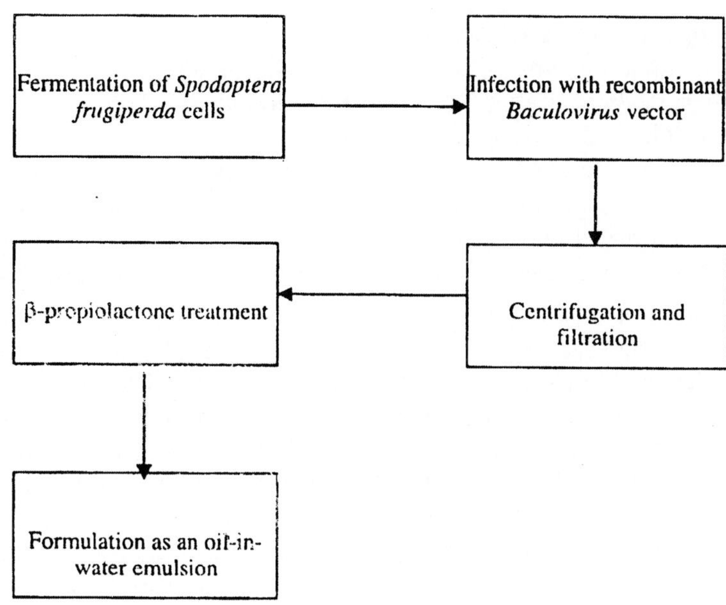

Fig. 5.12. Overview of the manufacture of the veterinary vaccine 'Porcilis pesti'.

Adjuvant Technology

Administration of many vaccines on their own stimulates a poor host immunological response. This is particularly true of the more recently developed subunit vaccines. An adjuvant is defined as any material that enhances the cellular and/or humoral immune response to an antigen. Adjuvants thus generally elicit an earlier, more potent and longer-lasting, immunological reaction against co-administered antigen. In addition, the use of adjuvants can often facilitate administration of reduced quantities of antigen to achieve an adequate immunological response. This implies consequent economic savings, as vaccines (particularly subunit and vector vaccines) are far more expensive to produce than the adjuvant.

A number of different adjuvant preparations have been developed. Most preparations also display some associated toxicity and, as a general rule, the greater the product's adjuvanticity, the more toxic it is likely to be. A few different adjuvants may be used in veterinary medicine; however (for safety reasons), aluminium-based products are the only adjuvants routinely used in human medicine. Application of many of the aggressive adjuvant materials is reserved for selected experimentation purposes in animals.

An ideal adjuvant should display several specific characteristics. These include:

1. Safety (no unacceptable local/systemic responses);
2. Elicit protective immunity, even against weak immunogens;
3. Be non-pyrogenic;
4. Be chemically defined (facilitates consistent manufacture and QC testing);
5. Be effective in infants/young children;
6. Yield stable formulation with antigen;
7. Be biodegradable;
8. Be non-immunogenic itself.

Adjuvant Mode of Action

Adjuvants are a heterogeneous family of substances, both in terms of their chemical structure and their mode of action. The observed adjuvanticity of any such substance may be due to one or more of the following factors:

1. Depot formation of antigen. This results in the subsequent slow release of the antigen from the site of injection, which, in turn, ensures its prolonged exposure to the immune system.
2. Enhanced antigen presentation to the cells of the immune system.
3. The direct induction of immunostimulatory substances, most notably interleukins and other cytokines.

Mineral-based Adjuvants

A number of mineral-based substances display an adjuvant effect. Although calcium phosphate, calcium chloride and salts of various metals (e.g. zinc sulfate and cerium nitrate) display some effect, aluminium-based substances are by far the most potent. Most commonly employed are aluminium hydroxide and aluminium phosphate. Their adjuvanticity, coupled to their proven safety, render them particularly valuable in the preparation of vaccines for young children. They have been incorporated into millions of doses of such vaccine products so far.

The principal method by which aluminium adjuvanted vaccines are prepared entails mixing the antigen in solution with a preformed aluminium phosphate (or hydroxide) precipitate under chemically defined conditions (e.g. of pH). Adsorption of the antigen to the aluminium-based gel ensues, with such preparations being generally termed '*aluminium-adsorbed vaccines*'; 1 mg of aluminium hydroxide will usually adsorb in the order of 50–200 μg of protein.

The major mode of action of such products appears to be depot formation at the site of injection. The antigen is only slowly released from the gel, ensuring its sustained exposure to immune surveillance. The aluminium compounds are also capable of activating complement. This can lead to a local inflammatory response, with consequent attraction of immunocompetent cells to the site of action.

Despite their popularity, aluminium-based adjuvants suffer from several drawbacks. They tend to stimulate only the humoral arm of the immune response effectively. They cannot be frozen or lyophylized, as either process promotes destruction of their gel-based structure. In addition, aluminium-based products display poor/no adjuvanticity when combined with some antigen (e.g. typhoid or *Haemophilus influenzae* type b capsular polysaccharides).

Oil-based Emulsion Adjuvants

The adjuvanticity of oil emulsions was first recognized in the early 1900s. However, the first such product to gain widespread attention was Freund's complete adjuvant (FCA), developed in 1937. This product essentially contained a mixture of paraffin (i.e. mineral) oil with dead mycobacteria, formulated to form a water-in-oil emulsion. Arlacel A (mannide mono-oleate) is usually added as an emulsifier.

Freund's incomplete adjuvant (FIA) is a similar product. It differs from FCA in that it lacks the mycobacterial component and, consequently, displays somewhat lesser adjuvanticity. The mode of action of FIA is largely attributed to depot formation. The mycobacterial components in FCA have additional direct immunostimulatory activities. Although it is one of the most potent adjuvant substances known, FCA is too toxic for human use.

Latterly, some oil-in-water adjuvants have been developed. Many are squalene-in-water emulsions. Emulsifiers most commonly used include polyalcohols, such as Tween and Span. In some cases, immunostimulatory molecules (including MDP and TDM) have also been incorporated in order to enhance adjuvanticity. These continue to be carefully assessed and may well form a future family of useful adjuvant preparations.

Bacteria/Bacterial Products as Adjuvants

Selected microorganisms have been identified that can trigger particularly potent immunological responses. The immunostimulatory properties of these cells have generated interest in their potential application as adjuvants. Examples include various mycobacteria, *Corynebacterium parvum*, *Corynebacterium granulosum* and *B. pertussis*. Although some such microorganisms are used as antigens in vaccines, they are considered too toxic to be used solely in the role of adjuvant. Researchers have thus sought to identify the specific microbial biomolecules responsible for the observed immunostimulatory activity. It was hoped that these substances, when purified, might display lesser/no toxic side effects while retaining their immunostimulatory capacity.

Fractionation of mycobacteria resulted in the identification of two cellular immunostimulatory components, namely TDM and MDPs. Both are normally found in association with the mycobacterial cell wall. TDM is composed of a molecule of trehalose (a disaccharide consisting of two molecules of α-D-glucose linked via an α 1-1 glycosidic bond), linked to two molecules of my- colic acid (a long-chain aliphatic hydrocarbon-based acid) found almost exclusively in association with mycobacteria. TDM, although retaining its adjuvanticity, is relatively non-toxic.

The structure of the native immunostimulatory MDPs was found to be *N*-acetyl muramyl-L-alanyl-D-isoglutamine. (*N*-Acetyl muramic acid is a base component of bacterial peptidoglycan.) Native TDM is a potent pyrogen and is too toxic for general use as an adjuvant. The molecular basis underlining MDP's adjuvanticity remains to be fully elucidated. Administration of MDP, however, is known to activate a number of cell types that play direct/indirect roles in immune function, and induces the secretion of various immunomodulatory cytokines.

A number of derivatives were synthesized in the hope of identifying a modified form that retained its adjuvanticity but displayed lesser toxicity. Some such derivatives, most notably threonyl-MDP, muramyl tripeptide and murabutide, display some clinical promise in this regard.

Threonlyn-MDP, for example, has been included in the formulation known as Syntex adjuvant formulation-1 (SAF-1). Animal studies suggest that this adjuvant is non-toxic and elicits a good B- and T-cell response.

An additional bacterial component displaying appreciable adjuvanticity is the *C. granulosum*-derived p40 particulate fraction. p40 is composed of fragments of cell wall peptidoglycan and associated glycoproteins.

Additional Adjuvants

In addition to the immunostimulatory substances discussed above, the adjuvanticity of a variety of other substances is also being appraised. These include saponins, liposomes and ISCOMs.

Saponins are a family of glycosides (sugar derivatives) widely distributed in plants. Each saponin consists of a sugar moiety bound to a 'sapogenin' (either a steroid or a triterpene). The immunostimulatory properties of the saponin fraction isolated from the bark of *Quillaja* (a tree) has been long recognized. Quil A (which consists of a mixture of related saponins) is used as an adjuvant in selected veterinary vaccines. However, its haemolytic potential precludes its use in human vaccines. Research efforts continue in an attempt to identify individual saponins (or derivatives thereof) that would make safe and effective adjuvants for use in human medicine.

Liposomes are membrane-based supramolecular particles that consist of a number of concentric lipid membrane bilayers separated by aqueous compartments. They were developed initially as carriers for therapeutic drugs. Initially, the bilayers were almost exclusively phospholipid based. More recently, non-phospholipid-based liposomes have been developed. The adjuvanticity of liposomes depends upon their composition, number of layers and charge characteristics. They act as effective adjuvants for both protein- and carbohydrate-based antigens and help stimulate both B- and T-cell responses. Their likely mode of action includes depot formation, but they also possibly increase/enhance antigen presentation to macrophages. The exact molecular mechanism(s) by which they stimulate a T-cell response remains to be elucidated, but it appears to be associated with their hydrophobicity. Liposomes are likely to gain more widespread use as adjuvants when technical difficulties, associated with their stability and consistent/ reproducible production, are resolved.

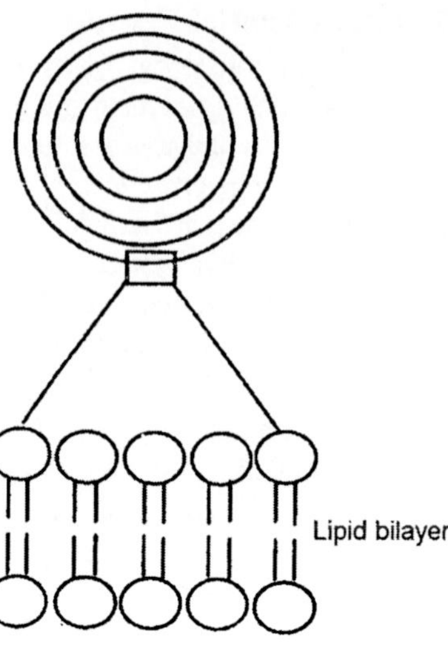

Fig. 5.13. Generalized liposome structure.

ISCOMs are stable (non-covalent) complexes composed of a mixture of Quil A, cholesterol and (an amphipathic) antigen. ISCOMs stimulate both humoral and cellular immune responses and have been used in the production of some veterinary vaccines. Their use in humans, however, has not been licensed so far, mainly due to safety concerns relating to the Quil A component. In summary, therefore, a whole range of adjuvants have thus far been identified/developed. Problems of toxicity have precluded the use of many of these adjuvants (particularly in humans). However, research efforts continue in an attempt to develop the next generation of safe and, hopefully, even more effective vaccine adjuvants.

6

Bioconversion of Penicillins

Biosynthesis of cephalosporins in *Cephalosporium acremonium* (syn. *Acremonium chrysogenum*) and *Streptomyces clavuligerus* proceeds through a biosynthetic pathway that includes expansion of the five-membered thiazolidine ring of the intermediate penicillin N into the six-membered dihydrothiazine ring of deacetoxycephalosporin C (DAOC). The ring-expansion step is catalyzed by the dioxygenase, DAOC synthase ("*expandase*"). Whereas the eukaryotic *C. acremonium* produces penicillin N and cephalosporin C, the prokaryote *S. clavuligerus* produces a variety of β-lactam antibiotics including clavulanic acid, penicillin N, and cephamycin C; cephamycins are 7-α-methoxycephalosporins. Expandase has been purified from both *S. clavuligerus* and *C. acremonium*. Its enzyme activity requires α-ketoglutarate, Fe^{2+}, and oxygen. In *C. acremonium*, the activity of expandase resides in a bifunctional enzyme that catalyzes not only ring expansion but also the hydroxylation of the methyl group of DAOC to deacetylcephalosporin C (DAC). In *S. clavuligerus* and in other prokaryotes, the two activities are associated with separate proteins. The properties of this synthase are very similar to those of other α-ketoglutarate-dependent dioxygenases, which incorporate one atom of oxygen into α-ketoglutarate to form succinate and the other atom into the product molecule. However, expandase differs in that no oxygen atom appears in its ring expansion product, DAOC.

Because of the effectiveness of cephalosporins against penicillin-resistant bacterial pathogens, understanding the substrate specificity, action, and regulation of expandase is of great scientific interest and practical importance.

Many investigators have reported that the enzyme, in cell-free extracts as well as after purification, has a narrow substrate specificity and no detectable activity on readily available and inexpensive penicillins (such as penicillin G and V) produced by *Penicillium chrysogenum*. Maeda et al. varied temperature, duration of reaction, buffers, and concentration of penicillin G, but without success. They were only able to observe ring expansion when the natural substrate penicillin N or its close relative D-carboxymethylcysteinyl-6-aminopenicillanic acid was used as substrate. Indeed, it is chemical ring expansion of penicillin G plus enzymatic removal of the phenylacetyl side chain that is used in industry to convert penicillin G to 7-aminodeacetoxycephalosporanic acid (7ADCA), an important intermediate for the manufacture of semisynthetic cephalosporins. However, the chemical process requires several steps, is expensive, and polluting. A simple biological route, requiring only two steps, i.e., enzymatic ring expansion and deacylation, might replace the chemical process, thereby reducing costs and environmental problems. Only recently have the conditions that allow some conversion of penicillin G to deacetoxycephalosporin G (DAOG) (phenylacetyl-7ADCA) been identified. Essentially, what was required were increased concentrations of iron and α-ketoglutarate.

Molecular Studies on Expandase Proteins and Genes

Ring expansion of penicillin N to DAOC was discovered by Kohsaka and Demain working with cell-free extracts of *C. acremonium*. The product of that reaction was identified as DAOC. The enzyme which catalyzed this reaction, expandase, exhibited properties of α-ketoglutarate-linked dioxygenases. Ring expansion activity was found to be markedly increased by ascorbic acid, Fe^{2+}, α-ketoglutarate, and oxygen. The enzyme showed an absolute requirement for α-ketoglutarate, and this co-substrate could not be replaced by chemically related compounds such as α-ketoadipate, pyruvate, oxaloacetate, glutamate, succinate, α-ketovalerate, or α-ketobutyrate.

The bifunctional expandase/hydroxylase of *C. acremonium* appeared to be a monomer with a molecular weight of 41,000 Da and an isoelectric point of 6.3. Both catalytic activities require α-ketoglutarate, Fe^{2+}, and oxygen and are stimulated by ascorbate, dithiothreitol (DTT), and ATP. Both activities were evident when Fe^{2+} was replaced by Fe^{3+} in the presence of a reducing agent; however, no activity was observed when Fe^{2+} was replaced by Mg^{2+}, Ca^{2+}, Cu^{2+}, Ni^{+2+} Co^{2+}, Zn^{2+}, Na^{+}, or K^{+}. The K_m value obtained for penicillin N was 29 μM, whereas for α-ketoglutarate it was 22 μM. Both activities were similarly sensitive to inhibition by metal chelators such as ethylene diaminetetraacetic acid (EDTA) or *o*-phenanthroline, as would be expected with chelators of Fe^{2+}. Inhibition by Zn^{2+} and sulfhydryl reagents such as *p*-hydroxymercuribenzoate (*p*-HMB), 5´-5´-dithiobis-2-nitrobenzoic acid (DTNB), or N-ethylmaleimide (NEM) suggests that at least one sulfhydryl group is essential for ring expansion activity. When isopenicillin N, penicillin G, penicillin V, ampicillin, carboxy-*n*-butyl penicillin, and 6-amino-penicillanic acid (6APA) were tested as substrate analogs, no ring expansion was observed.

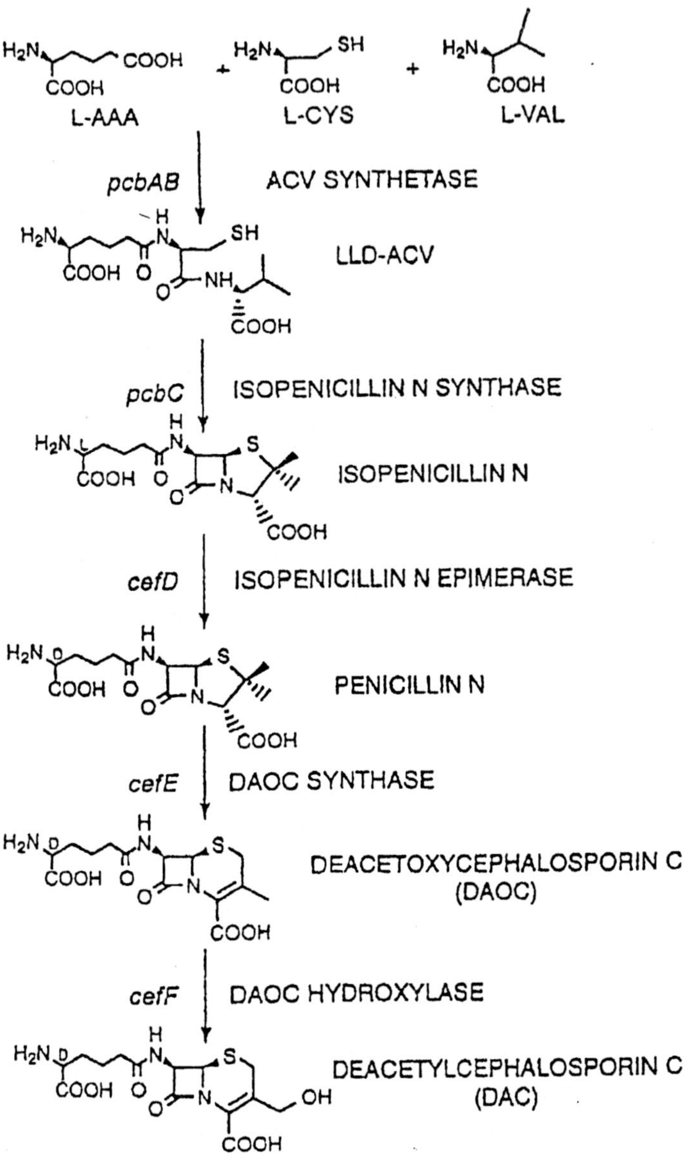

Fig. 6.1. Biosynthetic pathway to DAC.

Cloning of the expandase/hydroxylase gene (*cefEF*) from *C. acremonium* in *Escherichia coli* was achieved using probes based on amino acid sequences of fragments of the purified protein. The results obtained revealed an open reading frame (ORF) of 996 nt encoding a protein of 332 amino acids with a molecular weight of 40,000–41,000 Da. In this fungus, the cephalosporin genes are located in two different clusters on separate chromosomes. One of them is formed by the genes encoding the first two steps of the pathway, *pcbAB* and *pcbC*, found on chromosome VI, whereas the cluster containing the late genes (*cefEF* and *cefG*) was located on chromosome II. The two *cef* genes are oppositely oriented and expressed from divergent promoters located within a 938-bp intergenic region.

The *S. clavuligerus* expandase is a monomer of 34,600 Da with two isoelectric points of 6.1 and 5.3. Its catalytic activity requires α-ketoglutarate, Fe^{2+}, and oxygen, and it is stimulated by DTT and ascorbate but not by ATP. The synthase was equally active with Fe^{2+} or Fe^{3+} in the presence of ascorbate and DTT; however, these metal ions could not be replaced by Mg^{2+}, Ca^{2+}, Cu^{2+}, Ni^{2+}, Co^{2+}, Na^{+}, or K^{+}. As mentioned above for the fungal synthetase, the *S. clavuligerus* expandase activity is also very sensitive to metals chelators such as EDTA or *o*-phenanthroline, and to sulfhydryl reagents such as *p*-HMB, DTNB, and NEM. As was previously observed by other authors working with cell-free extracts, purified expandase was unable to expand isopenicillin N, penicillin G, penicillin V, ampicillin, or 6APA.

The crystal structure of the *S. clavuligerus* expandase has been recently reported and, based on it, a mechanism for the formation of the reactive ferryl species, a catalytic intermediate common to many nonheme oxygenases, was proposed. The apo-expandase, a crystallographic trimer, reacts first with the iron, which is ligated by three protein ligands (His 183, His 243, Asp 185) and three solvent molecules, causing dissociation of the apoenzyme into monomers, the catalytically active form. Then, the enzyme–Fe^{2+} complex reacts with α-ketoglutarate, whose binding replaces two solvent molecules around the iron, and with dioxygen. The ferryl form of expandase, which reacts with penicillin N, is created by the splitting of dioxygen and oxidative decarboxylation of α-ketoglutarate to succinate.

Based on a 22-residue amino-terminal sequence of the purified protein, the *cefE* gene coding for the *S. clavuligerus* expandase was cloned and expressed in *E. coli*. The gene contains an ORF of 933 nt encoding a protein of 311 amino acids with a molecular weight of 34,519 Da. Comparison of this gene and the *cefEF* gene of *C. acremonium* showed 67% similarity, whereas at the protein level there was a 57% similarity. The bacterial protein is 21 amino acids shorter than the fungal protein and its amino terminal group is not blocked. In this bacterium, the *cefE* gene is linked to the *cefD* gene (coding for the epimerase converting isopenicillin N to penicillin N) with an 81-bp intergenic region between them. Both genes are located 7 kb upstream of the *lat* gene (encoding lysine ε-aminotransferase) and are expressed from a large transcript.

The *Nocardia lactamdurans* expandase is a monomer which was initially reported to have a molecular weight of 27,000 Da. Cloning and expression of the *cefE* gene in *Streptomyces lividans* revealed an enzyme of 34,532 Da containing 314 amino acids and an isoelectric point of 4.9. This synthase behaves very similarly to the expandase of *S. clavuligerus* and requires α-ketoglutarate, Fe^{2+}, and oxygen, although it does not need ATP and ascorbate. A high specificity for the nature of the side chain in the penicillin substrate was also observed and only penicillin N was expanded, not isopenicillin N, penicillin G, or 6APA.

The *N. lactamdurans* gene has a high similarity to the *cefE* gene of *S. clavuligerus* (74.7%) and the *cefEF* gene of *C. acremonium* (69.2%). At the protein level, there is also a high similarity to the expandase of *S. clavuligerus* (70.4%) and with the expandase/hydroxylase of *C. acremonium* (59.5%). In *N. lactamdurans*, the *cefD* and *cefE* genes are clustered 0.7 kb upstream of the *lat* gene, lack any intergenic region, and are translationally coupled.

Recently, the gene cluster involved in cephabacin F (a 7-formylamino cephalosporin) biosynthesis in *Lysobacter lactamgenus* was characterized. This *cefE* gene encodes a protein of 319 amino acids with a molecular weight of 35,557 Da that shows 54% and 57% homology with the expandases of *S.*

clavuligerus and *C. acremonium*, respectively. The expandase gene is located just downstream of*pcbC* in a simple and compact cluster in which the genes encoding the four enzyme activities converting the tripeptide δ-(L-α-aminoadipyl)-L-cysteinyl-D-valine (ACV) to DAC are tightly linked within a 17-kb region of DNA in the same orientation.

Bioconversion of Penicillin G to DAOG

Resting Cells

S. clavuligerus NP1, a mutant that produces only trace levels of cephalosporins, was used, since the absence of significant levels of cephalosporins in this strain facilitates detection of cephalosporins produced by ring expansion from added penicillins. Mycelia were developed in two shaken stages of medium MST, containing 1% soluble starch, 3% trypticase soy broth without dextrose, and 90 mM 3-(N-morpholino)propanesulfonic acid (MOPS) buffer at pH 7.0. Mycelia were washed twice before being used for the reaction. The standard reaction mixture for expandase action was that described by Maeda et al. except that penicillin G replaced penicillin N. Additions were made in the order established by Shen et al. At various times during the shaking incubation, samples were taken, centrifuged to remove cells, and supernatant fluids assayed by the paper disk-agar diffusion bioassay, using *E. coli* Ess (a β-lactam supersensitive mutant). The formation of DAOG was determined by inclusion of penicillinase in the assay agar (this narrow-spectrum β-lactamase attacks penicillins but not cephalosporins) and measuring zones of growth inhibition.

Although previous attempts to expand the thiazolidine ring of penicillin G with cell-free extracts of *S. clavuligerus* had failed, success was achieved with resting cells. When $FeSO_4$, α-ketoglutarate, or ascorbic acid was absent, the amount of product was ~30% of that in the control. On the other hand, ATP, $MgSO_4$, KCl, and DTT did not play a significant role in the reaction with resting cells. The omission of DTT actually increased production by 50%.

Table 6.1. Effect of cofactors on the ring expansion of penicillin G using resting cells

Cofactor omitted	*μg DAOG/ml*
None	10.5
DDT (16 mM)	15.5
a-Ketoglutarate (1.28 mM)	3.7
$FeSO_4 \cdot 7H_2O$ (1.8 mM)	3.2
$MgSO_4 \cdot 7H_2O$ (8 mM)	10.1
KCl (8 mM)	11.5
Ascorbic acid (4 mM)	3.0
ATP (0.7 mM)	10.0

α-Ketoglutarate was known to be necessary as a cosubstrate for enzymatic ring expansion of penicillin N. Figure 6.2 shows that a doubling of activity of resting cells on penicillin G was observed when the α-ketoglutarate concentration was raised from the standard concentration of 0.64 mM to 1.28 mM. Figure 6.3 reveals that increasing concentrations of Fe^{2+} up to 1.8 mM increased ring expansion of penicillin G. This optimum concentration of Fe^{2+} was 45-fold higher than had been used for conversion of penicillin N by cell-free extracts. The optimum ascorbate concentration for conversion of penicillin G by resting cells was found to be 4-8 mM. Maeda et al. had used 5 mM ascorbate, and Lubbe et al. had used 4 mM ascorbate for cell-free conversion of penicillin N to DAOC. ATP did not improve resting cell activity on penicillin G, whereas cell-free extracts acting on penicillin N had been stimulated by ATP. Increasing cell mass enhanced the concentration of DAOG formed from penicillin G, the optimum concentration being 19 mg/ml. Higher cell concentrations inhibited the reaction, probably because oxygen supply was limiting under such conditions. In the studies of Cho et al., the buffer used for bioconversion was 50mM Tris-HCl [Tris = tris(hydroxy-methyl) aminomethane] at pH 7.4. It was later found that 50 mM MOPS buffer or 50 mM HEPES [N-(2-hydroxyethyl) piperazine-N´-(2-ethanesulfonic acid] buffer at pH 6.5 improved activity.

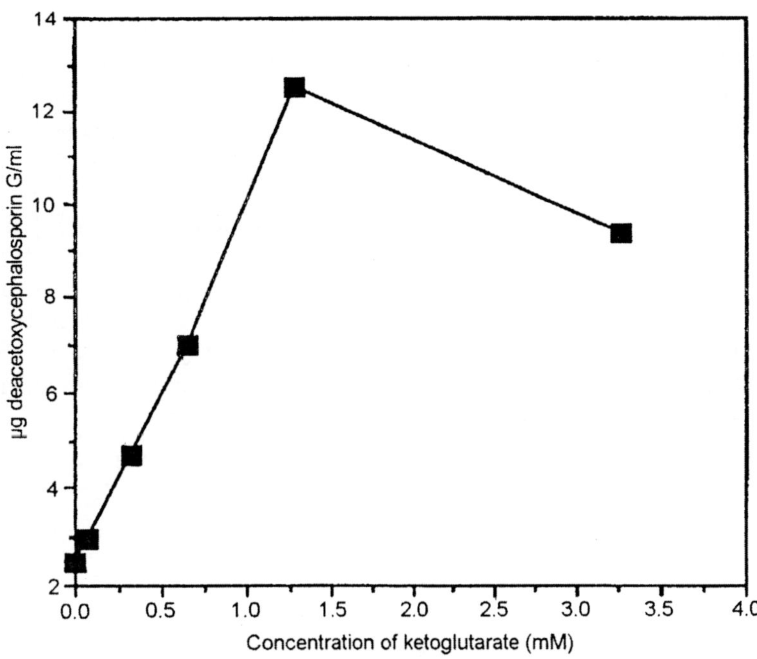

Fig. 6.2. Effect of α-ketoglutarate concentration on ring expansion of penicillin G by resting cells of Streptomyces clavuligerus.

To identify the products of the biotransformation, a system for the separation of penicillin G, DAOG, and deacetylcephalosporin G (DAG) was used. HPLC analysis of the 0-hr sample gave a profile showing several peaks. The peaks at 3.1 and 3.6 min corresponded to α-ketoglutarate and $FeSO_4$, respectively. The penicillin G peak eluted at 17 min. After 1 hr of incubation, two new peaks (3.65 and 15.3 min) appeared on the chromatogram. The 15.3-min peak was DAOG, but the 3.65-min peak was unidentified. During the subsequent 2 hr of biotransformation, these two peaks increased in size. No peak corresponding to DAG was detected during the reaction. The DAG peak would have eluted at 8 min. Thus, one of the products present in the biotransformation mixture was identified as DAOG. A new unidentified (more polar) peak with a retention time of 3.65 min was also produced. In *S. clavuligerus*, DAC is a precursor of three compounds: O-carbamoyldeacetylcephalosporin C, 7-α-hydroxy-O-carbamoyldeacetyl-cephalosporin C, and cephamycin C. The new unidentified peak might represent the phenylacetyl version of any one of these products.

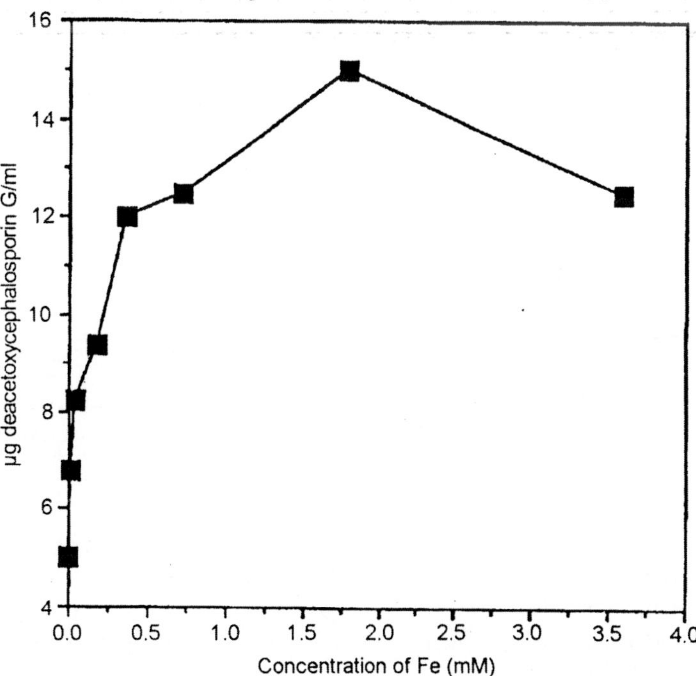

Fig. 6.3. Effect of $FeSO_4$ concentration on ring expansion of penicillin G by resting cells.

Cell-Free Extracts

To prepare cell-free extracts, broths were centrifuged and pellets were washed twice in 50 mM Tris-HCl supplemented with 0.1 mM DTT, and disrupted by sonication. After centrifugation, the resulting supernatant fluids were placed on ice and then used for the reaction. Reaction mixtures were incubated in tubes, and the reactions were stopped at various times by the addition of an equal volume of methanol. Using the high concentrations of $FeSO_4$ and α-ketoglutarate established for resting cell conversion of penicillin G to DAOG, activity was observed with cell-free extracts. Furthermore, high protein (6 mg/ml) and high substrate (5 mg/ml) concentrations increased the concentration of product made. Using the conditions employed earlier with penicillin N, in which protein concentration in the cell-free extracts was 1-2 mg/ml, only a low level of activity on penicillin G was observed. The penicillin G concentrations previously used by Maeda et al. were only 0.01–0.36 mg/ml. The importance of Fe^{2+}, α-ketoglutarate, and ascorbic acid and the lack of importance of ATP, $MgSO_4$, KCl, mentioned above with resting cells, were also observed with cell-free extracts acting on penicillin G. However, DTT did not decrease the activity of extracts on penicillin G, and was included in later experiments to protect the enzyme.

Table 6.2. Substrate specificity of expandase using cell-free extracts

Substrate	*Inhibition zone (mm)*
None	0
Adipyl-6APA	20.0
Ampicillin	17.0
Butyryl-6APA	17.5
Decanoyl-6APA	7.0
Heptanoyl-6APA	16.5
Hexanoyl-6APA	19.5
Nonanoyl-6APA	10.5
Octanoyl-6APA	16.0
Penicillin F	21.0
Penicillin G	29.0
Penicillin V	7.5
Penicillin mX	30.5
Penicillin X	30.5
2-Thiophenylacetyl-6APA	32.0
Valeryl-6APA	15.0

The substrate range of the expandase in cell-free extracts using the new conditions included all 15 penicillins tested. The largest bioassay zones of inhibition were produced by conversion of penicillins G, X, mX, and 2-thiophenylacetyl-6APA, whereas the smallest zones were obtained with decanoyl-6APA and penicillin V.

Early Cessation of the Reaction

As mentioned above, the extent of expansion by cell-free extracts increased with increases in concentration of both protein and substrate. However, in all cases, the concentration of product increased during the first 1-3 hr and then either remained stable or decreased. The extents of bioconversion were low, amounting to 0.61% at 1 mg/ml penicillin G, 0.32% at 2 mg/ml penicillin G, and 0.3 0% at 4 mg/ml penicillin G. To determine if the limiting factor after 2 hr was the exhaustion of one or more components of the reaction mixture, different concentrations and combinations of reaction constituents were added to the reaction tubes at 2 hr, but no additive was able to reactivate the system.

Even when additional extract protein was provided, no reactivation occurred. Only a very small increment in production was observed when both protein and cofactors were added.

Cell-free extracts were preincubated in buffer in the cold or at 30°C for 2 hr to assess the stability of the expandase over time. After 2 hr, the remaining components of the reaction mixture were added and the tubes were incubated under standard conditions for another 3 hr. In all cases, the initial rates were similar to that of the control (no preincubation) and amounts of product obtained were almost equal to the control value. Thus the lack of activity after 2-3 hr could not be attributed to enzyme instability during shaking at 30°C. When Fe^{3+} (as ferric sulfate) was substituted for Fe^{2+} in the reaction, activity was unaffected. Therefore, inactivation was apparently not due to oxidation of Fe^{2+}.

To determine whether one or more reaction mixture components might inactivate the enzyme, the cell-free extract was preincubated for 2 hr in the presence of different reaction components. After this preincubation, the remaining reaction components, including the penicillin G substrate, were added. The amount of product obtained was markedly different, depending on which component was present during preincubation. When buffer alone was present, the subsequent reaction yielded up to 95% of the amount of the product formed in the control reaction. When individual components were present during incubation, production remained between 64% and 85% of control. However, when preincubation was with Fe^{2+} plus ascorbic acid or Fe^{2+} plus α-ketoglutarate, no detectable product was obtained. Thus, a combination of Fe^{2+} with ascorbate or with α-ketoglutarate inactivated the enzyme during preincubation, and evidently did so during the reaction under standard conditions. The same phenomenon was seen with resting cells. As with extracts, inactivation was not merely due to the presence of oxidized Fe^{2+} because when the normal bioconversion reaction was carried out with Fe^{+3} (ferric sulfate) instead of Fe^{2+}, there was no inhibition.

The above studies done on cell-free extracts and resting cells revealed a very low bioconversion yield (based on added penicillin G), i.e., about 0.6%. To examine the dependence of product formation and bioconversion yield on substrate concentration, different concentrations of penicillin G were tested. The concentration of product formed was higher when higher concentrations of penicillin G were used, but the yield based on substrate added dramatically decreased. At 8 mg/ml of penicillin G, bioconversion was about 0.4%; at 2 mg/ml (the standard concentration), the yield was 1.0%; at 0.063 mg/ml, the yield was 9.0%; and at 0.015 mg/ml, the yield reached 16.5%.

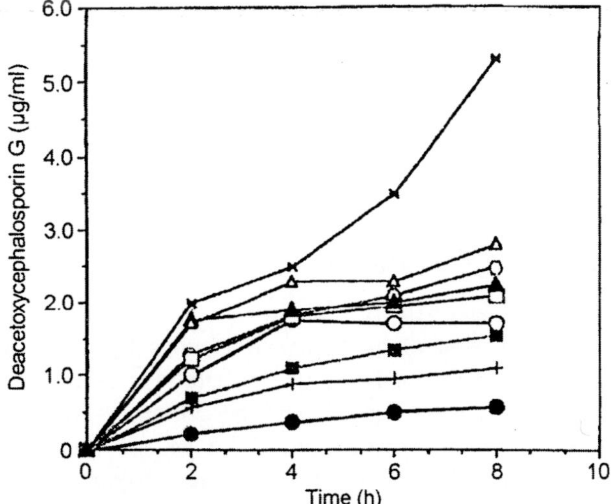

Fig. 6.4. Effect of substrate concentration on product formation.

Inactivation during aerobic incubation with Fe^{2+} plus ascorbic acid and/or α-ketoglutarate might have been due to formation of H_2O_2. As is the case for other α-ketoglutarate-dependent dioxygenases, expandase activity requires a reducing agent in addition to α-ketoglutarate and Fe^{2+}. This requirement can be fulfilled by several substances, although ascorbate is the most effective and is the reducing agent usually used with this type of enzyme. Its function may be that of keeping iron in the reduced form or, perhaps, to protect sulfhydryl groups on the enzyme. However, ascorbate can have adverse effects, since incubation of some enzymes with ascorbate and oxygen leads to rapid loss of enzymatic activity due to the production of H_2O_2 during autooxidation of this reducing agent.

Catalase is known to stimulate the activity of such enzymes, and Lübbe et al. reported this effect with expandase in both *C. acremonium* and *S. clavuligerus* using penicillin N as substrate. However, when 0.5-3 mg/ml of catalase was added to the preincubation mixture with cell-free extract, no protection from inactivation was observed. Nevertheless, when 15 mM H_2O_2 was added to a reaction mixture, activity was markedly reduced. If catalase (2 mg/ml) was also added, the inactivation due to peroxide was reversed, indicating that inactivation normally observed with Fe plus ascorbate was not due, at least exclusively, to formation of H_2O_2.

Fucci et al. described the oxygen-dependent inactivation of several key biosynthetic metabolic enzymes that involve mixed-function oxidation systems. These systems catalyze synthesis of H_2O_2 and reduction of Fe^{3+} to Fe^{2+} followed by oxidation of enzyme-bound Fe^{2+} to generate oxygen radicals (such as hydroxyl radicals or singlet oxygen) that attack a histidine (or other oxidizable amino acids) at the metal-binding site of the enzyme. In a recent study, Golan-Goldhirsh et al. reported that preincubation of different proteins in the presence of ascorbic acid and copper (or iron) led to their inactivation due to the autooxidation of ascorbic acid. In this reaction, four strong oxidant species are formed and, after preincubation, changes in the amino acid composition of all proteins studied were observed. In all of them, there was a major loss of histidine (His183 and His243) and methionine residues which ligate ferrous iron (with Asp185) to give a catalytically active form. Because inactivation of the expandase might be due to the formation of such "*activated oxygen*" species, the effects of different radical scavengers such as mannitol, dimethyl sulfoxide, and thiourea were examined. Participation of OH-radicals was contraindicated by the failure of these free-radical scavengers to prevent the inactivation of cell-free extract when preincubated with Fe^{2+} and ascorbate. Histidine inhibition of inactivation is considered presumptive evidence for a role of singlet oxygen in oxidase-catalyzed reactions. However, when this amino acid was added to the preincubation mixture containing Fe^{2+} and ascorbate, it failed to prevent inactivation. Also examined was the possible involvement of superoxide ion (O_2^- formed by a nonenzymatic reaction between ascorbate and iron) by adding different concentrations of superoxide dismutase (SOD) to the preincubation mixture containing extract, buffer, Fe^2 , ascorbate, and catalase; again no activity was observed after preincubation. Thus, "*activated oxygen*" species appear not to participate in the inactivation of expandase, since free-radical scavengers and SOD added during preincubation failed to protect enzyme activity.

Although DTT is not necessary in the enzymatic conversion of penicillin G, this compound is known to stimulate the expandase activity of frozen crude extracts of *S. clavuligerus* and *C. acremonium* on penicillin N. However, neither this reagent nor â-mercaptoethanol was able to stimulate the subsequent reaction with penicillin G when added during preincubation with $FeSO_4$ and ascorbate.

Effect of Growth in Alcohols

Production of antibiotic compounds by actinomycetes rarely takes place during periods of rapid growth in rich media. Rather, their biosyntheses occur best under conditions of nutrient imbalance, brought about by limitation of the carbon, nitrogen, or phosphorus source, and at low growth rates. In some cases, the expression of the genetic information for antibiotic biosynthesis has been linked to control mechanisms, such as the Pho system, responsible for detecting and adapting cells to available sources of nutrients present in the environment. The discovery of heat shock proteins (GroEL-like proteins), potentially important in antibiotic export and in the assembly of multienzyme complexes for polyketide antibiotic biosynthesis in a variety of streptomycetes, led to the first study of the relationship between non-nutritional stresses, such as heat shock or ethanol treatment, and antibiotic biosynthesis. In that study, jadomycin production was induced by ethanol or heat shock. Thus growth in the presence of alcohols was studied to determine the effect on resting cells of *S. clavuligerus* NP1 with regard to their ability to biotransform penicillin G into cephalosporin-type antibiotics. Cultures grown in control medium MST or MT (MST less starch) formed typical mycelial masses of tangled hyphae. However, in MT supplemented with ethanol, a different morphology was observed, depending on the alcohol concentration in the medium. In 1% ethanol the hyphae were somewhat more dispersed than in control medium, whereas in 2% ethanol the hyphae were extensively fragmented and dispersed.

In the presence of 1% ethanol or 1–2% methanol, growth was slightly less than in MT medium [2.9–3.4 mg/ml dry cell weight (DCW) in alcohol- supplemented cultures versus 3.6 mg/ml in MT]. With 2% ethanol, growth was severely restricted (0.9 mg/ml). Concentrations of alcohol higher that 2% totally inhibited growth. The omission of starch (MT medium) led to a slight increase in specific production of DAOG as compared to cells from MST medium. When MT medium was supplemented with 1% ethanol, there was a marked increase in specific production and a six- to sevenfold increase when 2% ethanol was added; much less of an effect was observed with methanol. Addition of ethanol or methanol at later times during growth (at 2, 6, and 12 hr) did not have any stimulatory effect on the bioconversion. The mechanism of alcohol stimulation of biotransformation of penicillin G to cephalosporins remains unknown, but it could be related to the known ability of ethanol treatment to trigger a heat-shock response. Alternatively, growth in alcohol might yield cells with increased membrane permeability, i.e., they might take up penicillin G or release DAOG more easily. The morphological effects observed when cells were grown in alcohol-supplemented media might reflect the latter mechanism.

Use of Immobilized Cells

For bioprocessing purposes, increase in the stability of biocatalysts is quite often achieved by immobilization of cells or enzymes. This technology is an attractive alternative to the use of expensive free enzymes and cofactors, and can coordinate multistep enzymatic processes into a single operation. Furthermore, fermentative biosynthesis of cephamycin C using immobilized cells of *S. clavuligerus* NRRL 3585 was accomplished by Freeman and Aharonowitz. Jensen et al. reported on the immobilization of β-lactam synthesizing enzymes from the same wild-type culture. None of these early studies used penicillin substrates other than the normal intermediate penicillin N, such as penicillin G.

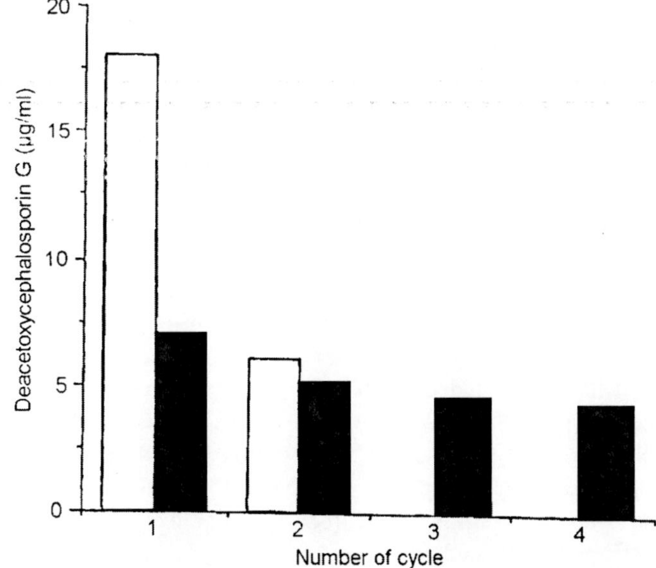

Fig. 6.5. Activity during sequential 2-hr cycles of incubation using free or immobilized cells. Cells were washed between cycles.

The oxidative ring expansion of penicillin G by free and entrapped resting cells of *S. clavuligerus* NP1 was compared, and immobilized cells were found to perform the expandase reaction albeit more slowly and less extensively than free cells. Both types of cells virtually ceased production at 2 hr. Different biomass amounts (2 g, 4 g, 6 g wet weight) were resuspended in 20 ml of polyethyleneimine-barium alginate solution and tested for ring expansion. Increased resting cell concentrations yielded increased product formation; again, the reaction markedly decreased in rate after 2 hr. To examine multiple cycles of ring expansion, free and immobilized resting cells were allowed to carry out oxidative ring expansion for 2 hr, followed by centrifugation in the cold for 5 min. The cells were washed with 50 mM MOPS (pH 6.5) buffer, and recentrifuged. The expandase reaction was again initiated. Two-hour cycles were carried out for up to four times with assays of product formation done at the end of each cycle. The activity of free cells was reduced by about 60% from the first to the second cycle, and was completely lost after the second cycle. In contrast, immobilized cells experienced only a small reduction of activity at each cycle and still had activity through four cycles. Other polymeric matrices such as agarose (4% w/v) and *k*-carrageenan (3% w/v) did not show activity. This may be due to reaction impedance due to strong diffusional limitations. Such external and internal barriers often reduce catalytic efficiency.

The above results demonstrated the capacity of resting cells entrapped in polyethyleneimine-barium alginate to perform repeated oxidative ring expansion of penicillin G to DAOG. Product formation rate was higher with free than with entrapped resting cells, probably due to strong diffusional limitations which prevent the expandase enzyme from binding the substrate and cofactors and/or preventing oxygen transfer to the interior of the beads. With free cells, diffusional limitation and mass transfer problems are less important than with immobilized systems. Similar behavior was reported by Freeman and Aharonowitz, who compared free and immobilized cells of *S. clavuligerus* NRRL 3585 in linear polyacrylamide gels for the fermentative formation of cephamycin C. They observed that free cells produced higher levels of cephamycin C than immobilized cells.

In vivo Construction of Hybrid Expandases by Homeologous Recombination

Homeologous recombination (recombination between partially homologous sequences) has been successfully used to produce novel antibiotics and functional hybrid proteins in *Streptomyces*. If partially homologous sequences are placed in tandem and in the same orientation, general recombination leads to excision of the duplicated genes as well as of the sequences lying between the sites of recombination. Because the *cefE* genes from *S. clavuligerus* and *N. lactamdurans* have a high degree of similarity at the nucleotide (74%) as well as at the amino acid (70%) sequence levels, it was of interest to determine whether recombination could take place at a significant frequency between these genes cloned in the same orientation on a plasmid. If so, hybrid expandases with potentially altered activity/specificity could be generated *in vivo* (Piret, Adrio, and Demain, unpublished data). As described below, chimeric *cefE* genes were obtained by recombination between the *cefE* genes from *S. clavuligerus* and *N. lactamdurans* in both *E. coli* and *Streptomyces* hosts.

Recombination of Expandase Genes in *E. coli*

To test whether recombination between the two *cefE* genes could take place on a plasmid, experiments were conducted in the *recA+ E. coli* strain ER1447. Plasmid pJALC was constructed from pCYB 160 (derived from pCYB1 by F. Feng), which carries the *cefE* gene from *N. lactamdurans*, to which was added a 3-kb *Bam*HI fragment from pULFJ32 containing the *cefE* (and part of *cefD*) gene from *S. clavuligerus* NRRL 3585. Following up to four rounds of growth in liquid culture, plasmid DNA was isolated from *E. coli* ER1447 carrying pJALC, digested with *Bgl*II, dephosphorylated, and used to transform *E. coli* DH5α (*recA*$^-$). Seventeen of the 63 (27%) resulting colonies contained an 8-kb plasmid, the size predicted after excision of the intervening region and one of the duplicated *cefE* genes. Indeed, treatment of these 17 plasmids with *Bgl*II, diagnostic for elimination of the region between the two *cefE* genes in pJALC, gave no digestion. Further restriction analysis revealed two major types of DNA rearrangements in these plasmids. Five of them gave two bands upon digestion with *Pst*I, indicating that both *Pst*I sites in pJALC were still present and that recombination had occurred downstream of the *Pst*I site located in the *N. lactamdurans cefE* gene. All of the remaining 12 plasmids gave a single band when digested with *Pst*I, indicating that one of the original *Pst*I sites had disappeared. Further analysis by restriction digestion showed that the *Pst*I site in the *cefE* gene from *N. lactamdurans* had been eliminated.

To analyze the crossover junctions in *E. coli*, representative recombination plasmids were sequenced and compared with then active *cefE* genes of *N. laciamdurans* and *S. clavuligerus*. In the five clones analyzed which had renamed both *Pst*I sites. recombination had occurred in one of two locations which encode fully conserved sequences of 12 bp in one case and 21 bp in the other. Similarly, in the clones retaining only one *Pst*I site, recombination had taken place in fully conserved sequence stretches of 2, 5, 11, 15, or 17 bp at five different positions within the first 550 bp of the chimeric *cefE* genes. Importantly, all clones analyzed had undergone in-frame recombination events.

Recombination of Expandase Genes in *Streptomyces*

Recombination was attempted in *S. lividans* 1326, a well-characterized laboratory host. To screen rapidly for recombination between the two *cefE* genes, the tyrosinase gene *melC* from *Streptomyces glauscescens* was used as a marker and inserted between the two *cefE* genes. Gene *melC* codes for the formation of the black pigment melanin; thus, screening for colonies containing a putative hybrid *cefE* gene was done by examination of colony color, since recombination should lead to loss of pigment production. A 2.3-kb *Kpn*I fragment from pMEA4 containing the tyrosinase gene from *S. glaucescens* was cloned into pSP73 to yield pJA73T-SP6. A 2.3-kb *Eco*RI-*Hind*III fragment from this plasmid was then ligated with pIJ487 to yield pJA487T. pJA487T was digested with *Bcl*I and the largest fragment (about 3 kb) was purified and ligated into the *Bgl*II site of pJALC to give pJALTC. pJALTC was digested with *Eco*RV and *Nsi*I and the 8.6-kb fragment, containing both *cefE* genes as well as the tyrosinase gene, was purified and inserted into the *Pst*I-*Ecl*136II-digested *S. lividans* vector pIJ680 to create pJA680.

Plasmid isolation from colonies grown on supplemented CG medium showed that all colonies producing a halo of black pigment (designated "B") contained a 12.5-kb plasmid, corresponding to pJA680. The 58 melanin-negative colonies (designated "W") analyzed carried plasmids of different sizes. Of these, 37 (64%) strains contained a 6.3-kb plasmid, the size expected to result from recombination between the two *cefE* genes. Plasmids of 5.8 kb (29%), 4 kb (3.5%), and 8 kb (3.5%), presumably due to unexpected, lower-frequency recombination events, were also found.

Plasmids from strains W21 and W64 (carrying 6.3-kb plasmids), W25 and W76 (8-kb plasmids), and B1 8 (pJA680) were analyzed with several restriction endonucleases. W21 and W64 gave identical restriction patterns and no digestion when treated with *Pst*I or *Xmn*I, meaning that *cefE* from *N. lactamdurans* was partially or fully deleted. Strains W25 and W76 showed no digestion when treated with *Pst*I but were cleaved when incubated with *Xmn*I, *Bam*HI, or *Sca*I, indicating that the *N. lactamdurans cefE* gene was truncated at its 32 end while *S. clavuligerus cefE* apparently remained intact. Sequencing of the hybrid junctions generated in *S. lividans* is now in progress.

Enzymatic Activities of Hybrid Expandases

To study the function of the chimeric *cefE* enzymes generated by recombination in *S. lividans*, the cell-free ring expansion abilities of several recombinants were determined. Three white strains, W21 (6.3-kb plasmid), W25 (8-kb) and W76 (8-kb) as well as the controls B11 and B18 (melanin-positive; pJA680) showed activity, producing inhibition zones in the agar diffusion bioassay. Although *S. clavuligerus* NP1 showed no activity when grown under the same culture conditions as the *S. lividans* strains, typical bioassay results were obtained when NP1 was grown as previously described. To ascertain that the inhibition zones were due to formation of DAOG, the samples were analyzed by HPLC. After 2 hr of incubation, a peak corresponding to DAOG was clearly present on the chromatograms.

Expansion of Adipylpenicillin

Reports on expansion of adipyl-6APA to adipyl-7ADCA in the literature are contradictory. Whereas Baldwin et al. claimed that partially purified extracts from *C. acremonium* were able to expand adipyl-

6APA, others did not observe expansion of this compound using crude extracts, semipurified preparations, or recombinant expandase preparations from *C. acremonium* or *S. clavuligerus*. However, researchers at Panlabs and Merck reported on the expansion of adipyl-6APA to adipyl-7-cephalosporanic acid (adipyl-7ACA) using whole cells. Their work was based on two previous reports which had demonstrated that feeding adipate to *P. chrysogenum* led to production of adipyl-6APA and that DAOC could be produced by *P. chrysogenum* transformants carrying the *S. clavuligerus cefE* (expandase) and *cefD* (epimerase) genes. Fungal plasmids harboring either the *S. clavuligerus cefE* (expandase) gene, the *C. acremonium cefEF* (expandase/hydroxylase) gene, or the fungal *cefEF* and *cefG* (acetyltransferase) genes were used to transform a high-titer penicillin-producing strain of *P. chrysogenum*. Transformants were grown in media containing adipic acid (1.7% disodium adipate) as side-chain precursor. When adipate was fed to the untransformed *P. chrysogenum* parent strain, adipyl-6APA was produced at 47% of the penicillin V titer produced by this strain when phenoxyacetate was used as sidechain precursor. One transformant (containing the bacterial expandase) produced up to 14% adipyl-6APA (relative to penicillin V titer) and 17% adipyl-7ADCA. Another recombinant clone containing the eukaryotic expandase/hydroxylase produced 15% adipyl-6APA, 2.6% adipyl-7ADCA, and 6.7% adipyl-7-aminodeacetylcephalosporanic acid. A third clone expressing the fungal expandase/hydroxylase and acetyltranferase activities was able to produce low amounts of adipyl-7ACA. The important cephalosporin intermediates, 7ADCA and 7ACA, were obtained by removing the adipyl side chain using a purified glutaryl acylase derived from a *Pseudomonas* strain.

Based on the work described by Crawford et al., researchers at Gist- Brocades transformed *P. chrysogenum* with plasmids containing either the *N. lactamdurans* or *S. clavuligerus cefE* genes under control of different promoters such as *penDE*, *pcbC*, and *gpdA* from *Aspergillus nidulans*. Transformants were grown in media containing adipate (0.5% v/v). Results showed that both expandases were active in *P. chrysogenum* and the highest adipyl-7-ADCA titers were obtained when the *pcbC* promoter was used. When other side-chain precursors were fed into fermentation media, transformants carrying the *cefE* gene from *S. clavuligerus* were able to incorporate these compounds into the corresponding cephalosporanic acids. The titers obtained (relative to the titer obtained with adipate) were 29.6% for carboxymethylpropionic acid, 25.1% for thiodipropionic acid, and 6.2% for phenylacetic acid.

The *cefE* genes from some cephalosporin-producing bacteria (*S. clavuligerus*, *N. lactamdurans*, *L. lactamgenus*) and the *cefEF* gene of *C. acremonium* have been cloned, sequenced, and expressed. All showed similar sizes, homology (ranging from 54 to 74%), and different locations in the cephalosporin gene clusters. The expandases, encoded by those genes, exhibited the properties of α-ketoglutarate-dependent dioxygenases and, in all cases, the presence of α-ketoglutarate, Fe^{2+}, and molecular oxygen was essential for their catalytic activity. All showed a high specificity for the nature of the side chain of the penicillin substrate and only penicillin N, the natural substrate, was expanded under the conditions employed. Success with resting cells acting on penicillin G allowed Cho et al. to demonstrate the ring expansion of penicillin G. By increasing the concentration of the substrate (penicillin G), cosubstrate (α-ketoglutarate), the chief cofactor, (Fe^{2+}), and cells, the conversion of penicillin G to DAOG was improved. Using such improved conditions, activity with cell-free extracts was also demonstrated on 14 other penicillins.

Incubation of *S. clavuligerus* cell-free extracts in the presence of $FeSO_4$ and either ascorbate or α-ketoglutarate for 2 hr led to elimination of subsequent expansion activity. It is clear that further work will have to be done to understand and overcome this intriguing case of inactivation. Growth of *S. clavuligerus* NP1 in the presence of ethanol resulted in an increase in DAOG production from penicillin G by resting cells. The mycelium produced in alcohol-supplemented medium was fragmented and dispersed as compared with growth in control (starch) medium.

The reaction of resting cells with penicillin G was rapid only for 1 hr and then proceeded at a very low rate. Preincubation of resting cells for 2 hr in buffer alone or with individual reaction components had only minor effects, whereas preincubation in the presence of combinations of Fe^{2+} and ascorbic acid or Fe^{2+} with α-ketoglutaric acid virtually eliminated activity. Similar results were obtained using cell-free extracts. The reaction yielded less than 1% conversion of added penicillin G. However, conversion yields as high as 16.5% were obtained by reducing the concentration of penicillin G. Immobilized cells of *S. clavuligerus* NP1, entrapped on a polymeric matrix, were able to perform oxidative ring expansion of penicillin G into DAOG. Cells entrapped in polyethyleneimine barium alginate (1.5%) were able to sustain activity for at least four 2-hr cycles, whereas free resting cells were inactive after the second cycle.

Homeologous recombination (recombination between partially homologous sequences) was used to produce novel, functional expandase enzymes (*in vivo*) which are hybrids of the *S. clavuligerus* and *N. lactamdurans* proteins. DNA sequencing of hybrids obtained in *E. coli* showed that recombination had occurred at several locations displaying conserved sequences as short as 2 bp. Hybrid genes obtained in a *Streptomyces* background produced expandases with altered activity on penicillin G, as confirmed by HPLC analysis. Additional novel bioprocesses for production of the cephalosporin intermediates 7ACA or 7ADCA have been developed. One process is based on a *P. chrysogenum* strain containing the expandase gene of *S. clavuligerus* or *N. lactamdurans*, or the expandase-hydroxylase gene of *C. acremonium*. The second involves the addition to the fermentation medium of adipic acid leading to the formation of adipylpenicillin, which is used as a substrate by the expandase to yield adipyl-7-cephalosporanic acids, including adipyl-7ADCA and adipyl-7ACA. Removal of the adipyl side chain is then carried out with a glutaryl acylase.

7

Plant-made Pharmaceutical Products

The future of pharmaceutical drugs in the United States is likely that of continuing economic growth, as there is increasing use of pharmaceutical drugs in the general population, with an estimated 43% of Americans using at least one pharmaceutical drug between 1999 and 2000. This fact, in conjunction with an aging population needing and demanding more and cheaper pharmaceutical drugs, with an average of 30 filled prescriptions for non-institutionalized Medicare enrollees aged 65 and older, suggests a need for alternative approaches to traditional "*vat-based*" mammalian cell-based production. Although such production approaches as animal-based "*pharming*" are promising, among the most promising of approaches is that of Plant-Made Pharmaceuticals (PMPs). These PMPs use genetically engineered plants, a technology used for over 20 years, to express substances that may be used to treat and cure such diseases as cancer, Alzheimer's, diabetes, HIV, heart disease, and others. By using naturally occurring processes in the plant, along with the ability to scale up production quickly, PMPs are a promising technology. However, as with any new technology, the potential pitfalls are plentiful, chief among which are the perceptions of the public, which is largely unaware of this technology, and whose perceptions place it on a threshold of acceptance or rejection, making it a "*boundary technology*".

PMPs may be considered a boundary technology for a variety of reasons. First, it is a subset of a relatively new technology, that of genetically engineered plants. As a result of its newness, risks from genetic engineering of plants are not well characterized. Although recent events suggest the potential risks, and the current inadequacy of the regulatory system to either prevent or respond to crises, from genetically engineered plants have not been tangibly experienced by the average American. Instead of actual events, characterized risks tend to exist as either extrapolations from laboratory experiments or as hypothetical events. Although laboratory experiments do provide a good deal of insight into the mechanisms by which events may occur, they do not replicate the reality of the fields in which PMPs may be grown with the field's dynamic, nonlinear, complex systems affected by multiple interacting factors such as weather, soil, cropping systems, chemical usage, and so on. Hypotheticals about PMPs tend to be extreme in nature and politically charged, with Cassandras of doom preaching worst-case scenarios and Candides of optimism trumpeting the best possible future. Neither perspective, however, appreciates the probabilistic nature of risk.

Here, risk is defined as hazard multiplied by exposure. And, in the words of Howard and Donnelly, "(I)n order for the risk to be zero, either the exposure or the hazard must be zero" , which, of course, is unlikely if not impossible, especially considering increased sensitivity of detection methods and understanding of the effect of different substances on different individuals. A second reason to consider PMPs as a boundary technology is that they promise to radically change public perceptions by drawing attention to the changed character of the plants themselves. It is here that hypothetical scenarios concerning PMPs make their mark, leading to acceptance or rejection of this technology. Although genetically engineered plants are currently a pervasive part of the agricultural landscape and consumed extensively, with the staple crops of corn and soybean grown in genetically engineered variants in the United States and comprising 45% and 85% of total acreage in 2004, respectively, there is little public awareness of their presence in the food supply, which is mainly a result of them being genetically engineered to express agronomic qualities, such as herbicide tolerance and pest resistance, which are typically not brought to the attention of the public. Although plants have long been used for medicinal purposes and food can have healing properties, genetically engineered plants, especially dealing with food crops, will likely draw public attention by underlining the transgenic nature of the products that span species and may even incorporate human DNA. Some precedent in public response to genetic engineering may be seen in "*second-g. neration*" food products with enhanced product quality, which, although offering useful characteristics, have yet to be economically successful.

The final reason PMPs may be considered a boundary technology derives from the previous reason. PMPs may be recognized as both a food and a medicinal application of genetic engineering. Although it is highly unlikely that the same plant will be processed for both food and pharmaceutical purposes, it is quite likely the public will perceive them as a unified technology. In terms of public response to date, there have been quite different paths in the reception of genetically engineered pharmaceuticals and medical products and that of genetically engineered plants. There has been little controversy over genetically engineered pharmaceutical products, likely because people are willing to accept risk when it comes to recovering the health they have lost, whereas people are likely to be risk averse when it comes to changing their diet, especially when they perceive nothing wrong with it. By exhibiting both characteristics, PMPs are likely to arouse ambiguity in response, depending on the personal salience of particular pharmaceutical products being developed.

Considering these reasons, this chapter will explore PMPs and their potential with an eye toward public response and policy actions. In this chapter, we first consider potential benefits of new products moving toward the market, such as enhanced access and decreased price. We next look at the risks of this boundary technology, especially adventitious presence in which PMPs might accidentally enter the food supply, which is illustrated by recounting three recent events in which the food chain was either breached or threatened by unapproved food products. We then consider public opinion toward PMPs, both in response to these incidents, as seen in comments to Federal Register changes, and through a regional survey of public opinion. Finally, we consider the federal regulations currently in place and recent political developments before drawing conclusions.

Benefits Offered by Plant-Made Pharmaceuticals (PMPs)

The benefits of PMPs have been well characterized and documented by proponents of this technology. Indeed, much of the research and development of this technology is driven by optimism that PMPs will have tremendous health benefits for an aging and growing population and the potential for economic gain, especially when compared with current production approaches. This outlook is bolstered by awareness of the sheer size of the pharmaceutical drug market. Of this market, an increasing proportion builds on genetic engineering.

According to Elbehri, three factors commend PMPs over current approaches to express pharmaceuticals, such as bacteria, yeast, and mammalian cells, and more recent technologies, such as insect cells and transgenic animals. These three factors are cost advantage, production scalability, and safety. The cost advantage of PMPs over the current use of mammalian cell cultures is great, with mammalian cell bioreactors ranging from $106–650 per gram of antibody, whereas PMPs would likely cost four to five times less for the same pharmaceutical.

The second factor is the capacity to more easily scale-up production than is currently the case with mammalian cell-based systems, which is based on the ability to increase production by growing more plants on added acreage in a short period of time, avoiding the need to build more production facilities with buildings, vats, and other associated capital costs. However, this benefit is offset by production being driven by growing seasons and the ability of plants to reproduce seeds enough to scale-up production. In other words, pharmaceuticals will be produced on the basis of an agricultural cycle, with the inherent difficulties of predicting weather, pest outbreaks, and other factors that influence natural systems. Although storage may not prove problematic, especially if the pharmaceutical is expressed in the seed (which might not be the case), predicting market demand is yet another difficult factor. Another difficulty with scaling up lies with enforcing regulatory controls. Expanding production acreage implies increased potential for inadvertent movement of the PMPs' genes, whether by cross-breeding with other plants or their being blown into neighboring fields, bringing with it legal liabilities for environmental and health damage if they occur. Therefore, expanded acreage implies expanded implementation of safeguards and increased surveillance.

The third and final factor is the belief that PMPs are safer than using proteins from recombinant microorganisms or cells, which is because "PMPs do not carry potentially harmful human or animal viruses into the drug", as plants do not serve as hosts for such human pathogens as HIV, prions, hepatitis, and so on. Furthermore, plants are typically constructed to express a portion of a pathogen or toxin, reducing possible infection or innate toxicity. This, however, does not alleviate concerns over potential allergenicity, which will be present in most pharmaceuticals.

In spite of the benefits offered, PMP development is still in its infancy, with retardation of its progress caused by reasons discussed in the next section. However, analysis of U.S. Department of Agriculture (USDA) data concerning release permits for "pharmaceuticals, industrial, and value-added proteins" over the last two years, during which time stricter regulatory standards were enforced, suggests a still-fertile field of research. Overall, 35 permits were applied for during 2004 and 2005, with permit applications increasing from 15 in 2004 to 20 in 2005, of which nearly 70% were granted and 60% were released into the fields.

Institutions doing research in PMPs tend to be dominated by small research companies. Although research universities, mainly Iowa State University (four applications) and the University of Kentucky and Washington State University (one application apiece), are involved in research, companies such as SemBioSys Genetics and Ventria (seven applications apiece), Planet Biotechnology and Prodigene (four applications), Large Scale Biology and Chlorogen, Inc. (three applications), and Garst (one application) are the mainstays of research currently being sent to the fields.

The five plants serving as hosts for the experimental activities reflect research realities. Tobacco is the preferred host, having nearly one third of the permit applications, reflecting its long-time use as a research plant in genetic engineering. Although corn has long history of experimentation and being used extensively in the field, and, as a result, is the second most popular plant for experimentation, the change in regulations in response to critiques of the regulatory system, and fears of it entering the food supply, has led to its reduced relevance in 2005, where only two university-based field trials were proposed, compared with its more extensive use (seven applications) in 2004. The remaining plants, safflower (seven applications), rice (six applications), and barley (two applications), might prove to be the preferred future host plants for PMPs and industrial products.

Examples of products being developed include Ventria BioScience's work on human recombinant lactoferrin and lysozyme, which may be used as an oral rehydration solution; SemBioSys has been developing PMP-based human insulin (to meet the needs of an increasing population of diabetics) and human APO IP, which reduces and stabilizes arterial plaque associated with "*acute coronary syndrome*" such as heart attacks and angina, as well as strokes; Planet Biotechnology's treatments of tooth decay by bacterial infection, hair loss through specific forms of chemotherapy, and treatment for the common cold by blocking infection by rhinovirus are likewise promising. Prodigene has brought to market recombinant trypsin, normally produced by the pancreas, which may be used in the production of insulin, human and veterinary vaccines, cell cultures, and wound care. It has also developed a vaccine targeting swine transmissible gastroenteritis. Finally, Chlorogen is developing a "*chloroplast transformation technology*" that would introduce genes into plants, allowing large-scale production without potential genetic transfer through pollen. These products and others promise increased product availability and a range of new products, with health benefits and economic growth implied.

Although the future of PMPs may, like any technology, be difficult to predict, the experimental activity concerning these plants appears to be relatively robust considering recent regulatory changes and increased public skepticism. Although the amount of permit applications are relatively small, especially compared with the sheer numbers of experimentation involving genetically engineered plants, PMPs and associated technologies appear to be growing in importance and in the fields. And given the benefits they offer in the production of new pharmaceutical drugs, this growth can be expected.

Threats Posed by Plant-made Pharmaceuticals (PMPs)

In spite of the benefits specifically offered by PMPs, and by genetically engineered plants generally, apprehension exists over their release into the environment. According to the National Research Council report "Bioconfinement of Genetically Engineered Organisms", three concerns exist over the unintentional movement of genes placed into target plants. The first is that the inserted genes will lead to the target plant or relatives cross-breeding and becoming weeds by obtaining benefits that enable it to overrun or disrupt ecosystems. The second concern is that wild relatives, especially those with economic, social, or moral values, will be at risk of extinction by either being outcompeted or through hybridization with genetically engineered plants. The third concern, that the genetic material will spread to other domesticated varieties, is perhaps one of the highest profile concerns for PMPs, especially when considering that many PMPs are currently being expressed in food plants. Although these concerns are currently being researched and will likely continue to pose a threat as genetically engineered plants dominate the commodity agriculture landscape, no evidence of these concerns coming to fruition have come to light to date.

Another major concern, if not the major concern, is that PMPs will somehow find their way into the food supply. As a result, it is feared the public will respond with decreased institutional trust and will make market decisions that negatively affect food producers. As a result, recent changes to the regulatory structure concerning agricultural biotechnology are occurring because of concerns "that the expansion in agricultural biotechnology increasingly will put pressure on seed production and commodity handling systems" to segregate and control its products. Specifically, concerns exist that the current regulatory scheme is not able to adequately address the amount and variety of new genetically engineered plants, with PMPs chief among them. Doubts over the agricultural biotechnology regulatory system have been raised by three recent events, calling into question the scientific basis for regulation, the effectiveness of regulatory enforcement, and the integrity of the food system.

StarLink Bt Corn

The first major event of focus national attention on the potential violability of the U.S. food chain occurred when StarLink corn made its way into the human food supply in 1999 and 2000. StarLink corn used the Cry9c variant of *Bacillus thuringiensis* (Bt), a protein that kills targeted insects by eating through their guts, leading to sepsis and the inability to digest food. StarLink corn was not deemed fit for either human consumption or export because of presumed possible human allergic reactions. As a result, it was to be used only for animal feed or nonfood industrial purposes.

In September and October of 2000, attention was drawn to the presence of StarLink corn in the food chain when the consumer group Genetically Engineered Foods Alert performed tests on taco shells and other corn-based products being sold in grocery stores and in fast food restaurants. Estimates by the USDA's Economic Research Service suggest 123.8 million bushels were co-mingled in 2000, whereas Aventis', the company responsible for StarLink, estimates that over 430 million bushels were co-mingled in 1999 and 2000 with an estimated 340,908 acres in 28 states planted with StarLink Bt corn. Overall, a total of nearly 300 products were recalled, including 70 types of corn chips, 80 types of taco shells, and almost 100 restaurant food products.

In an attempt to minimize economic loss and public concern, Aventis and USDA bought back existing grain supplies and recalled food containing StarLink corn. However, significant damage was done. In addition to illustrating the failure of the U.S. regulatory system concerning genetically engineered plants, there was disruption of the downstream food manufacturing marketplace with corn exports being affected. Indeed, within a single year, of 110,000 grain tests by federal inspectors, StarLink corn showed up in one-tenth. Although the complexity of market forces allows only estimation, a significant decrease in trade with Japan and South Korea occurred immediately after StarLink corn was found. Since then, the European Union has required labeling and tracing requirements for genetically engineered goods that are seen as greatly hindering U.S. farm product competitiveness, especially with respect to corn and soybean products. Overall, estimates suggest the StarLink event and the recall in its aftermath have cost the food industry $1 billion.

Prodigene PMP Corn

The second event, that of Prodigene's PMP corn, is one immediately relevant for PMP production. In September and October of 2002, in Iowa and Nebraska respectively, APHIS found "volunteer" corn plants genetically engineered to produce a pharmaceutical to prevent "traveler's diarrhea" growing in soybean fields in violation of permit conditions. Specifically, Prodigene did not abide by the conditions of their field release permit to eradicate all traces of the experimental crop from the fields, as small quantities of this corn ended up in soybean that was to be processed and sold for human consumption.

Although none of this corn made it into the food supply, this near miss drew attention to the regulatory system's lack of readiness in dealing with the next generation of genetically engineered crops, those producing pharmaceutical and industrial products. Prodigene had to pay a civil penalty of $250,000; destroy 500,000 bushels, or $2.7 million dollars worth, of soybean in Nebraska; and incinerate 155 acres of corn in Iowa because of concern that cross-pollination occurred, as well as posting a $1 million bond and accede to higher compliance standards for future field tests. Perhaps more important in terms of long-term political implications, the Grocery Manufacturers of America (GMA) and other food processing interest groups expressed concern over PMP field test regulations, with John R, Cady, CEO of the National Food Processors Association commenting "(it is) nothing short of alarming to know that at the earliest stages of development of crops for plant-made pharmaceuticals, the most basic preventative measures were not faithfully observed. This apparent violation of rules... very nearly placed the integrity of the food supply in jeopardy".

Syngenta Bt Corn

The third and most recent event came to light in March 2005 when the seed company Syngenta revealed that it had accidentally sold approximately 146,000 tons of experimental Bt-10 corn that had been approved for experimental use only by USDA but was grown on 37,000 acres over a four-year period (2001-2004). The antibiotic marker gene is often used in the experimental phase of many genetically engineered plant studies to test for the presence or absence of altered genetics. Although the fact that the Syngenta Bt-10 corn inadvertently entered the food chain raises questions about the effectiveness of the USDA regulatory system, especially after regulatory changes were put in place in response to the StarLink and Prodigene situations, the antibiotic marker gene entering the food supply has raised concern because of perceived problems with increased antibiotic resistance with human infections. Although many other factors contribute to antibiotic resistance, including their extensive use in farm animals, concern over the use of antibiotics in genetically engineered crops date back to the earliest days of genetically engineering when, in 1990, Calgene asked for an opinion concerning their use from FDA, and it was found that there was reasonable certainty no harm would result from its use. However, since that time, concerns are still being raised concerning their near ubiquitous use, whether in genetically engineered plants or in farm animals.

Although Syngenta officials argue that the release was relatively small, affecting 0.01% of all corn grown from 2001 to 2004, and has not appeared to affect U.S. consumers, response from abroad suggests that U.S. producers will be affected in the export marketplace. Specifically, on April 15, 2006, the European Union placed a temporary ban on U.S. corn imports unless they are proven to be Syngenta Bt-10-free; on May 25, 2006, they enforced this ban by impounding a U.S. shipment of corn gluten upon its arrival in Ireland when it was found to be tainted with Bt-10. Likewise, in South Korea, imports of U.S. corn are being investigated with certification of future shipments as Bt-10-free required for entry, while most recently, a shipment of corn to Japan found to be Bt-10-contaminated was found and held. As a result, Syngenta has been fined $375,000 and ordered to sponsor a compliance training conference by USDA. However, the regulatory response appears to be subdued at best, especially in light of previous failures by biotechnology companies to implement federal regulations.

According to the 1984 Coordinated Framework for the Regulation of Biotechnology, USDA, EPA, and FDA are responsible for regulating agricultural biotechnology. Although this framework has proved to be serviceable for most of its existence, recent events suggest it is not meeting the challenges posed by the increased volume and variety of genetically engineered crops. The instances discussed above illustrate some of the problems facing U.S. regulators, especially the reduced trust in institutions. However, what is most important for producers is that an inefficient and ineffective regulatory system might push consumers elsewhere.

Although critics argue that the above cases show the system is working by identifying flaws in the regulatory system and changing practices of both government agencies and industry, in the end, consumer trust is what matters most. Although lost consumer trust in domestic markets is a threat, with StarLink-tainted products being recalled from grocer's shelves in 2000, long-lasting effects in the U.S. market have not materialized, especially when the recent Syngenta Bt-10 corn case is considered. International trade disruption, however, has occurred in both StarLink and Syngenta cases and has been costly in terms of trade with the European Union and with Asian trade partners South Korea and Japan. Perhaps most important, trust in the U.S. regulatory system by our trade partners is waning, with a recent editorial title concerning the Syngenta case in the respected science journal *Nature* underscoring diminishing respect: "Don't rely on Uncle Sam".

Public Response to Plant-Made Pharmaceuticals (PMPs)

Public response to PMPs suggests they are of two minds concerning PMPs. On the one hand, PMPs promise to offer tangible benefits that directly enhance the quality of life by producing less expensive pharmaceutical drugs that may treat a broader range of ailments. This perspective is bolstered in a recent PEW report that showed a strong relationship between perception of PMPs as being a good use of genetic engineering and the likelihood of it having a positive impact on the respondent's family.

On the other hand, the risks of PMPs entering the food supply or remaining in the environment as weeds gives pause to critics of the technology. The StarLink and Syngenta Bt-10 cases stand out as examples of the regulatory and food systems' failure to prevent the unwanted presence of genetically engineered crops in the food supply. Although the Prodigene case was a near miss, it also focused attention on the flaws in the regulatory system and may have had a chilling effect on the development of both PMPs and PMIPs. Although these three cases reflect "growing pains" in regulating the technology as more plant products with a greater variety of uses enter the fields, the question remains as to whether this problem will be endemic or a "mere blip" that has been dealt with and will not recur.

Interested Public/Pressure Group Comments

The amount of comments in response to the 2003 Federal Register notices dealing with changes to the regulation of PMPs and PMIPs, which in turn are arguably in response to the Starlink and Prodigene incidents discussed in the previous section, reflect the new-found importance of the field release of genetically engineered plants to the public. The March 10, 2003 Federal Register notice concerning PMP and PMIP field testing requirements attracted at least 847 comments (of which 77 were late). In comparison, changes to the APHIS regulations in 1993 garnered 84 comments, whereas even more wide-ranging regulatory changes in 1997 attracted only 30 comments.

Although the numbers of comments received in response to PMP regulatory changes are exponentially higher than those received in response to prior Federal Register notices, multiple factors are responsible. E-government with electronic dockets easing comments on Federal rule-making has expanded public participation, especially with salient issues. For example, proposed organic standards posted in the Federal Register received an unprecedented 275,000 comments. Here, although the usual policy actors interested in genetically engineered plants are still involved, a high percentage of comments were sent by individuals and organizations not normally associated with this debate. As expected, support for the new technology came from biotechnology and biotechnology-related companies, agricultural organizations, state agricultural departments, universities, and agricultural sector pressure groups. Critiques were also received from those who appeared to have ties with the organic movement or environmental groups, as evidenced by the roughly 600 comments e-mailed as cut-and-paste forwards.

Unexpectedly, especially in comparison with previous regulatory changes, concerns were raised by other powerful groups. Namely, the GMA and affiliated groups expressed concern over uncontained field release of PMPs and PMIPs, especially in food and feed plants. Interestingly enough, concern by consumer groups and traditional biotechnology opponents was tempered, likely mitigated by the potential for medical benefits from this new technology.

Comments by the interested public in response to the changes to PMP regulations give insight into concerns the general public may have once their awareness of these new technologies are raised, especially if PMPs and PMIPs enter into widespread production. A few themes stand out when comments of those critiquing the proposed USDA regulations are analyzed. The first theme concerns the science used and its effectiveness in regulating the threats posed by PMPs and PMIPs to the food supply and the environment. The next two themes expand on institutional distrust suggesting that governmental institutions, namely USDA, are either negligent, showing disregard for American farmers and the public by allowing these "dangerous" plants to be grown, or have been captured by corporate interests and are doing their bidding despite the threat posed. The risk perceptions of those commenting on the regulations suggest this technology is unknown, unnatural, uncontrolled, and likely to end in disasters disproportionately affecting future generations. As can be expected by the foregoing responses, PMPs and PMIPs engender a good deal of fear and anger, emotional responses we deal with more systematically in the next section.

Public Opinion Concerning PMPs

Although the general public's opinion on PMPs is best analyzed through surveys, little research on their opinion has been carried out in the United States. In Canada, Einsiedel and Medlock carried out a series of focus groups analyzing attitudes toward PMPs and industrial products after providing information on plant molecular farming generally and five specific examples of this technology. Findings by them suggest greater support for novel medical products benefiting human health or the environment. Risk perceptions were driven by concerns over contamination of the food supply or the environment with higher risk seen as deriving from these products being grown outdoors in food plants that are able to go to seed or that flower, thus dispersing their genetic material to food plants that might be consumed by humans. When risk-benefit analyses were made, Einsiedel and Medlock found "acceptability is predicated on the idea that there are stringent approval processes and long-term measures in place to ensure safety".

One exception to the lack of systematic public opinion research on PMPs is a study carried out by Stewart and McLean using a telephone survey examining consumers living in Arkansas, Louisiana, Texas, Oklahoma, and New Mexico. This study was conducted between May 9 and June 10, 2004 by the Arkansas State University Center for Social Research using computer-assisted telephone interviewing (CATI) technology and had a very good response rate (a total of 680 interviews completed for a response rate of 61% and a margin of error of +/-3.5%).

Five questions were asked of participants and ascertained personal benefits, likelihood of PMPs entering the U.S. food supply, the likelihood of respondents eating food from PMPs, how worried the respondents would be if they ate food with PMPs in it, and how angry they would be if they ate it without their knowledge. PMPs were characterized as "plants genetically modified to produce pharmaceutical drugs. These are plants that are modified to produce compounds used in manufacturing vaccines for diarrhea, antibodies to fight cancer, and drugs to treat such illnesses as cystic fibrosis."

Findings suggest the respondents have mixed feelings about PMPs. Generally speaking, PMPs are seen as presenting personal benefits to respondents, with two-thirds seeing either "a great deal" or "some benefit". Of these, a plurality (36.5%) see a great deal of benefit for themselves, whereas only 12% see themselves as receiving no benefit at all from PMP-based products. Finally, only 12% had no opinion about PMPs.

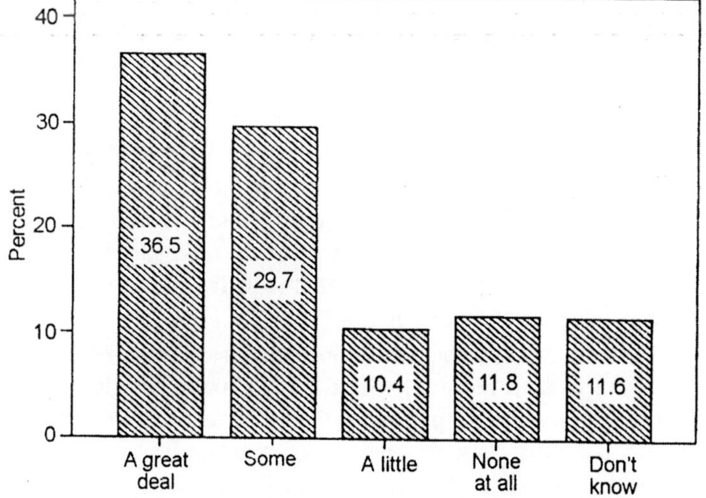

Fig. 7.1. How much benefit would you get from PMP GM plants?

Although respondents see benefits from PMPs, a majority see adventitious presence as likely to occur, with nearly 60% perceiving PMPs as accidentally entering the U.S. food supply. Only one fourth of respondents see this event as either "somewhat" or "very unlikely" to occur. Whether this pattern of response is because of the Starlink or Prodigene controversies discussed earlier in this chapter, because of a lack of faith in governmental and food production institutions to prevent this event from occurring, or the result of some other unspecified factor is not known; it may be assumed, however, that a relatively high level of public skepticism exists.

Although respondents see themselves as less likely to eat food with PMP components than see the potential for adventitious presence, those seeing it as either "very" or "somewhat likely" make up a substantial proportion of respondents, with a combined 45%. At the same time, 38% perceive themselves as able to avoid such foods, responding to the question that they are either "somewhat" or "very unlikely" to eat food coming from PMP plants.

Emotional response to eating food with PMPs in it suggests survey respondents are at least somewhat worried about the potential for it to occur. Overall, 23% are "very worried" and 13% are "quite a bit worried" about this event occurring. However, an increasing proportion of respondents show lesser levels of concern, with 16% "moderately worried," 19% "slightly worried," and 21% "not at all worried." Although levels of concern are not as high as can be expected, great potential exists for upsetting the public. The pattern of response suggests polarized opinions. Specifically, one-third of respondents state they would be "very angry" if they ate food with PMPs in it without their knowledge, whereas only one-fifth of respondents would be "not at all angry."

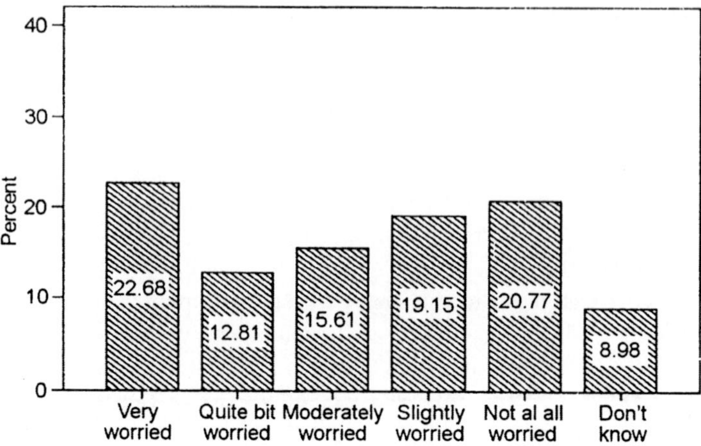

Fig. 7.2. How worried would you be if you ate food from PMP GM plants?

Conclusions

Research available concerning public attitudes towards PMPs emphasizes it's "boundary technology" nature. Great promise and great risk are inherent in PMPs because of the personal benefits of increased access to a wider array of pharmaceutical drugs balanced by their potential for accidental release into the food supply or the environment. These ambivalent feelings are likely to persist until either the benefits of PMPs are felt by their products entering the marketplace or an environmental or health catastrophe involving these products occurs. In either case, the absence of awareness of PMPs (and even genetically engineered plants) is a driving issue.

Regulation of Plant-made Pharmaceuticals (PMPs) in the Fields

The regulation of PMPs will establish a different, potentially more circuitous, path to the marketplace because of its "*boundary technology*" nature. Although, as a pharmaceutical, it will be regulated in a traditional manner by FDA, as a plant, it must adhere to standards set forth by USDA. As a genetically engineered plant, it triggers a set of regulations specific to this technology as a whole, and as a PMP specifically, as discussed below.

On the whole, the regulation of agricultural biotechnology has attracted relatively little public involvement until recently, which is most likely because of its highly technical nature and the downstream nature of most of its products, which have predominantly been concerned with replacing or reducing production inputs such as herbicides and pesticides. More recently, the promise of new products and dearth of experienced difficulties in the field experiments have led to relaxed regulations. However, recent events detailed above have publicized and politicized the regulation of agricultural biotechnology with stricter regulations and greater scrutiny by an expanding range of parties with economic and political clout.

To address the decreasing trust in the regulatory structure, the Office of Science and Technology Policy (OSTP) published "Proposed Federal Actions To Update Field Test Requirements for Biotechnology Derived Plants and To Establish Early Food Safety Assessments for New Proteins Produced by Such Plants" in August 2002. Specifically, the notice was published to provide guidance to USDA, EPA, and FDA to update field testing requirements for food and feed crop plants and establish early food safety assessments for new plant proteins, most specifically PMPs and PMIPs, in line with the 1986 Coordinated Framework. Three principles in the document are relied on in updating the Coordinated Framework: (1) The level of field test confinement should be consistent with the level of environmental, human, and animal health risk associated with the introduced proteins and trait(s); (2) if a trait or protein presents an unacceptable or undetermined risk, field test confinement requirements would be rigorous enough to restrict outcrossing or comingling of seed and, further, the occurrence of these gene or gene products from these field tests would be prohibited in commercial seed, commodities, and processed food and feed; and (3) even if these traits or proteins do not present a health or environmental risk, field test requirements should still minimize the occurrence of outcrossing and comingling of seed, although low levels of genes and gene products could be found acceptable based on meeting applicable regulatory standards.

In light of concerns raised by increased experimentation with PMPs and PMIPs, and addressed by OSTP in their notice, USDA's Animal and Plant Health Inspection Service (APHIS) changed rules concerning their field testing of PMPs in March 2003. Although the resulting regulations are expected to be modified further over the coming years, they currently incorporate significant changes in how PMPs and PMIPs are regulated. Specifically, for all plants genetically engineered to produce pharmaceutical or industrial compounds and field tested under permit, APHIS established seven conditions that can be grouped into three categories. The first considers field test siting, the second the dedication of equipment and facilities to their production, and the third considers procedural matters.

Field test siting regulations proposed by APHIS provide two conditions to be met, with special consideration for pharmaceutical corn. First, the perimeter fallow zone will be increased from 25 feet to 50 feet to prevent inadvertent comingling with plants to be used for food or feed. Second, production of food and feed plants at the field test site and perimeter fallow zone will be restricted for the following season to prevent inadvertent harvesting. Furthermore, specific permit conditions for pharmaceutical corn have been instituted, likely a result of corn being the organism of choice until the Prodigene event drew public concern and regulatory changes were put in place in its wake.

A second theme concerns the dedication of farm equipment and facilities to the production of such crops. First, APHIS requires planters and harvesters to be dedicated to the test site for the duration of the tests, and although tractors and tillage attachments do not have to be dedicated, they have to be cleaned in accordance with APHIS protocols. The equipment and regulated articles must be stored in dedicated facilities for the field test's duration.

The final three requirements from the proposed rules concern procedural aspects of dealing with field tests of PMPs and plants producing industrial compounds. First, APHIS requires submission of cleaning procedures to minimize risk of seed movement. Second, procedures for seed cleaning and drying are required to be submitted and approved to confine plant material and minimize risk of seed loss or spillage. Finally, permittees will be required to implement an APHIS-approved training program to successfully comply with the stated permit conditions.

A key factor in any regulatory arrangement is the ability to ensure that those regulated are complying with the requirements set forth. As a result of the potentially contentious nature of PMPs and plant-produced industrial compounds, APHIS plans to increase the number of field site inspections "to correspond with critical times relevant to the confinement measures". Therefore, in addition to maintaining records of activities related to meeting permitting conditions, and increasing the likelihood of auditing them to verify required permit conditions were met, APHIS might inspect permitted field tests up to five times during the growing season: once at pre-planting to evaluate the site location, once at the planting stage to verify site coordinates and adequate cleaning of planting equipment, at midseason to verify reproduction isolation protocols and distances, at harvest to verify cleaning of equipment and their appropriate storage, and again at postharvest to verify cleanup of the field site. In addition, two post-harvest inspections may occur to verify that the regulated articles do not persist in the environment. Finally, APHIS may inspect more frequently if deemed necessary. As a result of the potential for both PMPs and PMIPs entering into the food supply, and using the PMP regulatory changes as a starting point, APHIS took immediate action to remove the notification track option, requiring complete permit track review in their recent interim rule and request for comments.

The rationale given in the interim rule and request for comments was that although 14 field releases (9 notifications, 5 permits) had been carried out to date, the type of genetic engineering being carried out was to enhance such nutritional components as oil content. However, recent genetic modifications have been for "non-food traits with which APHIS has little regulatory experience or scientific familiarity". As such, the definition of PMIPs has three criteria: (1) the plants produce compounds new to the plant; (2) this compound has not normally been used in food or feed; and (3) the compound is being expressed for non-food/feed purposes.

An administrative reorganization of how USDA-APHIS regulates biotechnology created the Biotechnology Regulatory Services (BRS) to address concerns raised by PMPs and PMIPs specifically and genetically engineered organisms generally. According to USDA-APHIS, "Given the growing scope and complexity of biotechnology, now more than ever, APHIS recognizes the need for more safeguards and greater transparency of the regulatory process to ensure that all those involved in the field testing of GE crops understand and adhere to the regulations set forth by BRS."

Changes instituted by BRS include new training for APHIS inspectors in auditing and inspections of field trials, the use of new technologies such as global positioning systems, and analysis of historical trends to inform monitoring and inspection. According to APHIS, there are nine overarching goals that the changes will serve with key components being: (1) enhanced and increased inspections in which risk-based criteria, along with other factors, will be used to assess field test sites with higher-risk sites being inspected at least once a year, with other sites being randomly selected for yearly inspections; (2) auditing and verification of records of businesses and organizations to verify accuracy and implementation; (3) remedial measures to protect "agriculture, the food supply, and the environment in the event of compliance infraction" with the establishment of a "*first-responder*" group to deal with serious infractions; (4) standardized infraction resolution in which criteria will be established to determine the extent of an infraction and the response, whether further investigation, the issuance of a guidance letter, the issuance of a written warning, or referral to APHIS' Investigative and Enforcement Services (IES) unit for further action; (5) documentation, in which a database will be set up to track field test inspections and resulting compliance infractions, and transparency to keep stakeholders and the public informed on the regulatory decision- making process; (6) continuous process improvements where, as the science of biotechnology advances, so too will regulations and permit conditions to allow safe field testing; (7) an emergency response protocol, being developed with input from EPA and FDA, in which a quick response plan will be put in place "to counteract potential impacts on agriculture, the food supply, and the environment"; (8) training for field test inspectors in their dealings with PMP and PMIP field test sites, as well as the latest in auditing; and (9) certification concerning compliance with the highest level of auditing standards.

Although the reorganization can be seen as streamlining and focusing enforcement efforts, the potential for unduly high levels of workload stresses placed on this 26-member unit can be foreseen. First, BRS draws on APHIS inspectors to inspect field tests; however, more than 2600 of these agriculture quarantine inspectors have been transferred to the Department of Homeland Security. The current agreement between USDA-APHIS and DHS allows for continued access by APHIS and BRS, although it can be expected that problems might occur as a result of split responsibilities and duties. Implementation considerations are still an issue. Although thousands of field tests have been carried out in a variety of sites through the USDA-APHIS field permitting, notification, and petitioning program, these tend to be short-term tests, typically lasting for one growing season and collecting limited data that considers the ecological effect. Little work has been done in the way of long-term effects on the ecology of the regions in which they are sited.

Also, although genetically engineered plants have been in the fields for at least a decade, in the case of herbicide-tolerant and pest-resistant plants, their management has left something to be desired with large numbers of farmers not following federal regulatory standards. Although USDA states that of the 7402 field tests carried out between 1990 and 2001 and regulated by APHIS, only 115 resulted in compliance infractions and, for the most part, these were relatively minor infractions that did not raise public concern, concerns still exist. However, regarding PMPs, because of the regulations concerning them and the potential for controversy, it is likely that the regulations will be more stringently followed. The "*boundary technology*" nature of PMPs places it firmly into limbo in terms of social acceptability and, ultimately, economic viability. In terms of benefits, the opportunities afforded by this subset of genetic engineering of plants are in terms of increased diversity of products, reduced production costs, scalability on relatively short notice, and reduced potential for health risks of toxicity and pathogenicity because of less-easily crossed species barriers.

The risks of unintentional movement of genes into other plants or the entry of PMP products into the food supply, however unrealized to date, loom large. These threats are especially salient in light of likely scaling up of plantings of PMPs and greater diversity of PMP products. And when current regulatory difficulties are taken into account, it is an especially daunting challenge. Although the potential benefits of PMPs are large and the risks may be perceived as negligible, even if such products enter the food supply as feared, public opinion looms large in whether this boundary technology is accepted. Given that most Americans are not aware of their current consumption of genetically engineered foods and the extent of their market presence, PMPs entering the food supply would likely be their first "real" exposure to the risks of genetically engineered plants. The resulting response—apathy, hysteria, or somewhere in between—would have an extremely large impact on the future of PMPs and their growth, which is not to discount the effect of other factors that may hasten or retard the development of PMPs. Economic climate, government policies and regulations, international trade, and a slew of other factors will impact the future of PMPs. What remains is the question of how far and how fast this technology will develop.

8

Preservation of Pharmaceutical Products

Microbial spoilage of pharmaceutical products has been known for many years. Spoilage may result in the deterioration of the product due to loss of potency or to the initiation of an infection in the user. Sterile pharmaceutical products (single dose or multiple dose forms) require the addition of an antimicrobial preservative when they have been manufactured under aseptic conditions from presterilized ingredients. Where the products are subject to a terminal sterilization process, only the multiple dose category requires the addition of an antimicrobial agent. In the latter instance, the preservative is added to protect the product and end user against the consequences of microbial entry during use. Chemical antimicrobial agents are thus added to all multidose sterile formulations and to aqueous and aqueous-based non-sterile pharmaceuticals. Their function is to reduce the microbial load to a level, which is safe for the designated use of the product, and to maintain the numbers of viable microorganisms at or below that value for the storage and use life of the product. Preservatives must, therefore, be stable within the formulation for the shelf life of the product and be capable of dealing with all the abuses made to it by the consumer and user (i.e., contamination during use, incorrect storage etc).

For multidose sterile products, the preservative must be capable of reestablishing sterility between each use, whereas for a non-sterile topical cosmetic the function of the preservative might simply be to prevent growth. The associated toxicity of preservatives often limits the concentrations at which they can be employed; thus, lower concentrations are generally employed for opthalmic products and injectables. In choosing a preservative the likely capacity required, the rate of killing desired, and the ingredients and pH of the formulation must be borne in mind. The BP (1988) test for the "Efficacy of Preservatives in Pharmaceuticals" makes it quite clear that a preservative must in the first instance kill microorganisms and only accepts later that it will prevent growth. However, it does insist that there must be no outgrowth of the test organism, that is, the preservative possesses sufficient residual capacity to inhibit the growth of any survivors.

Definition of Terms

Disinfectants, antiseptics, and preservatives are chemicals that have the ability to destroy or inhibit the growth of microorganisms, and are used for this purpose. These and other terms commonly employed are defined as follows:

1. *Disinfectants*: Chemical agents or formulations that are too irritant or toxic on body surfaces, but are used to reduce the level of microorganisms from the surface of inanimate objects to one that is safe for a defined purpose.

2. *Antiseptics*: Chemical agents or formulations that can be used as an antimicrobial agents on body surfaces.
3. *Preservatives*: Chemical agents or formulations that are capable of reducing the number of viable microorganisms within an object or field to a level that is safe for its designated use and will maintain the numbers of viable microorganisms at or below a level for the use/shelf-life of the product.
4. *Bacteriostasis*: A state in which the growth of microorganisms is halted or inhibited.
5. *Bactericide*: A chemical antimicrobial agent that reduces the viability of a population of microorganisms exposed to it. This term is meaningless without specifying the concentration range over which this effect is obtained; such concentration ranges will vary between different species of microorganisms.
6. *Bacteriostat*: A chemical antimicrobial agent that can prevent the growth of microorganisms within an otherwise nutritious environment. This term is meaningless without specifying the concentration at which this effect is achieved. Bacteriostatic concentrations do vary between different species of microorganisms.

It should be noted that terms such as bactericide and bacteriostat should be discouraged in the USP and EP, the term "*antimicrobial agent*" has replaced these terms.

Preservative Ideals

At present there is no perfect preservative, and all materials are a compromise of a number of often contrary properties. The following are the properties of an ideal preservative compound and need to be considered when choosing a preservative.

1. *Definable in chemical terms*: Many of the existing preservatives, such as the quaternary ammonium compounds, are mixtures of various homologues. Often the activity obtained is a function of the mixture composition. Unless it is possible to define and control mixture composition, the performance of the agents will be variable, even if they conform to a pharmacopoeial specification.
2. *Broad spectrum of activity*: The compounds must possess a broad spectrum of antimicrobial activity against all species of microorganisms and also toward bacterial endospores. In practice, the only compounds that meet this requirement are formaldehyde, gluteraldehyde, hypochlorite, and ethylene oxide. All these compounds are highly irritant at sterilizing concentrations to be used in pharmaceutical products. Formaldehyde is, however, used at low concentrations in some shampoos; in these cases contact with the skin is short-lived and irritancy minimal. Agents such as quaternary ammonium compounds, phenolics, and the parabens group possess good activity against gram-positive bacteria but little or no activity toward spores. Certain gram-negative organisms such a *Pseudomonas aeruginosa* are virtually resistant to these agents. Generally, antifungal activity is difficult to obtain. Combinations of preservatives are sometimes employed to widen the spectrum of activity to include molds, bacteria, yeasts, and endospores.
3. *Effectiveness*: The compounds must be effective over a wide range of pH in order to be effective in all formulations. In practice, compounds are generally more active at either acid or alkaline pH. Thus, the pH of a formulation determines the types of preservative suitable for inclusion.
4. *Stablitity:* The compounds must be stable to light and elevated temperatures for the expected shelf life of the product. The effects of pH upon stability should be minimal. In this respect it is worth noting that the preservative Bronopol is stable only in the dark and at an acid pH. Under alkaline conditions are in the light it rapidly decomposes to give formaldehyde at concentrations that would be ineffective as a preservative. Instability to light can be protected against the packaging in a light-proof container. Storage tests must be performed on all formulations to ensure that adequate levels of preservative remain at the end of then expected shelf life of the product.

5. *Solubility*: Preservatives should ideally be used at concentrations much lower than that of the main constituents of the formulation. Their solubility ought to be such that it is possible to add them as a concentrated solution and where there is no danger of creating a saturated solution.
6. *Aesthetics*: Preservatives should have no perceptible odor, color, or taste, which might affect the aesthetic qualities of the final product. This can be of crucial importance for a cosmetic product but is less important for medical ones.
7. *Volatility*: Preservatives should be non-volatile. Thus, chloroform is not an ideal preservative as it is lost from the formulation each time it is exposed to air.
8. *Product incompatibility*: Preservatives should not be incompatible with any of the likely excipients within the product formulation. This would include incompatibilities with the container material and also the active ingredients. In practice this is very difficult to achieve.
9. *Toxicity*: At the concentrations employed, the preservative should be non-irritant, not cause hypersensitivity reactions, and be non-toxic. In this respect, the site of application is critical. Relatively few compounds are approved for use in opthalmic products due to their high sensitivity towards xenobiotics. Also, compounds safe for use on intact skin might be hazardous for inclusion in parenteral products.
10. *Solubility in oil*: Preservatives must not be too oil soluble as this can produce problems in two- and three-phase systems where the preservative accumulates in the oil and micellar phases and is unavailable for antimicrobial action in the biological (aqueous) phase. It is worth noting that the oil: water partition coefficient can alter as a function of pH and also as a function of the nature of the oil.
11. *Cost*: The preservative must be cost-effective in the context of the overall product positioning (i.e., cost of goods ratio).

Although a very large number of antimicrobial compounds have been examined for their suitability for preservation of pharmaceuticals, only a few (<20) are currently used in the majority of pharmaceutical products. Moreover, in many cases, the "least unsuitable" rather than the "optimum" preservative is selected for a particular product.

Dynamics of Preservation

The critical lethal parameters of the effectiveness of antimicrobial agents are the concentrations of the agents employed, the time of exposure, the types and numbers of organisms exposed, the pH of the environment or formulation, and the temperature of application. An understanding of the effects of these conditions upon the killing process and of the terms that describe such dependence is important to rationalize the use of preservatives in different situations and formulations.

Time of Contact

When exposed to lethal concentrations of a chemical antimicrobial agent, the viability of a bacterial population decreases exponentially with time. Such pseudo-first-order kinetics can be described by the equation

$$\frac{S}{S_0} = Ae^{-kt} \quad \ldots(1)$$

$$\log\frac{S}{S_0} = kt + \log A \quad \ldots(2)$$

where k is the rate constant, S is the number of surviving organisms at time t, and S_0 is the initial number of viable organisms within the population.

D-value is the time for 90% kill. That is,

$$\log S - \log S_0 = -1 \qquad \ldots(3)$$

and

$$D\text{-value} = 1/k \qquad \ldots(4)$$

In practice, such obedience to first-order kinetics is rare for chemical inactivation. More commonly, deviations from first-order kinetics are obtained, when there is either an initial lag in the rate of killing or when the rate of killing decreases with time of exposure. The former is commonly observed when the concentrations of preservative are minimally bactericidal and reflects the time required for injuries caused to the bacterial cells to assume lethal proportions. Such plateauing therefore decreases as concentrations of agent employed become greater and are inapparent at very high concentrations. The second effect reflects the presence of resistant organisms within the population, capacity effects on the action of the preservative, or failure of the neutralizer. In such cases commonly observed with quaternary ammonium compounds and biguanides, the levels of kill at the plateau value increase with increasing concentration of preservative. From these relationships, an estimate of the initial rate of killing (k) or the D-value (actual time to effect a 90% reduction in viability) can be made, but their predictive value must be questioned.

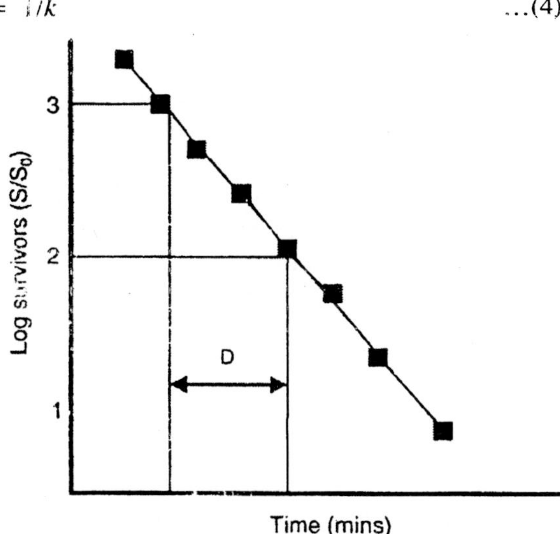

Fig. 8.1. Time survival kinetics for the inactivation of a bacterial population by treatment with a chemical agent. The D-value represents the time taken, at a given concentration of biocide, to reduce the surviving population by 90%.

Approximation to first-order kinetics implies that the sensitivity toward preservatives of a population of microorganisms is normally distributed. Decreases in the rate of killing with time often results from adsorptive loss of the preservative onto and into the killed cells, causing a decrease in the available concentration of the preservative for killing the surviving organisms. The susceptibility of preservatives to such adsorptive losses is described as its capacity.

Exponential decreases in viability with time mean that total elimination of all living cells cannot be guaranteed. Rather, knowing the initial size of the population and its susceptibility, the probability of having achieved sterility might be assigned to particular inactivation processes. Such assignments assume, often wrongly, that first-order kinetics are universally applicable.

Concentration of Preservatives

The efficacy of an antimicrobial agent varies as a direct function of its concentration. At very low concentrations the antimicrobial effect might be negligible, at intermediate concentrations the effects might be growth-inhibitory, whereas only at relatively high concentrations might they be bactericidal. Often different mechanisms of action are involved to bring about these different effects. For example, chlorhexidene inhibits growth through direct effects upon respiratory enzymes and ATP synthesis, but kills through causing gross permeability changes to the bacterial cell envelope. The minimum growth inhibitory concentration (MIC) of an agent gives little or no information about its bactericidal activity, but might indicate weaknesses in the overall antimicrobial spectrum of activity. Minimum lethal concentrations can range from 2 × MIC – 20 × MIC, dependent upon the antimicrobial substance and target organism. In the bactericidal range, the concentration exponent (η) describes the dependence of activity on concentration. This can be obtained as the slope of a graph of log D or k versus log concentration. Although these values vary slightly among organisms, they are fairly characteristic of compound groups and also often relate to mammalian toxicity. Thus, compounds with high concentration exponents more readily lose their biological activity when diluted upon parenteral administration than those with low exponents.

The concentration exponent gives no indication as to the level of activity of a particular agent, It only indicates the degree of dependence of activity upon concentration. If the $\log_{10}$ of a death time is plotted against the $\log_{10}$ of the concentration, a straight line is usually obtained, the slope of which is the concentration exponent. Given the D-value for a single concentration and concentration exponent, it is possible to calculate the activity at any other concentration. As different antimicrobial mechanisms are often involved ingrowth inhibition and killing, the use of concentration exponents to extrapolate MIC data to bactericidal situations should be avoided.

$$(\eta) = \frac{\log D \text{ at } C_2 - \log D \text{ at } C_1)}{\log C_1 - \log C_2} \qquad \text{...(5)}$$

The value of the concentration exponent also gives an indication of the susceptibility of the agent to inactivation by dilution and/or losses in activity through adsorption of the agent on organic debris or killed bacterial cells. The loss of an antimicrobial agent from solution in this manner relates to concentration in solution and absorptivity rather than to the inherent antimicrobial activity of the agent. The activity and concentration exponents of four hypothetical agents are described. Agents A & B and C & D have similar concentration exponents but different activities, whereas A & C and B & D have similar activities yet different concentration exponents. If isotoxic concentrations of each agent (equivalent D-value) are employed, and undergo a uniform drop in concentration through adsorption, the compounds with the higher activity will undergo the greatest loss of activity (A & C > B & D). For compounds of similar activity, the one with the higher concentration exponent will have the greatest activity loss (A > C and B > D). This can be generalized in the statement that capacity is inversely related to both the concentration exponent and activity. Preservatives used in sterile products generally have high concentration exponents and high activity. Such considerations are also helpful in determining inactivation conditions for the preservatives prior to sterility and preservative effectiveness tests.

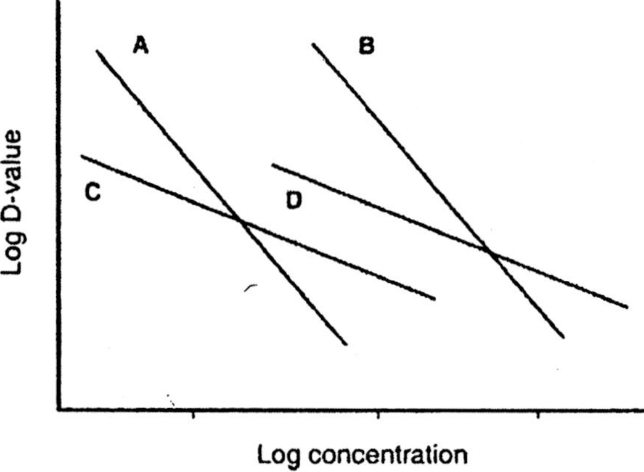

Fig. 8.2. Comparisons of the activity and concentration exponents of four hypothetical preservatives.

Temperature Effects

The rate of killing of an antimicrobial agent is directly dependent on the temperature of the interaction. This dependence is described by the temperature coefficient (Q or θ), which can be determined either from the slope of the graph relating the D-value or K and temperature, or from Eq. (6).

$$\text{Temp. Coefficient } [\theta_{t_1-t_2}] = \frac{D\text{ - value } t_2 (D_2)}{D\text{ - value } t_1 (D_1)} = \frac{kt_1}{kt_2} \qquad \text{...(6)}$$

The subscripts denote the temperature range over which the change in activity is defined. This is commonly given as the coefficient per 10°C rise (i.e., θ_{10} or Q_{10}), but is sometimes quoted for 1°C and 25°C changes. Although the temperature coefficients vary a little between organisms, they are characteristic for particular preservative groups. A high θ_{10} value renders a compound suitable for application at elevated temperatures but unsuitable for the preservation of formulations that might be stored over a wide temperature range. It should be noted that the temperature will also affect the degree of ionization in some circumstances; therefore, the concentration exponent for some compounds will be apparently affected by temperature.

Effect of pH

The degree of ionization of acidic and basic antimicrobial agents depends on pH. Some compounds are active only in the unionized state (e.g., phenolics) whereas others are preferentially active as either the anion or cation. It therefore follows that the activity of a particular concentration of an agent will be enhanced at a pH that favors the formation of the active species. Thus, cationic antibacterials such as acridines and quaternary ammonium compounds are more active under alkaline conditions. Conversely, phenols and benzoic acid are more active in an acid medium. Chlorbutol is less active above pH 5 and unstable above pH 6. Phenylmercuric nitrate is only active at above pH 6 whereas thiomersal is more active under acid conditions. The sporicidal activity of glutaraldehyde is considerably enhanced under alkaline conditions whereas hypochlorites are virtually ineffective at above pH 8.

Knowledge of the pK_a of a preservative allows the calculation of the fraction undissociated at any particular pH and hence (via the concentration exponent) the level of activity at that pH.

$$\text{Fraction of undissociated biocide} = \frac{1}{1} + \text{antilog}\,(\text{pH} - \text{pK}_a) \qquad \ldots(7)$$

The pH also affects activity by altering the net surface charge on the microorganisms. Thus, as pH is decreased, the surface becomes less negative and adsorption and thereby activity of cationic agents is reduced. These effects are greater for gram-negative than gram-positive bacteria.

Presence of Interfering Substances

In most instances, before an antibacterial agent can act on a cell, they must first combine. The presence of other materials, commonly referred to as organic matter, may reduce the effect of such an agent by adsorbing or inactivating it and thus reducing the amount available for combining with target cells. Extraneous matter may be able to form a protective coat around the cell, thereby preventing the penetration of the active agent to its site of action.

Preservation Interactions

Until the late 1930s, cosmetic and pharmaceutical formulations were stabilized with soaps. Although preservatives were often required, spoilage was only rarely a problem. With the advent of new materials for emulsion stabilization, preservation of the systems, or the lack of it, became a major problem. Nowadays we are aware of apparent incompatibilities between the new excipients and the established preservative agents and of the many interactions that can lead to preservative failure. No all-embracing set of rules have emerged to enable the "correct" preservative to be chosen for each formulation; only general guidelines exist.

The simplest form of interaction is one of adsorption/ adsorption of the preservative from the formulation into and onto container and excipients. In this respect, it is convenient to divide these into colloidal excipients, suspensions, metal ions, and polymers.

Colloids

1. *Gums*: Tragacanth, acacia, and plant polysaccharides such as agar and alginates are generally anionic in nature and will adsorb cationic preservatives such as chlorbutol, benzalkonium chloride, substituted phenols, phenylmercuric acetate, and merthiolates. Generally the adsorptive process increases with

the increase in concentration of the gum or polysaccharide. Colloidal solutions of tragacanth and acacia. but not agar or alginates. can often be preserved with cationic agents by increasing the concentration of the preservative to saturate the colloid. For preservatives such as parabens, the problem is exacerbated at alkaline pH when the preservative becomes fully ionized.

2. *Starches*: These bind substituted phenols but this can be overcome by increasing the concentration of the phenolic. Gelatin shows a slight interaction with the parabens group.
3. *Proteins*: These interact both with cationic and anionic preservatives depending on to the pH of the formulation and the net charge of the protein.
4. *Non-ionic surfactants*: Interactions with a range of preservatives are unpredictable. Cationic and anionic surfactants interact and are contraindicated with anionic and cationic preservatives respectively.
5. *Polyethylene glycols*: These interact particularly with the phenolic group of preservatives. The interaction increases with increase in molecular weight of the polymer. With increasing temperature, the extent of binding increases due to thermal desolving of the polymer and the creation of further binding sites.

Suspending Agents

These include clays, bentonite, kaolin, and talcs. They are generally anionic in nature and interact with most cationic agents. Inactivation depends on the pH of the system. Preservatives are only loosely associated with clays and therefore, desorb on dilution. The extent of these interactions are difficult to predict.

Container Materials

Nylon strongly adsorbs phenols and sorbic acid by covalent linkage. The degree of interaction depends on the pH, nature of the solvent, temperature, contact time, surface area, preservative concentration, and thickness of the nylon.

Acrylates and polyethylene affect most preservatives, including organic mercurials, phenolics, and benzoic acids. Leaching of hydroxyl ions from glass raises the pH and indirectly affects preservative activity. In this respect, glass must pass a "*limit-test*" for alkalinity.

Changing the container of a product from glass to plastic can alter its preservation. The container is as much a part of the formulation as is the product that is placed in it. Equally, adsorption and absorption into rubber closures can be significant, as exemplified by the phenolics.

Preservation of Two-phase Systems

When preservatives are added to two-phase oil-water systems, depending upon the hydrophilicity of the agent, they partition between the two phases. Bacteria will only grow within the aqueous phase or at the oil- water interface. Thus, preservative lost to the oil is unavailable for antibacterial action. Hence the concentration in the water phase is reduced, affecting the rate of kill, but the capacity of the system is unaffected as preservative lost by adsorption onto organic debris and bacteria is replaced from that held in the oil.

The distribution between the oil and water phases is easily predicted from the oil-water partition coefficient, K^0_w

$$K^0_w = \frac{\text{Concentration in oil}}{\text{Concentration in water}} \quad \ldots(8)$$

By knowing the concentration of preservative required for the necessary biological effect in the aqueous phase (C_w), the oil: water phase ratio (θ) and the K^0_w for the system, C, the concentration needed in the formulation, may be calculated from the expression

$$C_W = \frac{C(\theta+1)}{K_W^{0\,\theta+1}} \qquad \ldots(9)$$

It is also worth noting that altering the nature of the oil can affect partition coefficients quite dramatically, for example, the differences between vegetable and mineral oils.

If the preservative favors the oil, increasing the oil: water ratio dramatically decreases available concentration; if it favors the aqueous phase, the reverse occurs and can cause solubility problems. Unfortunately, both temperature and pH also affect K^0_W, in addition to the effects of pH directly on the activity of the preservative.

Preservation of Three-phase Systems

Most oil–water systems contain surfactants as emulgens in order to provide a stable emulsion. Some preservatives may associate directly with the surfactants whereas others may partition into the micellar phase of the surfactant, treating it as a third phase for partitioning. These effects can be calculated to some extent, where C_W depends not only on K^0_W but also on surfactant concentration. Initially it is assumed that the surfactant micelles form part of the aqueous phase. Thus, if K^0_W is the oil : aqueous phase partition coefficient and C_A the total aqueous concentration, then, as in Eq. (9),

$$C_A = \frac{C(\theta+1)}{K_A^{0\,\theta+1}} \qquad \ldots(10)$$

Now

$$C_W = \frac{C_A}{R}$$

where

$$R = C_A/C_W \text{ that is } C_A = RC_W$$

As

$$K^0_W = C_A/C_W \text{ and } C_0 = K^0_W C_W$$

substitution in Eq. (9) gives

$$C_A^W = \frac{C(\theta+1)}{C_0/C_A^{\theta+1}} \qquad \ldots(11)$$

and substituting once again for C_0,

$$C_A = \frac{C(\theta+1)}{\left(K_W^0 \frac{C_W}{C_A\theta}\right)+1} \qquad \ldots(12)$$

Substituting in Eq. (12) for $C_A = RC_W$ gives

$$RC_W = \frac{C(\theta+1)}{\left(K_W^0 C_W/RC_W\theta\right)+1} \qquad \ldots(13)$$

which then reduces to

$$C_W = \frac{C(\theta+1)}{[K_W^0\theta + R]} \qquad \ldots(14)$$

Eq. (14) allows the active concentration in the water phase to be calculated from C, the phase ratio (θ), K^0_W and R. This is useful as K^0_A varies with the concentration of the surfactant. R can be found from a graph relating C_A/C_W and surfactant concentration, where the slope of the line is k.

$$R = 1 + k \text{ [surfactant concentration]}$$

All preservative manufacturers provide values of k for a range of surfactants.

Toxicity and Safety Considerations

There are certain limitations on the use of antimicrobial preservatives based on their toxicity and potential side effects. The British Pharmacopeia recommends that the maximum quantity of an injection containing an antimicrobial preservative to be administered at a single occasion is 15 ml. The USP, on the other hand, recommends a maximum of 5 ml. These maximum volumes must be considered when toxicity data and concentrations of the agents included in the formulations are considered. The final concentration of any substance employed is a balance between its potential toxicity and antimicrobial activity. Additionally, because meninges are readily irritated, the inclusion of antimicrobial preservatives in any formulation that might gain access to the cerebrospinal fluid is precluded. Intracardiac and intraarterial injections must also not contain an antimicrobial preservative.

It is not surprising that preservatives sometimes prove toxic to humans. To assess the toxicity of any substance, it is necessary to know its acute and cumulative toxicity together with its "no effects levels" and also to be aware of its mutagenic, teratogenic, and carcinogenic potential. In addition, its local actions as well as its liability to cause hypersensitization might be important. Any new preservative must be subjected to a battery of such mandatory tests to provide these data as must a new application of an established biocide.

Acute Toxicity

Preservatives, for the most part, are used at very low concentrations and the question of their acute toxicity rarely arises. The margin of safety is not always very high, however.

Subacute and Chronic Toxicity

When substances are given repeatedly, manifestations of toxicity may differ, particularly if the compound is given at a rate faster than what the individual can detoxify or excrete. Some preservatives contain mercury and this may accumulate in the body.

Reproductive Toxicity

As part of the general safety testing of all preservatives, consideration is give to possible effects in higher animals on the fertility of either sex, the gestation or postnatal care, and development of the embryo. No direct causal relationships have been shown between any of the commonly used preservatives and. reproductive toxicity. However, indirect reproductive toxicity has been suggested, for example, benzoic acid as a preservative, increases blood salicylate levels, and may cause a significant increase in the teratogenic potential of aspirin. Organic mercury has been shown to be responsible for acongenital form of Minimata disease, but not at levels likely to be taken into the body through mercury-containing preservatives.

Carcinogenicity and Mutagenicity

Several preservatives have been scrutinized for being possible carcinogens, and their use regulated (e.g., chloroform and formaldehyde). Another possibility is that the preservative interacts with amines or amides to form carcinogenic nitrosamines. Published data on the mutagenicity of preservatives is limited as tests such as the Ames test can only be carried out at concentrations far less than those employed.

Preservative Combinations

The ideal properties expected from preservatives are not met by any of the current, established agents. All chemical agents have their limitations in terms of their antimicrobial activity, resistance to organic matter, stability, incompatibility, irritancy, or toxicity. It is also unlikely that new preservatives will be developed because of high costs of putting a new compound through toxicity tests and the likelihood of a new compound being impossible to cover by patent. More likely preservative combinations will be employed in the future, possibly to give synergistic combinations (e.g., hydrogen peroxide and peroxygen compounds, chlorhexidine and cetrimide). In this manner, preservative combinations may be used to extend the range and spectrum of preservation; for example, by combining a series of alkyl esters of 4-hydroxybenzoic acid, water solubility is decreased to such an extent that both the aqueous and oil phase of an emulsion are protected.

When acting simultaneously on a microbial population, combinations of preservatives may cause an increased, decreased or unchanged antimicrobial response when compared with their summed individual effects. A minimum requirement of any combination should be that it achieves at least the same level of protection overall as the individual components do. Ill-considered preservative combinations may lead to inclusion of irrelevant agents. In general, agents from the same chemical group or those having the same mode of action are likely to produce merely additive effects whereas those exhibiting different mechanisms or sites of action may serve either to reinforce (synergize) or reduce (antagonize) their individual activities. Such effects may be evaluated by preparing mixtures of the two preservatives being investigated and determining their growth inhibitory power by an MIC determination.

In general, synergistic effects can occur through three different mechanisms. The first mechanism is by inhibition of inactivation. Here, one compound increases the effective concentration of the other by inhibiting the microbial system responsible for its inactivation. To date, however, there are no reported observations of this mechanism with preservatives. The second synergistic mechanism is very common amongst preservatives and occurs when one compound increases the accessibility of targets to another. This usually occurs when one agent exerts its action by increasing the permeability of the cell wall or cell membrane. Besides damaging the cell in its own right, this can permit access (or increased access) of the second compound to targets that were previously concealed. An example of this type of synergy is seen in the cooperative action between benzalkonium chloride and thiomersal which disrupts the cytoplasmic membrane, thereby facilitating access of organomercurial agents that react with sulphydryl-containing enzymes in the cytoplasm. This type of synergy does not necessary require both compounds to possess significant antimicrobial activity. Finally, perhaps the broadest category of synergistic interactions is that in which two compounds act simultaneously at different targets, thereby significantly influencing the biochemistry of the cell. Although these targets must be different in order to produce synergy, they can be closely related. For example, the synergy between chlorocresol and 2-phenylethanol is thought to be through their respective effects on the generation and coupling of a proton gradient to active transport.

There are many significant practical benefits and advantages of preservative combinations. These include an increased spectrum of activity; the need for lower concentrations of each of the individual components, thereby possibly reducing potential toxicity; the prevention of resistance to individual preservatives; possible enhancement of antimicrobial activity beyond that expected by simple addition; an extended time course of preservation achieved by combining a labile, markedly biocidal preservative with a stable longer-acting ingredient. Furthermore, careful selection of individual agents for combination, based on their physicochemical properties, may serve to overcome microbiological problems created by the physical limitations of individual preservatives. In this respect, factors affecting preservative efficacy must be carefully considered.

9

Product Analysis

All pharmaceutical finished products undergo rigorous QC testing in order to confirm their conformance to predetermined specifications. Potency testing is of obvious importance, ensuring that the drug will be efficacious when administered to the patient. A prominent aspect of safety testing entails analysis of product for the presence of various potential contaminants.

The range and complexity of analytical testing undertaken for recombinant biopharmaceuticals far outweighs that undertaken with regard to 'traditional' pharmaceuticals manufactured by organic synthesis. Not only are proteins (or additional biopharmaceuticals such as nucleic acids) much larger and more structurally complex than traditional low molecular mass drugs, their production in biological systems renders the range of potential contaminants far broader. Recent advances in analytical techniques render practical the routine analysis of complex biopharmaceutical products. An overview of the range of finished-product tests of recombinant protein biopharmaceuticals is outlined below. Explanation of the theoretical basis underpinning these analytical methodologies is not undertaken, as this would considerably broaden the scope of the text.

Table 9.1 The range and medical significance of potential impurities present in biopharmaceutical products destined for parenteral administration

Impurity	*Medical consequence*
Microorganisms	Potential establishment of a severe microbial infection - septicaemia
Viral particles	Potential establishment of a severe viral infection
Pyrogenic substances	Fever response that, in serious cases, culminates in death
DNA	Significance is unclear - could bring about an immunological response
Contaminating proteins	Immunological reactions. Potential adverse effects if the contaminant exhibits an unwanted biological activity

Protein-Based Contaminants

Most of the chromatographic steps undertaken during downstream processing are specifically included to separate the protein of interest from additional contaminant proteins. This task is not an insubstantial one, particularly if the recombinant protein is expressed intracellularly.

In addition to protein impurities emanating directly from the source material, other proteins may be introduced during upstream or downstream processing. For example, animal cell culture media are typically supplemented with bovine serum/foetal calf serum (2–25 per cent), or with a defined cocktail of various regulatory proteins required to maintain and stimulate growth of these cells. Downstream processing of intracellular microbial proteins often requires the addition of endonuleases to the cell homogenate to degrade the large quantity of DNA liberated upon cellular disruption. (DNA promotes increased solution viscosity, rendering processing difficult. Viscosity, being a function of the DNA's molecular mass, is reduced upon nuclease treatment.)

Minor amounts of protein could also potentially enter the product stream from additional sources, e.g. protein shed from production personnel. Implementation of good manufacturing practice (GMP), however, should minimize contamination from such sources.

The clinical significance of protein-based impurities relates to (a) their potential biological activities and (b) their antigenicity. Whereas some contaminants may display no undesirable biological activity, others may exhibit activities deleterious to either the product itself (e.g. proteases that could modify/degrade the product) or the recipient patient (e.g. the presence of contaminating toxins).

Their inherent immunogenicity also renders likely and immunological reaction against protein-based impurities upon product administration to the recipient patient. This is particularly true in the case of products produced in microbial or other recombinant systems (i.e. most biopharmaceuticals). Although the product itself is likely to be non-immunogenic (usually being coded for by a human gene), contaminant proteins will be endogenous to the host cell, and hence foreign to the human body. Administration of the product can elicit an immune response against the contaminant. This is particularly likely if a requirement exists for ongoing, repeat product administration (e.g. administration of recombinant insulin). Immunological activation of this type could also potentially (and more seriously) have a sensitizing effect on the recipient against the actual protein product.

In addition to distinct gene products, modified forms of the protein of interest are also considered impurities, rendering desirable their removal from the product stream. Although some such modified forms may be innocuous, others may not. Modified product '*impurities*' may compromise the product in a number of ways, e.g.:

1. Biologically inactive forms of the product will reduce overall product potency;
2. Some modified product forms remain biologically active, but exhibit modified pharmacokinetic characteristics (i.e. timing and duration of drug action);
3. Modified product forms may be immunogenic.

Removal of Altered Forms of the Protein of Interest from the Product Stream

Modification of any protein will generally alter some aspect of its physicochemical characteristics. This facilitates removal of the modified form by standard chromatographic techniques during downstream processing. Most downstream procedures for protein-based biopharmaceuticals include both gel-filtration and ion-exchange steps. Aggregated forms of the product will be effectively removed by gel filtration (because they now exhibit a molecular mass greater by several orders of magnitude than the native product). This technique will also remove extensively proteolysed forms of the product. Glycoprotein variants whose carbohydrate moieties have been extensively degraded will also likely be removed by gel-filtration (or ion-exchange) chromatography. Deamidation and oxidation will generate product variants with altered surface charge characteristics, often rendering their removal by ion exchange relatively straightforward. Incorrect disulfide bond formation, partial denaturation and limited proteolysis can also alter the shape and surface charge of proteins, facilitating their removal from the product by ion exchange or other techniques, such as hydrophobic interaction chromatography.

The range of chromatographic techniques now available, along with improvements in the resolution achievable using such techniques, renders possible the routine production of protein biopharmaceuticals which are in excess of 97–99 per cent pure. This level of purity represents the typical industry standard with regard to biopharmaceutical production.

A number of different techniques may be used to characterize protein-based biopharmaceutical products. and to detect any protein-based impurities that may be present in that product. Analysis for non-protein-based contaminant is described in subsequent sections.

Product Potency

Any biopharmaceutical must obviously conform to final product potency specifications. Such specifications are usually expressed in terms of 'units of activity' per vial of product (or per therapeutic dose, or per milligram of product). A number of different approaches may be undertaken to determine product potency. Each exhibits certain advantages and disadvantages.

Bioassays represent the most relevant potency-determining assay, as they directly assess the biological activity of the biopharmaceutical. Bioassay involves applying a known quantity of the substance to be assayed to a biological system that responds in some way to this applied stimulus. The response is measured quantitatively, allowing an activity value to be assigned to the substance being assayed.

All bioassays are comparative in nature, requiring parallel assay of a 'standard' preparation against which the sample will be compared. Internationally accepted standard preparations of most biopharmaceuticals are available from organizations such as the World Health Organization (WHO) or the United States Pharmacopeia. An example of a straightforward bioassay is the traditional assay method for antibiotics. This usually entailed measuring the zone of inhibition of microbial growth around an antibiotic-containing disc, placed on an agar plate seeded with the test microbe. Bioassays for modern biopharmaceuticals are generally more complex. The biological system used can be whole animals, specific organs or tissue types, or individual mammalian cells in culture.

Bioassays of related substances can be quite similar in design. Specific growth factors, for example, stimulate the accelerated growth of specific animal cell lines. Relevant bioassays can be undertaken by incubation of the growth-factor-containing sample with a culture of the relevant sensitive cells and radiolabelled nucleotide precursors. After an appropriate time period, the level of radioactivity incorporated into the DNA of the cells is measured. This is a measure of the bioactivity of the growth factor. The most popular bioassay of EPO involves a mouse-based bioassay (EPO stimulates red blood cell production, making it useful in the treatment of certain forms of anaemia; Chapter 10). Basically, the EPO-containing sample is administered to mice along with radioactive iron (^{57}Fe). Subsequent measurement of the rate of incorporation of radioactivity into proliferating red blood cells is undertaken. (The greater the stimulation of red blood cell proliferation, the more iron taken up for haemoglobin synthesis.)

One of the most popular bioassay for interferons is termed the 'cytopathic effect inhibition assay'. This assay is based upon the ability of many interferons to render animal cells resistant to viral attack. It entails incubation of the interferon preparation with cells sensitive to destruction by a specific virus. That virus is then subsequently added. and the percentage of cells that survive thereafter is proportional to the levels of interferon present in the assay sample. Viable cells can assimilate certain dyes, such as neutral red. Addition of the dye followed by spectrophotometric quantitation of the amount of dye assimilated can thus be used to quantitate percentage cell survival. This type of assay can be scaled down to run in a single well of a microtitre plate. This facilitates automated assay of large numbers of samples with relative ease. Although bioassays directly assess product potency (i.e. activity), they suffer from a number of drawbacks, including:

1. *Lack of precision*. The complex nature of any biological system, be it an entire animal or individual cell, often results in the responses observed being influenced by factors such as metabolic status of individual cells. or (in the case of whole animals) subclinical infections, stress levels induced by human handling, etc.

2. *Time*. Most bioassays take days, and in some cases week, to run. This can render routine bioassays difficult, and impractical to undertake as a quick QC potency test during downstream processing.
3. *Cost*. Most bioassay systems, in particular those involving whole animals, are extremely expensive to undertake.

Because of such difficulties alternative assays have been investigated, and sometimes are used in conjunction with, or instead of, bioassays. The most popular alternative assay system is the immunoassay.

Immunoassays employ monoclonal or polyclonal antibody preparations to detect and quantify the product. The specificity of antibody–antigen interaction ensures good assay precision. The use of conjugated radiolabels (RIA) or enzymes (EIA) to allow detection of antigen–antibody binding renders such assays very sensitive. Furthermore, when compared with a bioassay, immunoassays are rapid (undertaken in minutes to hours), inexpensive, and straight-forward to undertake. The obvious disadvantage of immunoassays is that immunological reactivity cannot be guaranteed to correlate directly to biological activity. Relatively minor modifications of the protein product, although having a profound influence on its biological activity, may have little or no influence on its ability to bind antibody. For such reasons, although immunoassays may provide a convenient means of tracking product during downstream processing, performing a bioassay on at the very least the final product is usually necessary to prove that potency falls within specification.

Determination of Protein Concentration

Quantification of total protein in the final product represents another standard analysis undertaken by QC. A number of different protein assays may be potentially employed.

Table 9.2. Common assay methods used to quantitate proteins. The principle upon which each method is based is also listed

Method	*Principle*
Absorbance at 280 nm (A_{280}; UV method)	The side chain of selected amino acids (particularly tyrosine and tryptophan) absorbs UV at 280 nm
Absorbance at 205 nm (far-UV method)	Peptide bonds absorb UV at 190–220 nm
Biuret method	Binding of copper ions to peptide bond nitrogen under alkaline conditions generates a purple colour
Lowry method	Lowry method uses a combination of the Biuret copper-based reagent and the 'Folin–Ciocalteau' reagent, which contains phosphomolybdic-phosphotungstic acid. Reagents react with protein, yielding a blue colour that displays an absorbance maximum at 750 nm
Bradford method	Bradford reagent contains the dye Coomassie blue G-250 in an acidic solution. The dye binds to protein, yielding a blue colour that absorbs maximally at 595 nm
Bicinchonic acid method	Copper-containing reagent that, when reduced by protein, reacts with bicinchonic acid yielding a complex that displays an absorbance maximum at 562 nm
Peterson method	Essentially involves initial precipitation of protein out of solution by addition of trichloroacetic acid. The protein precipitate is redissolved in NaOH and the Lowry method of protein determination is then performed
Silver-binding method	Interaction of silver with protein – very sensitive method

Detection and quantification of protein by measuring absorbency at 280 nm is perhaps the simplest such method. This approach is based on the fact that the side chains of the amino acids tyrosine and tryptophan absorb at this wavelength. The method is popular, as it is fast, easy to perform and is non-destructive to the sample. However, it is a relatively insensitive technique, and identical concentrations of different proteins will yield different absorbance values if their content of tyrosine and tryptophan vary to any significant extent. Hence, this method is rarely used to determine the protein concentration of the final product, but it is routinely used during downstream processing to detect protein elution off chromatographic columns, and hence track the purification process.

Measuring protein absorbance at lower wavelengths (205 nm) increases the sensitivity of the assay considerably. Also, as it is the peptide bonds that are absorbing at this wavelength, the assay is subject to much less variation due to the amino acid composition of the protein.

The most common methods used to determine protein concentration are the dye-binding procedure using Coomassie brilliant blue, and the bicinchonic-acid-based procedure. Various dyes are known to bind quantitatively to proteins, resulting in an alteration of the characteristic absorption spectrum of the dye. Coomassie brilliant blue G-250, for example, becomes protonated when dissolved in phosphoric acid, and has an absorbance maximum at 450 nm. Binding of the dye to a protein (via ionic interactions) results in a shift in the dye's absorbance spectrum, with a new major peak (at 595 nm) being observed. Quantification of proteins in this case can thus be undertaken by measuring absorbance at 595 nm. The method is sensitive, easy and rapid to undertake. Also, it exhibits little quantitative variation between different proteins.

Protein determination procedures using bicinchonic acid were developed by Pierce Chemicals, who hold a patent on the product. The procedure entails the use of a copper-based reagent containing bicinchonic acid. Upon incubation with a protein sample, the copper is reduced. In the reduced state it reacts with bicinchonic acid, yielding a purple colour that absorbs maximally at 562 nm.

Silver also binds to proteins, an observation that forms the basis of an extremely sensitive method of protein detection. This technique is used extensively to detect proteins in electrophoretic gels, as discussed in the next section.

Detection of Protein-based Product Impurities

SDS polyacrylamide gel electrophoresis (SDS-PAGE) represents the most commonly used analytical technique in the assessment of final product purity. This technique is well established and easy to perform. It provides high-resolution separation of polypeptides on the basis of their molecular mass. Bands containing as little as 100 ng of protein can be visualized by staining the gel with dyes such as Coomassie blue. Subsequent gel analysis by scanning laser densitometry allows quantitative determination of the protein content of each band (thus allowing quantification of protein impurities in the product).

The use of silver-based stains increases the detection sensitivity up to 100 fold, with individual bands containing as little as 1ng of protein usually staining well. However, because silver binds to protein non-stoichiometrically, quantitative studies using densitometry cannot be undertaken.

SDS-PAGE is normally run under reducing conditions. Addition of a reducing agent such as β-mercaptoethanol or dithiothreitol (DTT) disrupts interchain (and intrachain) disulfide linkages. Individual polypeptides held together via disulfide linkages in oligomeric proteins will thus separate from each other on the basis of their molecular mass.

The presence of bands additional to those equating to the protein product generally represent protein contaminants. Such contaminants may be unrelated to the product or may be variants of the product itself (e.g. differentially glycosylated variants, proteolytic fragment, etc.). Further characterization may include western blot analysis. This involves eluting the protein bands from the electrophoretic gel onto a nitrocellulose filter. The filter can then be probed using antibodies raised against the product. Binding of the antibody to the '*contaminant*' bands suggests that they are variants of the product.

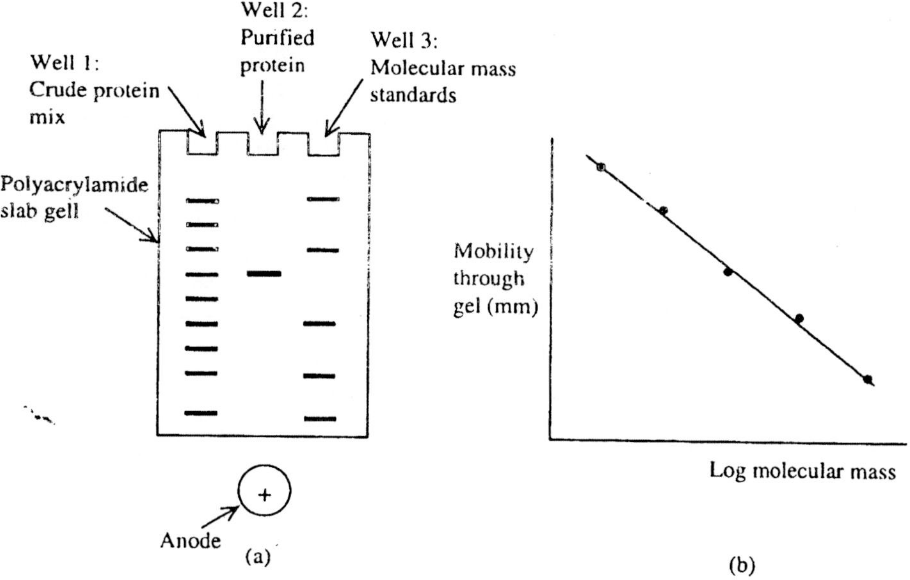

Fig. 9.1. Separation of proteins by SDS-PAGE.

One concern relating to SDS -PAGE-based purity analysis is that contaminants of the same molecular mass as the product will go undetected as they will co-migrate with it. Two-dimensional electrophoretic analysis would overcome this eventuality in most instances. Two-dimensional electrophoresis is normally run so that proteins are separated from each other on the basis of a different molecular property in each dimension. The most commonly utilized method entails separation of proteins by isoelectric focusing in the first dimension, with separation in the second dimension being undertaken in the presence of SDS, thus promoting band separation on the basis of protein size. Modified electrophoresis equipment that renders two- dimensional electrophoretic separation routine is freely available. Application of biopharmaceutical finished products to such systems allows rigorous analysis of purity.

Isoelectric focusing entails setting up a pH gradient along the length of an electrophoretic gel. Applied proteins will migrate under the influence of an electric field until they reach a point in the gel at which the pH equals the protein's isoelectric point pI (the pH at which the protein exhibits no overall net charge; only species with a net charge will move under the in- fluence of an electric field). Isoelectric focusing thus separates proteins on the basis of charge characteristics. This technique is also utilized in the biopharmaceutical industry to determine product homogeneity. Homogeneity is best indicated by the appearance in the gel of a single protein band, exhibiting the predicted pI value. Interpretation of the meaning of multiple bands, however, is less straightforward, particularly if the protein is glycosylated (the bands can also be stained for the presence of carbohydrates). Glycoproteins varying slightly in their carbohydrate content will vary in their sialic acid content and, hence, exhibit slightly different pI values. In such instances, isoelectric focusing analysis seeks to establish batch-to-batch consistency in terms of the banding pattern observed. Isoelectric focusing also finds application in analysing the stability of biopharmaceuticals over the course of their shelf life. Repeat analysis of samples over time will detect deamidation or other degradative processes that alter protein charge characteristics.

. Capillary Electrophoresis

Capillary electrophoresis systems are also likely to play an increasingly prominent analytical role in the QC laboratory. As with other forms of electrophoresis, separation is based upon different rates of protein migration upon application of an electric field. As its name suggests, in the case of capillary electrophoresis, this separation occurs within a capillary tube. Typically, the capillary will have a diameter of 20–50 μm and be up to a 1 m long (it is normally coiled to facilitate ease of use and storage). The dimensions of this system yield greatly increased surface area:volume ratio (compared with slab gels), hence greatly increasing the efficiency of heat dissipation from the system. This, in turn, allows operation at a higher current density, thus speeding up the rate of migration through the capillary. Sample analysis can be undertaken in 15–30 min, and on-line detection at the end of the column allows automatic detection and quantification of eluting bands.

The speed, sensitivity, high degree of automation and ability to quantitate protein bands directly render this system ideal for biopharmaceutical analysis.

High-performance Liquid Chromatography

HPLC occupies a central analytical role in assessing the purity of low molecular mass pharmaceutical substances. It also plays an increasingly important role in analysis of macromolecules, such as proteins. Most of the chromatographic strategies used to separate proteins under 'low pressure' (e.g. gel filtration, ion exchange, etc.) can be adapted to operate under high pressure. Reverse-phase-, size-exclusion- and, to a lesser extent, ion-exchange-based HPLC chromatography systems are now used in the analysis of a range of biopharmaceutical preparations. On-line detectors (usually a UV monitor set at 220 or 280 nm) allows automated detection and quantification of eluting bands. HPLC is characterized by a number of features that render it an attractive analytical tool. These include:

1. Excellent fractionation speeds (often just minutes per sample);
2. Superior peak resolution
3. High degree of automation (including data analysis);
4. Ready commercial availability of various sophisticated systems.

Reverse-phase HPLC (RP-HPLC) separates proteins on the basis of differences in their surface hydophobicity. The stationary phase in the HPLC column normally consists of silica or a polymeric support to which hydrophobic arms (usually alkyl chains, such as butyl, octyl or octadecyl groups) have been attached. Reverse-phase systems have proven themselves to be a particularly powerful analytical technique, capable of separating very similar molecules displaying only minor differences in hydrophobicity. In some instances a single amino acid substitution or the removal of a single amino acid from the end of a polypeptide chain can be detected by RP-HPLC. In most instances, modifications such as deamidation will also cause peak shifts. Such systems, therefore, may be used to detect impurities, be they related or unrelated to the protein product. RP-HPLC finds extensive application in, for example, the analysis of insulin preparations. Modified forms, or insulin polymers, are easily distinguishable from native insulin on reverse-phase columns.

Although RP-HPLC has proven its analytical usefulness, its routine application to analysis of specific protein preparations should be undertaken only after extensive validation studies. HPLC in general can have a denaturing influence on many proteins (especially larger, complex proteins). Reverse-phase systems can be particularly harsh, as interaction with the highly hydrophobic stationary phase can induce irreversible protein denaturation. Denaturation would result in the generation of artifactual peaks on the chromatogram. Size-exclusion HPLC (SE-HPLC) separates proteins on the basis of size and shape. As most soluble proteins are globular (i.e. roughly spherical in shape), separation is essentially achieved on the basis of molecular mass in most instances. Commonly used SE-HPLC stationary phases include silica-based supports and cross-linked agarose of defined pore size. Size-exclusion systems are most often used to analyse product for the presence of dimers or higher molecular mass aggregates of itself, as well as proteolysed product variants.

Calibration with standards allows accurate determination of the molecular mass of the product itself, as well as any impurities. Batch-to-batch variation can also be assessed by comparison of chromatograms from different product runs. Ion-exchange chromatography (both cation and anion) can also be undertaken in HPLC format. Though not as extensively employed as reverse-phase or size-exclusion systems, ion-exchange-based systems are of use in analysing for impurities unrelated to the product, as well as detecting and quantifying deamidated forms.

Mass Spectrometry

Recent advances in the field of mass spectrometry now extend the applicability of this method to the analysis of macromolecules such as proteins. Using electrospray mass spectrometry, it is now possible to determine the molecular mass of many proteins to within an accuracy of ± 0.01 per cent. A protein variant missing a single amino acid residue can easily be distinguished from the native protein in many instances. Although this is a very powerful technique, analysis of the results obtained can sometimes be less than straightforward. Glycoproteins, for example, yield extremely complex spectra (due to their natural heterogeneity), making the significance of the findings hard to interpret.

Immunological Approaches to Detection of Contaminants

Most recombinant biopharmaceuticals are produced in microbial or mammalian cell lines. Thus, although the product is derived from a human gene, all product-unrelated contaminants will be derived from the producer organism. These non-self proteins are likely to be highly immunogenic in humans, rendering their removal from the product stream especially important. Immunoassays may be conveniently used to detect and quantify non-product-related impurities in the final preparation (immunoassays generally may not be used to determine levels of product-related impurities, as antibodies raised against such impurities would almost certainly cross-react with the product itself).

The strategy usually employed to develop such immunoassays is termed the 'blank run approach'. This entails constructing a host cell identical in all respects to the natural producer cell, except that it lacks the gene coding for the desired product. This blank producer cell is then subjected to upstream processing procedures identical to those undertaken with the normal producer cell. Cellular extracts are subsequently subjected to the normal product purification process, but only to a stage immediately prior to the final purification steps. This produces an array of proteins that could co- purify with the final product. These proteins (of which there may be up to 200 as determined by two-dimensional electrophoretic analysis) are used to immunize horses, goats or other suitable animals. Therefore, polyclonal antibody preparations capable of binding specifically to these proteins are produced. Purification of the antibodies allows their incorporation in radioimmunoassay or enzyme-based immunoassay systems, which may subsequently be used to probe the product. Such multi-antigen assay systems will detect the sum total of host-cell-derived impurities present in the product. Immunoassays identifying a single potential contaminant can also be developed.

Immunoassays have found widespread application in detecting and quantifying product impurities. These assays are extremely specific and very sensitive, often detecting target antigen down to parts per million levels. Many immunoassays are available commercially, and companies exist that will rapidly develop tailor-made immunoassay systems for biopharmaceutical analysis.

Application of the analytical techniques discussed thus far focuses upon detection of proteinaceous impurities. A variety of additional tests are undertaken that focus upon the active substance itself. These tests aim to confirm that the presumed active substance observed by electrophoresis, HPLC, etc. is indeed the active substance, and that its primary sequence (and, to a lesser extent, higher orders of structure) conform to licensed product specification. Tests performed to verify the product identity include amino acid analysis, peptide mapping, N-terminal sequencing and spectrophotometric analyses.

Amino Acid Analysis

Amino acid analysis remains a characterization technique undertaken in many laboratories, in particular if the product is a peptide or small polypeptide (molecular mass ≤10 kDa). The strategy is simple. Determine the range and quantity of amino acids present in the product and compare the results obtained with the expected (theoretical) values. The results should be comparable.

The peptide/polypeptide product is usually hydrolysed by incubation with 6 mol l^{-1} HCl at elevated temperatures (110°C), under vacuum, for extended periods (12–24 h). The constituent amino acids are separated from each other by ion-exchange chromatography and identified by comparison with standard amino acid preparations. Reaction with ninhydrin allows subsequent quantification of each amino acid present.

Although this technique is relatively straightforward and automated amino acid analysers are commercially available, it is subject to a number of disadvantages that limits its usefulness in biopharmaceutical analysis. These include:

1. Hydrolysis conditions can destroy/modify certain amino acid residues, in particular tryptophan, but also serine, threonine and tyrosine;
2. The method is semi-quantitative rather than quantitative;
3. Sensitivity is at best moderate; low-level contaminants may go undetected (i.e. not significantly alter the amino acid profile obtained), particularly if the product is a high molecular mass protein.

These disadvantages, along with the availability of alternative characterization methodologies, limit application of this technique in biopharmaceutical analysis.

Peptide Mapping

A major concern relating to biopharmaceuticals produced in high-expression recombinant systems is the potential occurrence of point mutations in the product's gene, leading to an altered primary structure (i.e. amino acid sequence). Errors in gene transcription or translation could also have similar consequences. The only procedure guaranteed to detect such alterations is full sequencing of a sample of each batch of the protein, which is a considerable technical challenge. Although partial protein sequencing is normally undertaken, the approach most commonly used to detect alterations in amino acid sequence is peptide (fingerprint) mapping.

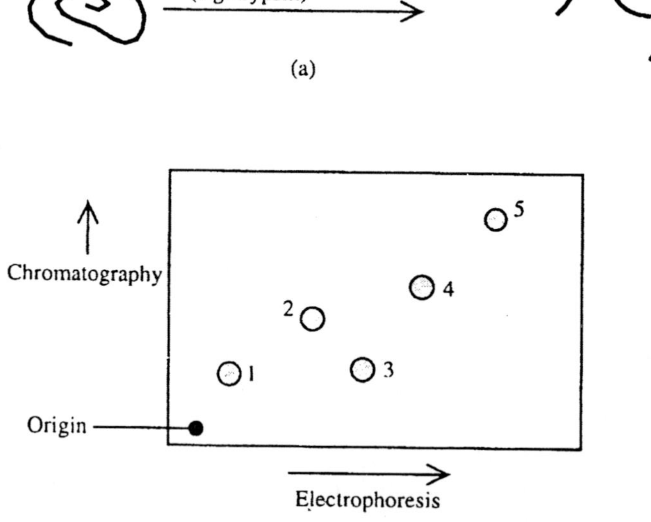

Fig. 9.2. Generation of a peptide map.

Peptide mapping entails exposure of the protein product to a reagent that promotes hydrolysis of peptide bonds at specific points along the protein backbone. This generates a series of peptide fragments. These fragments can be separated from each other by a variety of techniques, including one- or two-dimensional electrophoresis, and RP-HPLC in particular. A standardized sample of the protein product when subjected to this procedure will yield a characteristic peptide fingerprint, or map, with which the peptide maps obtained with each batch of product can subsequently be compared. If the peptides generated are relatively short, then a change in a single amino acid residue is likely to alter the peptide's physicochemical properties sufficiently to alter its position within the peptide map. In this way, single (or multiple) amino acid substitutions, deletions, insertions or modifications can usually be detected. This technique plays an important role in monitoring batch-to-batch consistency of the product, and also obviously can confirm the identity of the actual product. The choice of reagent used to fragment the protein is critical to the success of this approach. If a reagent generates only a few very large peptides, a single amino acid alteration in one such peptide will be more difficult to detect than if it occurred in a much smaller peptide fragment. On the other hand, generation of a large number of very short peptides can be counterproductive, as it may prove difficult to resolve all the peptides from each other by subsequent chromatography. Generation of peptide fragments containing an average of 7–14 amino acids is most desirable.

The most commonly utilized chemical cleavage agent is cyanogen bromide (it cleaves the peptide bond on the carboxyl side of methionine residues). V8 protease, produced by certain staphylococci, along with trypsin are two of the more commonly used proteolytic-based fragmentation agents. Knowledge of the full amino acid sequence of the protein usually renders possible pre-determination of the most suitable fragmentation agent for any protein. The amino acid sequence of hGH, for example, harbours 20 potential trypsin cleavage sites. Under some circumstances it may be possible to use a combination of fragmentation agents to generate peptides of optimal length.

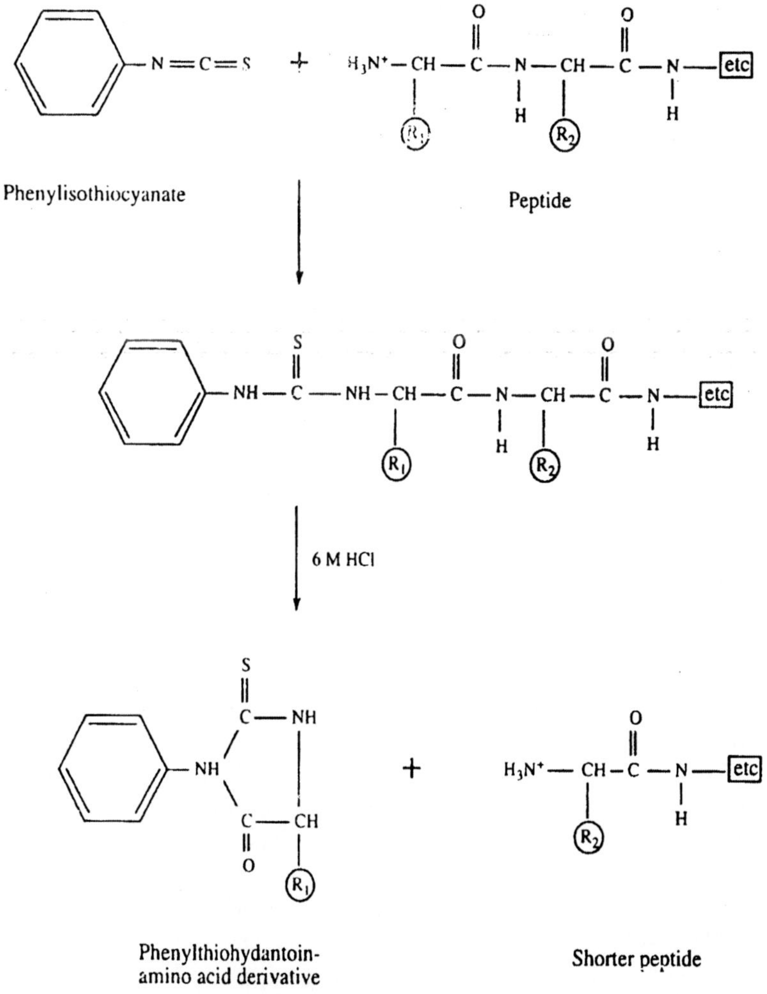

N-terminal Sequencing

N-terminal sequencing of the first 20–30 amino acid residues of the protein product has become a popular quality control test for finished biopharmaceutical products. The technique is useful, as it:

1. Positively identifies the protein;
2. Confirms (or otherwise) the accuracy of the amino acid sequence of at least the N-terminus of the protein;
3. Readily identifies the presence of modified forms of the product in which one or more amino acids are missing from the N-terminus.

Fig. 9.3. The Edman degradation method, by which the sequence of a peptide/polypeptide may be elucidated.

N-terminal sequencing is normally undertaken by Edman degradation. Although this technique was developed in the 1950s, advances in analytical methodologies now facilitate fast and automated determination of up to the first 100 amino acids from the N-terminus of most proteins, and usually requires a sample size of less than 1 μmol to do so. Analogous techniques facilitating sequencing from a polypeptide's C-terminus remain to be satisfactorily developed. The enzyme carboxypeptidase C sequentially removes amino acids from the C-terminus, but often only removes the first few such amino acids. Furthermore, the rate at which it hydrolyses bonds can vary, depending on what amino acids have contributed to bond formation. Chemical approaches based on principles similar to the Edman procedure have been attempted. However, poor yields of derivatized product and the occurrence of side reactions have prevented widespread acceptance of this method.

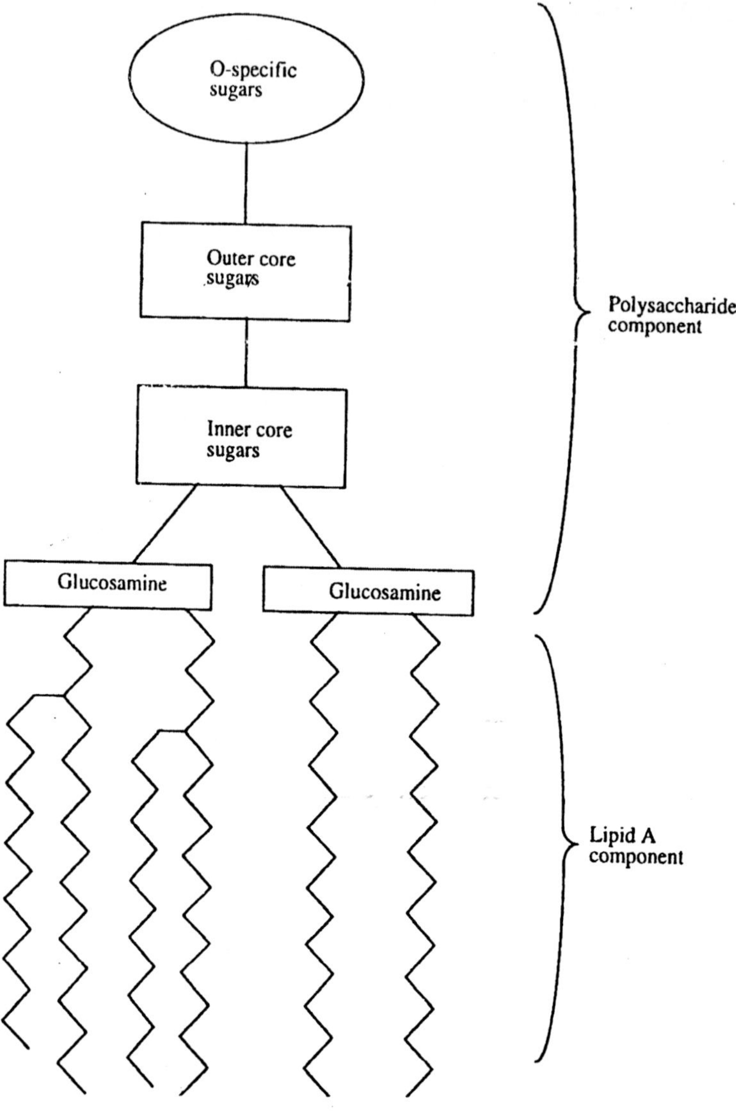

Fig. 9.4. Structure of a generalized LPS molecule.

Analysis of Secondary and Tertiary Structure

Analyses such as peptide mapping, N-terminal sequencing or amino acid analysis yield information relating to a polypeptide's primary structure, i.e. its amino acid sequence. Such tests yield no information relating to higher-order structures (i.e. secondary and tertiary structure of polypeptides, along with quaternary structure of multi-subunit proteins). Although a protein's three-dimensional conformation may be studied in great detail by X-ray crystallography or NMR spectroscopy, routine application of such techniques to biopharmaceutical manufacture is impractical, both from a technical and an economic standpoint. Limited analysis of protein secondary and tertiary structure can, however, be more easily undertaken using spectroscopic methods, particularly far-UV circular dichroism. More recently proton-NMR has also been applied to studying higher orders of protein structure.

Endotoxin and other Pyrogenic Contaminants

Pyrogens are substances that, when they enter the blood stream, influence hypothalamic regulation of body temperature, usually resulting in fever. Medical control of pyrogen-induced fever proves very difficult, and in severe cases results in patient death. Pyrogens represent a diverse group of substances, including various chemicals, particulate matter and endotoxin (LPS), a molecule derived from the outer membrane of Gram-negative bacteria. Such Gram-negative organisms harbour 3–4 million LPS molecules on their surface, representing in the region of 75 per cent of their outer membrane surface area. Gram-negative bacteria clinically significant in human medicine include *E. coli*, *Haemophilus influenzae*, *Salmonella enterica*, *Klebsiella pneumoniae*, *Bordetella pertussis*, *Pseudomonas aeruginosa*, *Chylamydia psittaci* and *Legionella pneumophila*.

In many instances the influence of pyrogens on body temperature is indirect. For example, entry of endotoxin into the bloodstream stimulates the production of IL-1 by macrophages. It is the IL-1 that directly initiates the fever response (hence its alternative name, '*endogenous pyrogen*').

Although entry of any pyrogenic substance into the bloodstream can have serious medical consequences, endotoxin receives most attention because of its ubiquitous nature. Therefore, it is the pyrogen most likely to contaminate parenteral (bio)pharmaceutical products. Effective implementation of GMP minimizes the likelihood of product contamination by pyrogens. For example, GMP dictates that chemical reagents used in the manufacture of process buffers be extremely pure. Such raw materials, therefore, are unlikely to contain chemical contaminants displaying pyrogenic activity. Furthermore, GMP encourages filtration of virtually all parenteral products through a 0.45 or 0.22 μm filter at points during processing and prior to filling in final product containers (even if the product can subsequently be sterilized by autoclaving). Filtration ensures removal of all particulate matter from the product. In addition, most final product containers are rendered particle free immediately prior to filling by an automatic pre-rinse using WFI. As an additional safeguard, the final product will usually be subject to a particulate matter test by QC before final product release. The simplest format for such a test could involve visual inspection of vial contents, although specific particle detecting and counting equipment is more routinely used.

Contamination of the final product with endotoxin is more difficult to control because:

1. Many recombinant biopharmaceuticals are produced in Gram-negative bacterial systems; thus, the product source is also a source of endotoxin.
2. Despite rigorous implementation of GMP, most biopharmaceutical preparations will be contaminated with low levels of Gram-negative bacteria at some stage of manufacture. These bacteria shed endotoxin into the product stream, which is not removed during subsequent bacterial filtration steps. This is one of many reasons why GMP dictates that the level of bioburden in the product stream should be minimized at all stages of manufacture.
3. The heat stability exhibited by endotoxin means that autoclaving of process equipment will not destroy endotoxin present on such equipment.
4. Adverse medical reactions caused by endotoxin are witnessed in humans at dosage rates as low as 0.5 ng per kilogram body weight.

Endotoxin, the Molecule

As its name suggests, LPS consists of a complex polysaccharide component linked to a lipid (lipid A) moiety. The polysaccharide moiety is generally composed of 50 or more monosaccharide units linked by glycosidic bonds. Sugar moieties often found in LPS include glucose, glucosamine, mannose and galactose, as well as more extensive structures such as L-glycero-mannoheptose. The polysaccharide component of LPS may be divided into several structural domains. The inner (core) domains vary relatively little between LPS molecules isolated from different Gram-negative bacteria. The outer (O-specific) domain is usually bacterial-strain specific. Most of the LPS biological activity (pyrogenicity) is associated with its lipid A moiety. This usually consists of six or more fatty acids attached directly to sugars such as glucosamine. Again, as is the case in relation to the carbohydrate component, lipid A moieties of LPS isolated from different bacteria can vary somewhat. The structure of *E coli*'s lipid A has been studied in the greatest detail; its exact structure has been elucidated and it can be chemically synthesized.

Pyrogen Detection

Pyrogens may be detected in parenteral preparations (or other substances) by a number of methods. Two such methods are widely employed in the pharmaceutical industry.

Historically, the rabbit pyrogen test constituted the most widely used method. This entails parenteral administration of the product to a group of healthy rabbits, with subsequent monitoring of rabbit temperature using rectal probes. Increased rabbit temperature above a certain point suggests the presence of pyrogenic substances. The basic rabbit method, as outlined in the European Pharmacopoeia, entails initial administration of the product to three rabbits. The product is considered to have passed the test if the total (summed) increase of the temperature of all three animals is less than 1.15°C. If the total increase recorded is greater than 2.65°C then the product has failed. However, if the response observed falls between these two limits the result is considered inconclusive, and the test must be repeated using a further batch of animals.

This test is popular because it detects a wide spectrum of pyrogenic substances. However, it is also subject to a number of disadvantages, including:

1. It is expensive (there is a requirement for animals, animal facilities and animal technicians);
2. Excitation/poor handling of the rabbits can affect the results obtained, usually prompting a false positive result;
3. Subclinical infection/poor overall animal health can also lead to false positive results;
4. Use of different rabbit colonies/breeds can yield variable results.

Another issue of relevance is that certain biopharmaceuticals (e.g. cytokines such as lL-1 and TNF) themselves induce a natural pyrogenic response. This rules out use of the rabbit- based assay for detection of exogenous pyrogens in such products. Such difficulties have led to the increased use of an *in vitro* assay; the *Limulus* ameobocyte lysate (LAL) test. This is based upon endotoxin-stimulated coagulation of amoebocyte lysate obtained from horseshoe crabs. This test is now the most widely used assay for the detection of endotoxins in biopharmaceutical and other pharmaceutical preparations.

Development of the LAL assay was based upon the observation that the presence of Gram- negative bacteria in the vascular system of the American horseshoe crab, *Limulus polyphemus*, resulted in the clotting of its blood. Tests on fractionated blood showed that the factor responsible for coagulation resided within the crab's circulating blood cells, i.e. the amoebocytes. Further research revealed that the bacterial agent responsible of initiation of clot formation was endotoxin.

The endotoxin molecule activates a coagulation cascade quite similar in design to the mammalian blood coagulation cascade. Activation of the cascade also requires the presence of divalent cations such as calcium or magnesium. The final steps of this pathway entail the proteolytic cleavage of the polypeptide coagulogen, forming coagulin, and a smaller peptide fragment. Coagulin molecules then interact non-covalently, forming a 'clot' or 'gel'.

The LAL-based assay for endotoxin became commercially available in the 1970s. The LAL reagent is prepared by extraction of blood from the horseshoe crab, followed by isolation of its amoebocytes by centrifugation. After a washing step, the amoebocytes are lysed and the lysate dispensed into pyrogen-free vials. The assay is normally performed by making a series of 1:2 dilutions of the test sample using (pyrogen-free) WFI(and pyrogen-free test tubes). A reference standard endotoxin preparation is treated similarly. LAL reagent is added to all tubes, incubated for 1 h, and these tubes are then inverted

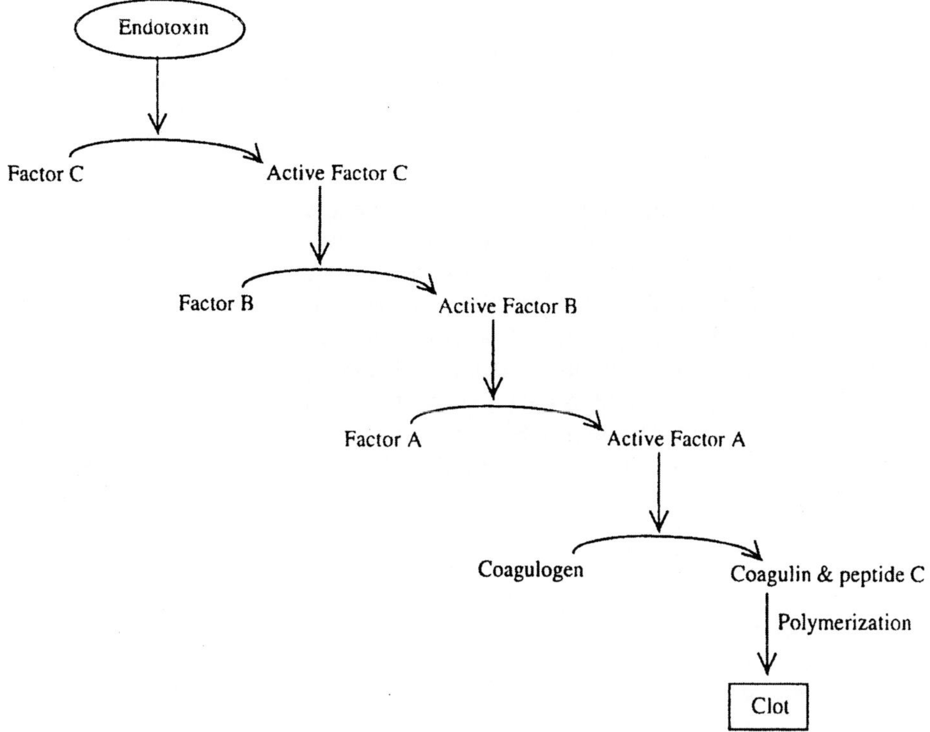

Fig. 9.5. Activation of clot formation by endotoxin.

to test for gel (i.e. clot) formation, which would indicate presence of endotoxin. More recently, a colorimetric-based LAL procedure has been devised. This entails addition to the LAL reagent of a short peptide, susceptible to hydrolysis by the LAL clotting enzyme. This synthetic peptide contains a chromogenic tag (usually *para*-nitroaniline, pNA) which is released free into solution by the clotting enzyme. This allows spectrophotometric analysis of the test sample, facilitating more accurate end-point determination. The LAL system displays several advantages when compared with the rabbit test, most notably:

1. Sensitivity – endotoxin levels as low as a few picograms per millilitre of sample assayed will be detected;
2. Cost – the assay is far less expensive than the rabbit assay;
3. Speed – depending upon the format used, the LAL assay may be conducted within 15–60 min.

Its major disadvantage is its selectivity: it only detects endotoxin-based pyrogens. In practice, however, endotoxin represents the pyrogen that is by far the most likely to be present in pharmaceutical products. The LAL method is used extensively within the industry. It is used not only to detect endotoxin in finished parenteral preparations, but also in WFI and in biological fluids, such as serum or cerebrospinal fluid. Before the LAL assay is routinely used to detect/quantify endotoxin in any product, its effective functioning in the presence of that product must be demonstrated by validation studies. Such studies are required to prove that the product (or, more likely, excipients present in the product) do not interfere with the rate/extent of clot formation (i.e. are neither inhibitors nor activators of the LAL-based enzymes). LAL enzyme inhibition could facilitate false-negative results upon sample assay. Validation studies entail, for example, observing the effect of spiking endotoxin-negative product with know quantities of endotoxin, or spiking endotoxin with varying quantities of product, before assay with the LAL reagents. All ancillary reagents used in the LAL assay system (e.g. WFI, test tubes, pipette tips for liquid transfer, etc.) must obviously be endotoxin free. Such items can be rendered endotoxin free by heat. Its heat-stable nature, however, renders very vigorous heating necessary in order to destroy contaminant endotoxin. A single autoclave cycle is insufficient, with total destruction requiring three consecutive autoclave cycles. Dry heat may also be used (180°C for 3 h or 240°C for 1 h).

GMP requires that, where practicable, process equipment coming into direct contact with the biopharmaceutical product stream should be rendered endotoxin free (depyrogenated) before use. Autoclaving, steam or dry heat can effectively be used on many process vessels, pipework, etc., which are usually manufactured from stainless steel or other heat-resistant material. Such an approach is not routinely practicable in the case of some items of process equipment, such as chromatographic systems. Fortunately, endotoxin is sensitive to strongly alkaline conditions; thus, routine cleaning in place of chromatographic systems using 1 mol l^{-1} NaOH represents an effective depyrogenation step. Gentler approaches, such as exhaustive rinsing with WFI (until an LAL test shows the eluate to be endotoxin free), can also be surprisingly effective. It is generally unnecessary to introduce specific measures aimed at endotoxin removal from the product during downstream processing. Endotoxin present in the earlier stages of production is often effectively removed from the product during chromatographic fractionation. The endotoxin molecule's highly negative charge often facilitates its effective removal from the product stream by ion-exchange chromatography. Gel-filtration chromatography also serves to remove endotoxin from the product. Although individual LPS molecules exhibit an average molecular mass of less than 20 kDa, these molecules aggregate in aqueous environments and generate supramolecular structures of molecular mass 100–1000 kDa.

The molecular mass of most biopharmaceuticals is considerably less than 100 kDa. The proteins would thus elute from gel-filtration columns much later than contaminating endotoxin aggregates. Should the biopharmaceutical exhibit a molecular mass approaching or exceeding 100 kDa, then effective separation can still be achieved by inclusion of a chelating agent such as EDTA in the running buffer. This promotes depolymerization of the endotoxin aggregates into monomeric (20 kDa) form. Additional techniques capable of separating biomolecules on the basis of molecular mass (e.g. ultrafiltration) may also be used to remove endotoxin from the product stream.

DNA

The clinical significance of DNA-based contaminants in biopharmaceutical products remains unclear. The concerns relating to the presence of DNA in modern biopharmaceuticals focus primarily upon the presence of active oncogenes in the genome of several producer cell types (e.g. monoclonal antibody production in hybridoma cell lines). Parenteral administration of DNA contaminants containing active oncogenes to patients is considered undesirable. The concern is that uptake and expression of such DNA in human cells could occur. There is some evidence to suggest that naked DNA can be assimilated by some cells at least, under certain conditions. Guidelines to date state that an acceptable level of residual DNA in recombinant products is of the order of 10 pg per therapeutic dose.

DNA hybridization studies (e.g. the '*dot blot*' assay) utilizing radiolabelled DNA probes allows detection of DNA contaminants in the product, to levels in the nanogram range. The process begins with isolation of the contaminating DNA from the product. This can be achieved, for example, by phenol and chloroform extraction and ethanol precipitation. The isolated DNA is then applied as a spot (i.e. a 'dot') onto nitrocellulose filter paper, with subsequent baking of the filter at 80°C under vacuum. This promotes (a) DNA denaturation, yielding single strands, and (b) binding of the DNA to the filter. A sample of total DNA derived from the cells in which the product is produced is then radiolabelled with ^{32}P using the process of nick translation. It is heated to 90°C (promotes denaturation, forming single strands) and incubated with the baked filter for several hours at 40°C. Lowering the temperature allows reannealing of single strands via complementary base-pairing to occur. Labelled DNA will reanneal with any complementary DNA strands immobilized on the filter. After the filter is washed (to remove non-specifically bound radiolabelled probe) it is subjected to autoradiography, which allows detection of any bound probe.

Quantification of the DNA isolated from the product involves concurrent inclusion in the dot blot assay of a set of spots, containing known quantities of DNA, and being derived from the producer cell. After autoradiography, the intensity of the test spot is compared with the standards. In many instances there is little need to incorporate specific DNA removal steps during downstream processing. Endogenous nucleases liberated upon cellular homogenization come into direct contact with cellular DNA, resulting in its degradation. Commercial DNase's are sometimes added to crude homogenate to reduce DNA-associated product viscosity. Most chromatographic steps are also effective in separating DNA from the product stream. Ion-exchange chromatography is particularly effective, as DNA exhibits a large overall negative charge (due to the phosphate constituent of its nucleotide backbone).

Microbial and Viral Contaminants

Finished-product biopharmaceuticals, along with other pharmaceuticals intended for parenteral administration, must be sterile (the one exception being live bacterial vaccines). The presence of microorganisms in the final product is unacceptable for a number of reasons:

1. Parenteral administration of contaminated product would likely lead to the establishment of a severe infection in the recipient patient.
2. Microorganisms may be capable of metabolizing the product itself, thus reducing its potency. This is particularly true of protein-based biopharmaceuticals, as most microbes produce an array of extracellular proteases.
3. Microbial-derived substances secreted into the product could adversely affect the recipient's health. Examples include endotoxin secreted from Gram-negative bacteria, or microbial proteins that would stimulate an immune response.

Terminal sterilization by autoclaving guarantees product sterility. Heat sterilization, however, is not a viable option in the case of biopharmaceuticals. Sterilization of biopharmaceuticals by filtration, followed by aseptic filling into a sterile final-product container, inherently carries a greater risk of product contamination. Finished-product sterility testing of such preparations thus represents one of the most critical product tests undertaken by QC. Specific guidelines relating to sterility testing of finished products are given in international pharmacopoeias.

Biopharmaceutical products are also subjected to screening for the presence of viral particles prior to final product release. Although viruses could be introduced, for example, via infected personnel during downstream processing, proper implementation of GMP minimizes such risk. Any viral particles found in the finished product are most likely derived from raw material sources. Examples could include HIV or hepatitis viruses present in blood used in the manufacture of blood products. Such raw materials must be screened before processing for the presence of likely viral contaminants.

A variety of murine (mouse) and other mammalian cell lines have become popular host systems for the production of recombinant human biopharmaceuticals. Moreover, most monoclonal antibodies used for therapeutic purposes are produced by murine-derived hybridoma cells. These cell lines are sensitive to infection by various viral particles. Producer cell lines are screened during product development studies to ensure freedom from a variety of pathogenic advantageous agents, including various species of bacteria, fungi, yeast, mycoplasma, protozoa, parasites, viruses and prions. Suitable microbiological precautions must subsequently be undertaken to prevent producer cell banks from becoming contaminated with such pathogens. Removal of viruses from the product stream can be achieved in a number of ways. The physicochemical properties of viral particles differ greatly from most proteins, ensuring that effective fractionation is automatically achieved by most chromatographic techniques. Gel-filtration chromatography, for example, effectively separates viral particles from most proteins on the basis of differences in size.

In addition to chromatographic separation, downstream processing steps may be undertaken that are specifically aimed at removal or inactivation of viral particles potentially present in the product stream. Significantly, many are 'blanket' procedures, equally capable of removing known or potentially likely viral contaminants and any uncharacterized/undetected viruses. Filtration through a 0.22 μm filter effectively removes microbial agents from the product stream, but fails to remove most viral types. Repeat filtration through a 0.1 μm filter is more effective in this regard. Alternatively, incorporation of an ultrafiltration step (preferably at the terminal stages of downstream processing) also proves effective. Incorporation of downstream processing steps known to inactivate a wide variety of viral types provides further assurance that the final product is unlikely to harbour active virus. Heating and irradiation are amongst the two most popular such approaches. Heating the product to between 40 and 60°C for several hours inactivates a broad range of viruses. Many biopharmaceuticals can be heated to such temperatures without being denatured themselves. Such an approach has been used extensively to inactivate blood-borne viruses in blood products. Exposure of product to controlled levels of UV radiation can also be quite effective, while having no adverse effect on the product itself.

Viral Assays

A range of assay techniques may be used to detect and quantify viral contaminants in both raw materials and finished-biopharmaceutical products. No generic assay exists that is capable of detecting all viral types potentially present in a given sample. Viral assays currently available will detect only a specific virus, or at best a family of closely related viruses. The strategy adopted, therefore, usually entails screening product for viral particles known to be capable of infecting the biopharmaceutical source material. Such assays will not normally detect newly evolved viral strains, or uncharacterized/ unknown viral contaminants. This fact underlines the importance of including at least one step in downstream processing that is likely to inactivate or remove viruses indiscriminately from the product. This acts as a safety net. Current viral assays fall into one of three categories:

- Immunoassays;
- Assays based on viral DNA probes;
- Bioassays.

Generation of antibodies that can recognize and bind to specific viruses is straightforward. A sample of live or attenuated virus, or a purified component of the viral caspid, can be injected into animals to stimulate polyclonal antibody production (or to facilitate monoclonal antibody production by hybridoma technology). Harvested antibodies are then employed to develop specific immunoassays that can be used to screen test samples routinely for the presence of that specific virus. Immunoassays capable of detecting a wide range of viruses are available commercially. The sensitivity, ease, speed and relative inexpensiveness of these assays render them particularly attractive. An alternative assay format entails the use of virus-specific DNA probes. These can be used to screen the biopharmaceutical product for the presence of viral DNA. The assay strategy is similar to the dot blot assays used to detect host-cell-derived DNA contaminants, as discussed earlier. Viral bioassays of various different formats have also been developed. One format entails incubation of the final product with cell lines sensitive to a range of viruses. The cells are subsequently monitored for cytopathic effects or other obvious signs of viral infection. A range of mouse-, rabbit- or hamster-antibody production tests may also be undertaken. These bioassays entail administration of the product to a test animal. Any viral agents present will elicit production of antiviral antibodies in that animal. Serum samples (withdrawn from the animal approximately 4 weeks after product administration) are screened for the presence of antibodies recognizing a range of viral antigens. This can be achieved by enzyme immunoassay, in which immobilized antigen is used to screen for the virus-specific antibodies. These assay systems are extremely sensitive, as minute quantities of viral antigen will elicit strong antibody production. A single serum sample can also be screened for antibodies specific to a wide range of viral particles. Time and expense factors, however, militate against this particular assay format.

Miscellaneous Contaminants

In addition to those already discussed, biopharmaceutical products may harbour other contaminants, some of which may be intentionally added to the product stream during the initial stages of downstream processing. Examples could include buffer components, precipitants (ethanol or other solvents, salts, etc.), proteolytic inhibitors, glycerol, anti-foam agents, etc. In addition to these, other contaminants may enter the product during downstream processing in a less controlled way. Examples could include metal ions leached from product-holding tanks/pipework, or breakdown products leaking from chromatographic media. The final product containers must also be chosen carefully. They must be chemically inert and be of suitable quality to eliminate the possibility of leaching of any substance from the container during product storage. For this reason, high-quality glass vials are often used.

In some instances it may be necessary to demonstrate that all traces of specific contaminants have been removed prior to final product filling. This would be true, for example, of many proteolytic inhibitors added during the initial stages of downstream processing to prevent proteolysis by endogenous proteases. Some such inhibitors may be inherently toxic, and many could (inappropriately) inhibit endogenous proteases of the recipient patient.

Demonstration of absence from the product of breakdown products from chromatographic columns may be necessary in certain instances. This is particularly true with regard to some affinity chromatography columns. Various chemical-coupling methods may be used to attach affinity ligands to the chromatographic support material. Some such procedures entail the use of toxic reagents, which, if not entirely removed after coupling, could leach into the product. In some cases ligands can also subsequently leach from the columns, particularly after sustained usage or overvigorous sanitation procedures. Improvements in the chemical stability of modern chromatographic media, however, have reduced such difficulties, and most manufacturers have carried out extensive validation studies regarding the stability of their product.

Sophisticated analytical methodologies facilitate detection of vanishingly low levels of many contaminants in biopharmaceutical preparations. The possibility exists, however, that uncharacterized contaminants may persist, remaining undetected in the final product. As an additional safety measure, finished products are often subjected to 'abnormal toxicity' or '*general safety*' tests. Standardized protocols for such tests are outlined in various international pharmacopoeias. These normally entail parenteral administration of the product to at least five healthy mice. The animals are placed under observation for 48 h and should exhibit no ill effects (other than expected symptoms). The death or illness of one or more animals signals a requirement for further investigation, usually using a larger number of animals. Such toxicity testing represents a safety net, designed to expose any unexpected activities in the product that could compromise the health of the recipient.

Validation Studies

Validation can be defined as 'the act of proving that any procedure, process, equipment, material, activity or system leads to the expected results'. Routine and adequate validation studies form a core principle of GMP as applied to (bio)pharmaceutical manufacture, as such studies help assure the overall safety of the finished product. All validation procedures must be carefully designed and fully documented in written format. The results of all validation studies undertaken must also be documented, and retained in the plant files. As part of their routine inspection of manufacturing facilities, regulatory personnel will usually inspect a sample of these records, to ensure conformance to GMP.

Validation studies encompass all aspects of (bio)pharmaceutical manufacture. All new items of equipment must be validated before being routinely used. Initial validation studies should be comprehensive, with follow-up validation studies being undertaken at appropriate time intervals (e.g. daily, weekly or monthly). It is considered judicious to validate older items of equipment with increased frequency. Such studies can forewarn the manufacturer of impending equipment failure. Some validatory studies are straightforward, e.g. validation of weighing equipment simply entails weighing of standardized weights. Autoclaves may be validated by placing external temperature probes at various points in the autoclave chamber during a routine autoclave run. Validation studies should confirm that all areas within the chamber reach the required temperature for the required time.

Periodic validation of clean room air (HEPA) filters is also an essential part of GMP. After their installation, HEPA filters are subjected to a leak test. Particle counters are also used to validate cleanroom conditions. A particle counter is a vacuum-cleaner-like machine capable of sucking air from its surroundings at constant velocity and passing it through a counting chamber. The number of particles per cubic metre of air tested can easily be determined. Furthermore, passage of the air through a 0.2 μm filter housed in the counter will trap all airborne microorganisms. By placing the filter on the surface of a nutrient-agar-containing Petri dish, trapped microorganisms will grow as colonies, allowing determination of the microbial load per cubic metre of air.

In addition to equipment, many processes/procedures undertaken during pharmaceutical manufacture are also subject to periodic validation studies. Validation of biopharmaceutical aseptic filling procedures is amongst the most critical. The aim is to prove that the aseptic procedures devised are capable of delivering a sterile finished product, as intended.

Aseptic filling validation entails substituting a batch of final product with nutrient broth. The broth is subject to sterile filtration and aseptic processing. After sealing the final product containers, they are incubated at 3 0–37 °C, which encourages growth of any contaminant microorganisms. (Growth can be easily monitored by subsequently measuring the absorbance at 600 nm.) Absence of growth validates the aseptic procedures developed.

Contaminant-clearance validation studies are of special significance in biopharmaceutical manufacture. Downstream processing must be capable of removing contaminants such as viruses, DNA and endotoxin from the product steam. Contaminant-clearance validation studies normally entail spiking the raw material (from which the product is to be purified) with a known level of the chosen contaminant and subjecting the contaminated material to the complete downstream processing protocol. This allows determination of the level of clearance of the contaminant achieved after each purification step, and the contaminant reduction factor for the overall process.

Viral clearance studies, for example, are typically undertaken by spiking the raw material with a mixture of at least three different viral species, preferably ones that represent likely product contaminants, and for which straightforward assay systems are available. Loading levels of up to 1×10^{10} viral particles are commonly used. The cumulative viral removal/inactivation observed should render the likelihood of a single viral particle remaining in a single therapeutic dose of product being greater that one in a million. A similar strategy is adopted when undertaking DNA clearance studies. The starting material is spiked with radiolabelled DNA and then subjected to downstream processing. The level of residual DNA remaining in the product stream after each step can easily be determined by monitoring for radioactivity. The quantity of DNA used to spike the product should ideally be somewhat in excess of the levels of DNA normally associated with the product prior to its purification. However, spiking of the product with a vast excess of DNA is counterproductive, in that it may render subsequent downstream processing unrepresentative of standard production runs.

For more comprehensive validation studies, the molecular mass profile of the DNA spike should roughly approximate to the molecular mass range of endogenous contaminant DNA in the crude product. Obviously, the true DNA clearance rate attained by downstream processing procedures (e.g. gel filtration) will depend to some extent on the molecular mass characteristics of the contaminant DNA. Other manufacturing procedures requiring validation include cleaning, decontamination and sanitation (CDS) procedures developed for specific items of equipment/processing areas. Of particular importance is the ability of such procedures to remove bioburden. This may be assessed by monitoring levels of microbial contamination before and after application of CDS protocols to the equipment item in question.

10

Antifungal and Antiparasitic Drugs

In addition to bacteria and viruses, several parasitic microorganisms may produce infections in humans. In particular, certain species of fungi, protozoa, and helminths (worms) frequently cause infections in humans. Although some types of parasitic infections are limited or unknown in developed nations such as the United States, parasitic infections generally represent the most common form of disease worldwide. These infections are especially prevalent in tropical and subtropical environments and in impoverished areas of the world where sanitation and hygiene are inadequate. In addition, the incidence of serious fungal and other parasitic infections has been increasing in industrialized nations because of the increased susceptibility of immunocompromised patients, such as patients with acquired immunodeficiency syndrome (AIDS), to these infections. Hence, the effective pharmacologic treatment of these infections remains an important topic in the global management of disease.

The pharmacologic treatment of parasitic infections is a complex and extensive topic. In this limited space, it is difficult to describe the many species of each parasite, all the diseases caused by parasites, and the chemical methods currently available to selectively destroy various fungi, protozoa, and helminths in humans. Consequently, the general aspects of each type of parasitic infection are reviewed briefly, followed by the primary drugs used to treat specific fungal, protozoal, and helminthic infections. This discussion will acquaint physical therapists and occupational therapists with the nature of these types of infections and the basic chemotherapeutic techniques and agents that are used to treat these problems.

Antifungal Agents

Fungi are plantlike microorganisms that exist ubiquitously throughout the soil and air and in plants and animals. Although abundant in nature (about 100,000 species exist), only a few species produce serious infections in humans. A disease caused by fungal infection is also referred to as a *mycosis*. Some fungal infections are relatively local or superficial, affecting cutaneous and mucocutaneous tissue. Examples of common superficial fungal infections include the tinea (ringworm) infections that cause problems such as athlete's foot. Common mucocutaneous fungal infections include candidiasis and yeast infections of vaginal tissues. Other fungal infections are deeper or more systemic. For instance, fungal infections may affect the lungs, central nervous system (CNS), or other tissues and organs throughout the body.

Often, fungal infections are relatively innocuous because they can be destroyed by the body's normal immune defense mechanisms. However, some infections require pharmacologic treatment, especially if the patient's endogenous defense mechanisms are compromised in some way. For instance, patients undergoing immunosuppressive drug treatment with glucocorticoids or certain antibiotics may develop systemic fungal infections. In addition, diseases that attack the immune system, such as AIDS, leave the patient vulnerable to severe fungal infections. Fungal infections that are relatively easy to treat in the immunocompetent person may become invasive and life threatening in those who lack adequate immune function. Hence, there is a significant need for effective systemic antifungal agents in certain high-risk patients. Certain drugs can be administered systemically to treat infections in various tissues. Other agents are more toxic; their use is limited to local or topical application for fungal infections in the skin and mucous membranes.

Systemic Antifungal Agents

The antifungal agents that can be administered systemically by oral or intravenous routes are listed here. These agents are often used to treat invasive (deep) fungal infections in the body, or they can be administered systemically to treat more superficial infections that have disseminated over a large area of the skin or subcutaneous tissues. The clinical use, mechanism of action, and potential adverse effects of these drugs are addressed here.

Amphotericin B

Clinical use. Amphotericin B (Amphocin, Fungizone Intravenous) is one of the primary drugs used to treat severe systemic fungal infections. This drug is often chosen to treat systemic infections and meningitis caused by *Candida*, *Cryptococcus*, and several other species of pathogenic fungi. Amphotericin is also effective against certain protozoal infection such as leishmaniasis. Typically, this drug is administered by slow intravenous infusion. Local and topical administration may also be used to treat limited infections caused by susceptible fungi.

Several newer forms of amphotericin B (Abelcet, AmBisome, Amphotec) have also been developed. These drugs are encapsulated in small lipid spheres (liposomes) and then injected slowly by intravenous infusion. The lipid-based preparations appear to deliver higher doses of amphotericin B to the site of fungal infections more directly, thereby reducing the risk of adverse effects such as renal toxicity. Clinical studies suggest that these lipid forms can therefore be used to treat serious fungal infections while reducing the risk of nephrotoxicity and other side effects.

Mechanism of action. Amphotericin B appears to work by binding to specific steroid-like lipids (sterols) located in the cell membrane of susceptible fungi. This binding causes increased permeability in the cell membrane, leading to a leaky membrane and loss of cellular components.

Adverse effects. The effectiveness of amphotericin B against serious systemic fungal infections is tempered somewhat by a high incidence of side effects. Most patients experience problems such as headache, fever, muscle and joint pain, muscle weakness, and gastrointestinal distress (nausea, vomiting, stomach pain or cramping). As indicated, nephrotoxicity may also occur in some patients, but the use of the lipid-based formulations of this drug may reduce this risk. Considering the life-threatening nature of some fungal infections such as meningitis, certain side effects of amphotericin B must often be tolerated while the drug exerts its antifungal actions.

Fluconazole

Clinical use. Fluconazole (Diflucan) can be administered orally to treat serious systemic fungal infections. This drug is often the primary treatment for urinary tract infections, pneumonia, and infections of the mouth and esophagus caused by the *Candida* species of fungus. This agent may also be used to treat cryptococcal meningitis and may help prevent recurrence of cryptococcal infections in patients with AIDS. Fluconazole is somewhat less toxic than more traditional agents such as amphotericin B, and can be administered orally, which is an advantage over amphotericin B. There is some concern, however, about fluconazole's effectiveness in treating deep, systemic fungal infections in severely ill patients. Hence, this drug can be combined with other antifungals such as amphotericin B to provide optimal treatment for certain cases of candidiasis and other severe fungal infections.

Mechanism of action. Fluconazole and similar agents (itraconazole, ketoconazole) inhibit certain enzymes in fungal cells that are responsible for the synthesis of important sterols. A deficiency of these sterols results in impaired membrane function and other metabolic abnormalities within the fungal cell. Fluconazole also directly damages the fungal membrane by destroying certain membrane components such as triglycerides and phospholipids. Loss of normal membrane structure and function results in the destruction of the fungus.

Adverse effects. Hepatotoxicity is the most serious adverse effect of fluconazole; this drug should be used cautiously in patients with impaired liver function. Other common side effects include headache and gastrointestinal disturbances (abdominal pain, nausea, vomiting).

Flucytosine

Clinical use. The antifungal spectrum of flucytosine (Ancobon) is limited primarily to the *Candida* and *Cryptococcus* species. This drug is used systemically to treat endocarditis, urinary tract infections, and the presence of fungi in the bloodstream (fungemia) during candidiasis. Flucytosine is also used to treat meningitis and severe pulmonary infections caused by cryptococcosis. This drug is often combined with amphotericin B to provide optimal effects and to decrease the chance of fungal resistance.

Mechanism of action. Flucytosine is incorporated into susceptible fungi, where it undergoes enzymatic conversion to fluorouracil, which acts as an antimetabolite during RNA synthesis in the fungus. Fluorouracil is incorporated into RNA chains but acts as a false nucleic acid. This event ultimately impairs protein synthesis, thus disrupting the normal function of the fungus.

Adverse effects. Flucytosine may cause hepatotoxicity and may also impair bone marrow function, resulting in anemia, leukopenia, and several other blood dyscrasias. This drug may also produce severe gastrointestinal disturbances, including nausea, vomiting, diarrhea, and loss of appetite.

Griseofulvin

Clinical use. Griseofulvin (Fulvicin, Grisactin, other names) is used primarily in the treatment of common fungal infections of the skin known as tinea, or ringworm. For example, this drug is administered to treat fungal infections of the feet (tinea pedis, or "athlete's foot"), infections in the groin area (tinea cruris, or "jock rash"), and similar infections of the skin, nails, and scalp. Griseofulvin is administered orally.

Mechanism of action. Griseofulvin enters susceptible fungal cells and binds to the mitotic spindle during cell division. This binding impairs the mitotic process, thus directly inhibiting the ability of the cell to replicate itself.

Adverse effects. Common side effects of griseofulvin administration include headaches—which may be severe—and gastrointestinal disturbances (nausea, vomiting, diarrhea). Some individuals may exhibit hypersensitivity to this drug as evidenced by skin rashes. Skin photosensitivity (increased reaction to ultraviolet light) may also occur.

Itraconazole

Clinical use. Itraconazole (Sporanox) is an azole antifungal agent that is effective against many systemic fungal infections. For example, this drug is used to treat blastomycosis and histoplasmosis infections in the lungs and other tissues, especially in patients with a compromised immune system. Itraconazole may also be used as the primary or alternative treatment for other fungal infections, such as aspergillosis, chromomycosis, coccidioidomycosis, and various infections caused by the *Candida* species. Like fluconazole, itraconazole can be administered orally and can be given intravenously in severe systemic infections.

Mechanism of action. Itraconazole works like fluconazole and similar azoles. These drugs disrupt membrane function of the fungal cell by inhibiting the synthesis of key membrane components such as sterols. and by directly damaging other membrane components such as phospholipids. Impaired membrane function leads to metabolic abnormalities and subsequent death of the fungal cell.

Adverse effects. Side effects associated with itraconazole include headache, gastrointestinal disturbances (nausea, vomiting), and skin rash.

Ketoconazole

Clinical use. Ketoconazole (Nizoral) is used to treat a variety of superficial and deep fungal infections. This drug can be administered orally to treat pulmonary and systemic infections in candidiasis, coccidioidomycosis, histoplasmosis, and several other types of deep fungal infections. Oral administration is also used to treat tinea infections of the skin, scalp, and other body areas. Ketoconazole is available in topical preparations for the treatment of tinea infections and other relatively localized infections, including certain vaginal infections.

Mechanism of action. Ketoconazole selectively inhibits certain enzymes that are responsible for the synthesis of important sterols in fungal cells. A deficiency of sterols results in impaired membrane function and other metabolic abnormalities within the fungal cell. At higher concentrations, ketoconazole may also directly disrupt the cell membrane, resulting in the destruction of the fungus.

Adverse effects. Gastrointestinal disturbances (nausea, vomiting, stomach pain) are the most common adverse effects when ketoconazole is administered systemically. Some degree of hepatotoxicity may occur, and severe or even fatal hepatitis has been reported on rare occasions. In large, prolonged dosages, this drug may also impair testosterone and adrenocorticosteroid synthesis, resulting in breast tenderness and enlargement (gynecomastia) and decreased sex drive in some men. Because of these side effects, other drugs such as itraconazole have largely replaced systemic use of ketoconazole.

Echinocandins

Clinical use. Echinocandins comprise a relatively new group of antifungals that includes drugs such as caspofungin (Cancidas) and micafungin (Mycamine). These drugs are administered intravenously to treat severe esophageal infections caused by *Candida.* Caspofungin is also used to treat systemic aspergillosis infections in patients who cannot tolerate other drugs such as amphotericin B or fluconazole. Other echinocandin drugs are currently being developed, and their use may expand in the future if newer agents reach the market.

Mechanism of action. These drugs inhibit the glucan synthase enzyme that is responsible for the biosynthesis of beta-D-glucan—a component of the fungal cell membrane. Loss of this membrane component disrupts the integrity of the fungal cell wall, resulting in death of the fungus.

Adverse Effects. Primary side effects of caspofungin and micafungin include gastrointestinal disturbances (nausea, vomiting) and headache. Some local irritation may also occur at the injection site when these drugs are administered intravenously.

Terbinafine

Clinical use. Terbinafine (Lamisil) is effective against a broad spectrum of fungi and can be administered systemically to treat infections in the toenails and fingernails (onychomycosis) that are caused by various fungi. Oral administration of this drug may also be useful in treating ringworm infections such as tinea corporis, tinea capitis (ringworm of the scalp), and tinea cruris, especially if these infections do not respond to topical treatment. Terbinafine is likewise available in creams and solutions for topical treatment of various tinea infections, including tinea pedis and tinea versicolor.

Mechanism of action. Terbinafine inhibits a specific enzyme (squalene epoxidase) that is responsible for sterol synthesis in the fungal cell membrane. This action impairs cell wall synthesis, with subsequent loss of cell membrane function and integrity. Inhibition of this enzyme causes squalene to accumulate in the fungal cell, which can also impair cell function and lead to death of the fungus.

Adverse effects. Systemic administration of terbinafine may cause a hypersensitivity reaction (skin rashes, itching) and gastrointestinal problems such as nausea, vomiting, and diarrhea. This drug may also cause a change or loss of taste, an effect that may last several weeks after the drug is discontinued. Topical administration is generally well tolerated, although signs of local irritation (itching, redness, peeling skin) may indicate a need to discontinue this drug.

Voriconazole

Clinical use. Voriconazole (Vfend) is similar chemically to other azole antifungals such as fluconazole. Voriconazole has a broad antifungal spectrum, and is administered systemically to treat aspergillosis and other serious fungal infections caused by *Scedosporium apiospermum* and *Fusarium*.

Mechanism of action. Voriconazole inhibits sterol biosynthesis in fungal cell membranes. That is, this drug acts like fluconazole and similar agents to impair membrane synthesis, which results in membrane integrity loss and death of the fungal cell.

Adverse effects. Skin rashes and vision disturbances (blurred vision, seeing bright spots) are common during voriconazole administration, but these side effects are usually transient and fairly uneventful. Serious problems, such as liver toxicity and cardiac arrhythmias, may occur in susceptible patients.

Topical Antifungal Agents

As mentioned earlier, certain antifungals are too toxic to be administered systemically, but these drugs can be applied topically to treat fungal infections in the skin and mucous membranes. These drugs are therefore commonly used to treat various fungal infections in the skin (dermatophytosis), including tinea infections such as tinea pedis and tinea cruris. These drugs can also be applied locally to treat *Candida* infections in the mucous membranes of the mouth, pharynx, and vagina.

Topical azole antifungals

Clinical use. These drugs are related to the systemic azoles (fluconazole, itraconazole, ketoconazole; see earlier) and share a common chemical background, mechanism of action, and antifungal spectrum. The topical azoles, however, are too toxic for systemic use and are therefore restricted to local application. Nonetheless, these drugs are valuable in controlling fungal infections in the skin and mucocutaneous tissues. For example, azoles such as butoconazole, clotrimazole, miconazole, terconazole, and tioconazole can be applied via creams, ointments, and suppositories to treat vaginal *Candida* infections. Other agents such as econazole, oxiconazole, and sulconazole can be applied via creams, solutions, or powders to treat tinea infections that cause athlete's foot (tinea pedis) and jock rash (tinea cruris). Certain azoles can also be applied locally via lozenges or elixirs (syrups) to treat oral candidiasis infections that occur in patients with a compromised immune system. Hence, these agents are used to treat local mycoses that occur in a variety of clinical situations.

Mechanism of action. Like the systemic azoles, clotrimazole and other topical antifungal azoles work by inhibiting the synthesis of key components of the fungal cell membrane; that is, these drugs impair production of membrane sterols, triglycerides, and phospholipids. Loss of these components results in the membrane's inability to maintain intracellular homeostasis, leading to death of the fungus.

Adverse effects. There are relatively few side effects when these drugs are applied locally. Gastrointestinal distress (cramps, diarrhea, vomiting) can occur if azole lozenges are swallowed. Other problems associated with topical use include local burning or irritation of the skin or mucous membranes.

Other topical agents

Clinical use. Other topical antifungals include nystatin (Mycostatin, Nilstat, others), naftifine (Naftin), butenafine (Mentax), and tolnaftate (Aftate, Tinactin, other names). Nystatin has a wide spectrum of activity against various fungi, but is not used to treat systemic infections because it is not absorbed from the gastrointestinal tract. Therefore, nystatin is administered via several topical preparations to treat cutaneous, oropharyngeal, or vaginal candidiasis. Topical and local (oropharyngeal) use of nystatin is especially important in treating candidiasis in immunocompromised patients, including patients with AIDS.

Naftifine, tolnaftate, and butenafine are used primarily to treat local and superficial cases of tinea infection. These agents are found in several over-the- counter products that are administered topically to treat tinea infections such as tinea pedis and tinea cruris.

Mechanism of action. Nystatin exerts its antifungal effects in a manner similar to that of amphotericin B: that is, this drug binds to sterols in the cell membrane, which causes an increase in membrane permeability and a loss of cellular homeostasis. Naftifine and butenafine inhibit a fungal enzyme (squalene epoxidase) that is responsible for the synthesis of a key membrane component (ergosterol), resulting in the loss of membrane integrity and death of the fungus. Tolnaftate appears to stunt the growth of fungal cell bodies, but the exact mechanism of this drug is unknown.

Adverse effects. Nystatin is generally well tolerated when applied locally. Systemic absorption through mucous membranes may cause some gastrointestinal disturbances (nausea, vomiting, diarrhea), but these side effects are generally mild and transient. Topical use of butenafine, naftifine, and tolnaftate is likewise safe, although local burning and irritation of the skin may occur in some individuals.

Antiprotozoal Agents

Protozoa are single-celled organisms that represent the lowest division of the animal kingdom. Of the several thousand species of protozoa, approximately 35 represent a threat of parasitic infection in humans.

One relatively common disease caused by protozoal infection is malaria. Malaria is caused by several species of a protozoan parasite known as plasmodia. Although this disease has been virtually eliminated in North America and Europe, malaria continues to be a primary health problem throughout many other parts of the world. Individuals who live in these areas, as well as those traveling to parts of the world where malaria is prevalent, must often undergo antimalarial chemotherapy. Hence, drugs that prevent and treat malaria are extremely important.

In addition to malaria, several other serious infections may occur in humans due to parasitic invasion by protozoa. Severe intestinal infections (dysentery) produced by various protozoa occur quite frequently, especially in areas where contaminated food and drinking water are prevalent. Infections in tissues such as the liver, heart, lungs, brain, and other organs may also occur because of protozoal infestation. As mentioned in this chapter's introduction, individuals with a compromised immune system may be especially susceptible to these intestinal and extraintestinal infections. Drugs that are primarily used to treat and prevent malaria are grouped together, followed by drugs that are used to treat other types of protozoal infections (intestinal and extraintestinal infections).

Antimalarial Agents

Chloroquine

Clinical use. Historically, chloroquine (Aralen) has been one of the primary antimalarial drugs. This drug provides a safe, effective, and relatively inexpensive method for treating malaria, and is also administered routinely to individuals who are traveling to areas of the world where they may be exposed to malaria infection. Resistance to this drug, however, has emerged in many areas of the world where malaria is prevalent. That is, the parasite that causes this disease (the *Plasmodium* amoeba) has developed mechanisms that render this drug ineffective. If these chloroquine-resistant strains are encountered, other antimalarial drugs such as quinine or artemisinin derivatives must be used.

Chloroquine is also used for the treatment of conditions other than malaria. This drug is effective against other types of protozoal infections such as amebiasis and may be used with iodoquinol or emetine to treat infections in the liver and pericardium. Chloroquine is effective in rheumatoid disease and is used in the treatment of conditions such as rheumatoid arthritis and systemic lupus erythematosus. However, the reasons why this antiprotozoal agent is also effective against rheumatoid disease are unclear. Chloroquine is administered orally.

Mechanism of action. Although the exact mechanism is unknown, chloroquine may impair metabolic and digestive function in the protozoa by becoming concentrated within subcellular vacuoles and raising the pH of these vacuoles. This effect may inhibit the ability of the parasite to digest hemoglobin from the blood of the host erythrocytes. Impaired hemoglobin digestion leads to the accumulation of toxic heme by-products in the protozoa, which subsequently leads to death of this parasite. Chloroquine may also bind directly to DNA within susceptible parasites and inhibit DNA/RNA function and subsequent protein synthesis. The ability to impair protein synthesis may contribute to the antiprotozoal actions of this drug.

Adverse effects. The most serious problem associated with chloroquine is the possibility of toxicity to the retina and subsequent visual disturbances. This issue is usually insignificant, however, when this drug is used for short periods in relatively low doses. Other relatively mild side effects may occur, including gastrointestinal distress (nausea, vomiting, stomach cramps, diarrhea), behavior and mood changes (irritability, confusion, nervousness, depression), and skin disorders (rashes, itching, discoloration).

Hydroxychloroquine

Hydroxychloroquine (Plaquenil) is derived chemically from chloroquine and is similar to it in clinical use, mechanism of action, and adverse effects. Hydroxy-chloroquine does not have any distinct therapeutic advantages over chloroquine, but it may be substituted in certain individuals who do not respond well to chloroquine.

Mefloquine

Clinical use. Mefloquine (Lariam) has emerged as one of the most important antimalarial agents. This drug is especially important in the prevention and treatment of malaria that is resistant to traditional antimalarial drugs such as chloroquine and quinine. Mefloquine is often the drug of choice for antimalarial prophylaxis, especially in areas of the world where chloroquine-resistant strains of malaria are common. Mefloquine can be used alone, but combining this drug with other antimalarials such as an artemisinin derivative may provide more effective treatment against malaria.

Mechanism of action. Although the drug's exact mechanism of action is unknown, mefloquine may exert antimalarial effects similar to chloroquine; that is, these drugs inhibit hemoglobin digestion in malarial parasites, thus causing heme by-products to accumulate within the protozoa and cause toxicity and death of this parasite.

Adverse effects. Mefloquine is safe and well tolerated when used at moderate doses to prevent malarial infection. At higher doses, such as those used to treat infection, mefloquine may cause dizziness, headache, fever, joint and muscle pain, and gastrointestinal problems (abdominal pain, nausea, vomiting, diarrhea). These side effects, however, may be difficult to distinguish from the symptoms associated with malaria. Although rare, neuropsychiatric symptoms such as confusion, psychosis, and seizures may occur, especially when this drug is used at higher dosages for prolonged periods.

Primaquine

Clinical use. Primaquine is typically used to treat the relapses of specific forms of malaria, and is generally administered in acute or severe exacerbations, or when other drugs (chloroquine, mefloquine) are ineffective in suppressing malarial attacks. Primaquine may also be used to prevent the onset of malaria in individuals who are especially at risk because of prolonged exposure to the disease. This drug is administered orally.

Mechanism of action. Primaquine appears to impair DNA function in susceptible parasites. The exact manner in which this occurs is unknown.

Adverse effects. Gastrointestinal disturbances (nausea, vomiting, abdominal pain), headache, and visual disturbances may occur during primaquine therapy. A more serious side effect, acute hemolytic anemia, may occur in patients who have a specific deficiency in the enzyme glucose-6-phosphate dehydrogenase. This enzymatic deficiency is genetic, and is more common in certain individuals of African, Mediterranean, and Asian descent; hence there is an increased risk of hemolytic anemia in these groups. People with specific cases of this enzyme deficiency should be identified so that alternative antimalarial drugs can be used.

Pyrimethamine

Clinical use. When used alone, pyrimethamine (Daraprim) is only of minor use in treating and preventing malaria. However, the antimalarial effectiveness of pyrimethamine is increased dramatically by combining it with the antibacterial drug sulfadoxine. The combination of these two drugs (known commercially as Fansidar) has been used to prevent or treat certain forms of chloroquine-resistant malaria. Regrettably, resistance to pyrimethamine/ sulfadoxine treatment has also increased in many areas to the point where this drug combination is no longer effective.

Pyrimethamine may also be combined with other antimalarials such as artemisinin derivatives, but these regimens should only be used if the malarial parasites are not resistant to the specific drugs in the regimen. Pyrimethamine can also be combined with a sulfonamide drug such as dapsone, sulfadiazine, or sulfamethoxazole to treat protozoal infections that cause toxoplasmosis, or fungal infections that cause *Pneumocystis* pneumonia. These agents are administered orally.

Mechanism of action. Pyrimethamine blocks the production of folic acid in susceptible protozoa by inhibiting the function of the dihydrofolate reductase enzyme. Folic acid helps catalyze the production of nucleic and amino acids in these parasites. Therefore, this drug ultimately impairs nucleic acid and protein synthesis by interfering with folic acid production. These agents also inhibit folic acid synthesis in certain bacterial and protozoal cells.

Adverse effects. The incidence and severity of side effects from pyrimethamine-sulfadoxine are related to the dosage and duration of therapy. Toxicity is fairly common when these drugs are given in high dosages for prolonged periods, and adverse effects include gastrointestinal disturbances (vomiting, stomach cramps, loss of appetite), blood dyscrasias (agranulocytosis, leukopenia, thrombocytopenia), CNS abnormalities (tremors, ataxia, seizures), and hypersensitivity reactions (skin rashes, anaphylaxis, liver dysfunction). As indicated above, resistance may also occur during repeated use, and this drug strategy may be ineffective in certain strains of malaria that have already developed resistant mechanisms. Hence, pyrimethamine-sulfadoxine is usually administered on a very limited basis, such as a single dose at the onset of malarial symptoms.

Quinine

Clinical use. Quinine is one of the oldest forms of antimalarial chemotherapy, having been obtained from the bark of certain South American trees as early as the 1600s. Although quinine was the principal method of preventing and treating malaria for many years, the use of this drug has diminished somewhat because it is relatively toxic and expensive to produce. Hence, the routine use of this drug has largely been replaced by newer, safer agents such as mefloquine and artemisinin derivatives. Quinine, however, remains one of the most effective antimalarial drugs and is currently used to treat severe malaria that is resistant to other drugs. Quinine sulfate is administered orally, and quinine dihydrochloride is administered by slow intravenous infusion.

Mechanism of action. The exact mechanism of quinine is not known. This drug probably exerts antimalarial effects similar to those of chloroquine—that is, inhibition of hemoglobin digestion and subsequent accumulation of toxic heme by-products that lead to death in susceptible protozoa.

Adverse effects. Quinine is associated with many adverse effects involving several primary organ systems. This drug may produce disturbances in the CNS (headache, visual disturbances, ringing in the ears), gastrointestinal system (nausea, vomiting, abdominal pain), and cardiovascular system (cardiac arrhythmias). Problems with hypersensitivity, blood disorders, liver dysfunction, and hypoglycemia may also occur in some individuals.

Other antimalarials: Use of artemisinin derivatives

Clinical use. Artemisinin derivatives are naturally occurring compounds that appear to be effective against many forms of the protozoa that cause malaria. These drugs consist of the parent compound (artemisinin) and several products that can be synthesized from artemisinin such as artesunate, artemether, and dihydroartemisinin. It does not appear that any one derivative is superior to another in treating malaria, hence the term artemisinin derivative can be used to collectively describe this group. These agents act rapidly and appear to be effective against all malarial parasites that infect humans. Moreover, resistance to artemisinin derivatives has not yet emerged, so these drugs have moved to the forefront as primary antimalarial agents, especially in parts of the world where resistance to traditional drugs is problematic. Artemisinin derivatives can likewise be used alone or combined with other antimalarials (e.g., mefloquine or piperaquine) to improve efficacy and reduce the chance of drug resistance.

Mechanism of action. Artemisinin derivatives appear to work by a two-step process occurring within the malarial parasite. In the first step, the drug is activated when it is cleaved by the heme-iron component within the protozoa. This cleavage forms a highly reactive free radical that, in the second step, reacts with and destroys essential protozoal proteins. Destruction of these proteins results in the loss of cellular function and subsequent death of the protozoa.

Adverse effects. Because these drugs are fairly new, the potential for side effects remains to be determined fully. Studies on animals suggested that these drugs may be neurotoxic, but this effect has not been proven conclusively in humans. Future research should help determine the relative risks and benefits of these agents, as well as how artemisinin derivatives can complement other drugs in the antimalarial armamentarium.

Drugs Used to Treat Protozoal Infections in the Intestines and Other Tissues

Atovaquone

Clinical use. Atovaquone (Mepron) is used primarily to treat the protozoon that causes toxoplasmosis and the fungus that causes pneumocystis pneumonia in immunocompromised patients. This drug is not typically the primary treatment for pneumocystis, but is often reserved for patients who cannot tolerate more traditional treatments using sulfamethoxazole and trimethoprim or pentamidine. Atovaquone can also be used to prevent and treat resistant cases of malaria, and the antimalarial effects of this drug seem especially useful when combined with proguanil.

Mechanism of action. Atovaquone appears to selectively inhibit electron transport in susceptible microorganisms. This inhibition directly decreases production of ATP in the microorganism and may interfere with nucleic acid synthesis, ultimately resulting in death of the parasite.

Adverse effects. Atovaquone may cause side effects such as fever, skin rash, cough, headache, and gastrointestinal problems (nausea, vomiting, diarrhea).

Emetine and dehydroemetine

Clinical use. Emetine and dehydroemetine (Mebadin) are used primarily to treat protozoal infections in the intestinal tract and extraintestinal sites such as the lungs and liver. These drugs are powerful amebicides and are generally reserved for severe, acute cases of intestinal amebiasis (dysentery). Because of the potential for adverse effects, these drugs are no longer marketed in the United States, and safer agents like metronidazole are often used in their place. Emetine and dehydroemetine are typically administered by deep subcutaneous injection or intramuscular injection.

Mechanism of action. These drugs exert a direct effect on susceptible protozoa by causing degeneration of subcellular components such as the nucleus and reticular system within the parasite.

Adverse effects. As indicated earlier, the effectiveness of emetine and dehydroemetine is limited by a number of potentially serious side effects. In particular, problems with cardiotoxicity may occur, as reflected by arrhythmias, palpitations, and other changes in cardiac conduction and excitability. Gastrointestinal disturbances such as diarrhea, nausea, and vomiting are also quite common. Generalized muscular aches and weakness may occur, as well as localized myositis near the site of administration. Hence, these drugs are administered under close medical supervision and are withdrawn as soon as the amebicidal effects are apparent.

Iodoquinol

Clinical use. Iodoquinol (Diquinol, Yodoxin, other names) is used primarily to treat protozoal infections within the intestinal tract, and it is often combined with a second tissue amebicide, which kills protozoa at extraintestinal sites. For instance, iodoquinol may be combined with metronidazole to ensure the destruction of parasites throughout the body. Iodoquinol is usually administered orally. Because iodoquinol is relatively toxic, the routine use of this drug has been replaced somewhat by other agents such as paromomycin, which may be somewhat safer.

Mechanism of action. The mechanism of action of iodoquinol as an amebicide is unknown.

Adverse effects. Iodoquinol is neurotoxic and may produce optic and peripheral neuropathies when administered in large dosages for prolonged periods. Problems with muscle weakness and ataxia may also occur because of the neurotoxic effects of this drug. Other adverse effects include gastrointestinal distress (nausea, vomiting, cramps) and various skin reactions (rashes, itching, discoloration), but these effects are relatively mild and transient.

Metronidazole

Clinical use. Metronidazole (Flagyl, Protostat, other names) is effective against a broad spectrum of protozoa and is often the primary agent used against protozoal infections in intestinal and extraintestinal tissues. Metronidazole is often the drug of choice for treating several intestinal infections (amebiasis, giardiasis) and amebic abscesses in other tissues such as the liver. Metronidazole is also the primary drug used to treat trichomoniasis, a sexually transmitted protozoal disease affecting the vagina and male genitourinary tract.

Metronidazole has bactericidal effects and is used in certain gram-negative bacterial infections. This drug may be administered orally or intravenously. Other agents have also been developed that are structurally and functionally similar to metronidazole. Tinidazole (Tindamax), for example, can be used in cases where metronidazole is not tolerated or is ineffective.

Mechanism of action. The exact mechanism of action of metronidazole is not known. It is believed that this drug is reduced chemically within the parasitic cell to a metabolite that impairs nucleic acid and DNA synthesis. The exact nature of this metabolite, however, and other features of the cytotoxic effects of this drug remain to be determined.

Adverse effects. Gastrointestinal disturbances including nausea, vomiting, diarrhea, stomach pain, and an unpleasant taste in the mouth are relatively common with metronidazole. Other adverse effects such as hypersensitivity reactions, peripheral neuropathy, hematologic abnormalities, and genitourinary problems have been reported, but their incidence is relatively low.

Nitazoxanide

Clinical use. Nitazoxanide (Alinia) is a relatively new agent that is used primarily to treat diarrhea caused by intestinal cryptosporidia and giardia infections. This drug is approved for use in children aged 1 to 11, and is administered orally.

Mechanism of action. Nitazoxanide appears to inhibit electron transport in susceptible protozoa, thus inhibiting energy metabolism in these parasites. This drug may have other antiprotozoal effects that remain to be determined.

Adverse effects. This drug is generally well tolerated. Gastrointestinal disturbances (vomiting, diarrhea) and headache have been reported, but these effects may be due to the intestinal infection rather than the drug.

Paromomycin

Clinical use. Paromomycin (Humatin) is an aminoglycoside antibacterial that is used primarily to treat mild to moderate intestinal infections (amebiasis). This drug may also be used as an adjunct to other amebicides during the treatment of more severe protozoal infections. Paromomycin is also effective against some bacteria and tapeworms, and may be used as a secondary agent in certain bacterial or helminthic infections. This drug is administered orally.

Mechanism of action. Paromomycin acts selectively on protozoa within the intestinal lumen and destroys these parasites by a direct toxic effect.

Adverse effects. Paromomycin is not absorbed from the intestine to any great extent, so adverse effects are fairly limited. Nonetheless, problems with gastrointestinal distress (nausea, vomiting, abdominal pain) may occur as this drug exerts amebicidal effects within the intestine.

Pentamidine

Clinical use. Pentamidine (Nebupent, Pentam, other names) is effective against several types of extraintestinal protozoal infections, including certain forms of trypanosomiasis (African sleeping sickness) and visceral infections caused by Leishmania protozoa. Typically, pentamidine is reserved as a secondary agent in treating these infections and is used when the principal drug in each case is not available or is tolerated poorly. Use of this drug as a primary agent has increased, however, in the treatment of pneumocystis infections in patients with AIDS. This drug is usually administered by parenteral routes such as deep intramuscular injection or slow intravenous infusion. Pentamidine may also be administered by oral inhalation to treat lung infections, and this strategy is now commonly used as prophylaxis and treatment of pneumocystis pneumonia in patients with AIDS.

Mechanism of action. The exact mechanism of this drug is not clear, and pentamidine may affect different parasites in different ways. Some possible antiprotozoal actions of this drug include the inhibition of protein and nucleic acid synthesis, cellular metabolism, and oxidative phosphorylation in susceptible parasites.

Adverse effects. The primary adverse effect of systemic pentamidine administration is renal toxicity. Renal function may be markedly impaired in some patients, but kidney function usually returns to normal when the drug is withdrawn. Other adverse effects include hypotension, hypoglycemia, gastrointestinal distress, blood dyscrasias (leukopenia, thrombocytopenia), and local pain and tenderness at the site of injection. Adverse effects are reduced substantially when the drug is given by inhalation, and this method of administration is desirable when pentamidine is used to prevent pneumocystis pneumonia in patients with human immunodeficiency virus (HIV) disease.

Other Antiprotozoal Drugs

Several additional agents have been developed to treat intestinal and extraintestinal infections caused by various protozoa. These agents include melarsoprol, nifurtimox, sodium stibogluconate, and suramin. The use and distribution of these drugs, however, is quite different from the agents described previously. In the United States, these additional drugs are usually available only from the Centers for Disease Control (CDC), in Atlanta, Georgia. At the request of the physician, the CDC dispenses the drug to the physician, who then provides the agent to the patient.

In general, these drugs are reserved for some of the more serious or rare types of protozoal infections. As might be expected, adverse side effects of these drugs are quite common. However, these drugs may be lifesaving in some of the more severe infections, which is why the CDC controls their distribution.

ANTHELMINTICS

Infection from helminths, or parasitic worms, is the most common form of disease in the world. There are several types of worms that may invade and subsist from human tissues. Common examples include tapeworms (cestodes), roundworms (nematodes), and flukes (trematodes). Worms can enter the body by various routes but often are ingested as eggs in contaminated food and water. Once in the body, the eggs hatch, and adult worms ultimately lodge in various tissues, especially the digestive tract. Some types (flukes) may also lodge in blood vessels such as the hepatic portal vein. Depending on the species, adult worms may range from a few millimeters to several meters in length. The adult worms begin to steal nutrients from their human host and may begin to obstruct the intestinal lumen or other ducts if they reproduce in sufficient numbers. These agents are often very effective; a single oral dose is usually sufficient to selectively destroy the parasite. Brief descriptions of the basic pharmacologic effects and possible adverse effects of the primary anthelmintic agents are presented below.

Albendazole

Albendazole (Albenza) is primarily used to treat infections caused by the larval form of certain cestodes (tapeworms). These infections often cause cysts (hydatid disease) in the liver, lungs, and other tissues; albendazole is used as an adjunct to the surgical removal of these cysts or as the primary treatment if these cysts are inoperable. This drug is also effective against many gastrointestinal roundworms and hookworms, and is typically used as a secondary agent if other anthelmintics are not effective in treating these infections.

Albendazole exerts its anthelmintic effects by acting on the intestinal cells of parasitic worms and by inhibiting glucose uptake and glycogen storage by these parasites. This effect ultimately leads to lack of energy production, degeneration of intracellular components, and subsequent death of the parasite. Albendazole is usually well tolerated when used for short-term treatment of infections in gastrointestinal or other tissues. Long-term treatment for conditions such as hydatid disease may result in abnormal liver function tests (e.g., increased serum aminotransferase activity), and liver function should therefore be monitored periodically to prevent hepatotoxicity if this drug is used for extended periods.

Diethylcarbamazine

Diethylcarbamazine (Hetrazan) is used to treat certain roundworm infections of the lymphatics and connective tissues, including loiasis, onchocerciasis, and *Bancroft filariasis*. This agent immobilizes immature roundworms (microfilariae) and facilitates the destruction of these microfilariae by the body's immune system. Diethylcarbamazine is also effective against the adult forms of certain roundworms.

but the mechanism of this anthelmintic action against mature nematodes is not known. Side effects associated with diethylcarbamazine include headache, malaise, weakness, and loss of appetite. More severe reactions (fever, acute inflammatory response) may also occur following diethylcarbamazine use, but these reactions may be caused by the release of antigenic substances from the dying roundworms rather than from the drug itself.

Ivermectin

Ivermectin (Mectizan, Stromectol) is the primary treatment for filarial nematode infections (onchocerciasis) that invade ocular tissues and cause loss of vision (river blindness). Ivermectin may also be used in filarial infections in other tissues (lymphatics, skin). This drug is a secondary agent for treating intestinal nematodes such as strongyloidosis.

Ivermectin binds to chloride ion channels in parasitic nerve and muscle cells, thereby increasing membrane permeability to chloride. Increased intracellular chloride results in hyperpolarization of nerve and muscle tissues, which results in paralysis and death of the parasite. Ivermectin is well tolerated during short- term use in mild-to-moderate infections. Administration in more severe infections may cause swollen or tender lymph glands, fever, skin rash, itching, and joint and muscle pain, but these reactions may be caused by the death of the infectious parasites rather than by the drug itself.

Mebendazole

Mebendazole (Vermox) is effective against many types of roundworms and a few tapeworms that parasitize humans. Like albendazole, this drug selectively damages intestinal cells in these worms, thus inhibiting the uptake and intracellular transport of glucose and other nutrients into these parasites. This activity leads to the destruction of the epithelial lining and subsequent death of the parasite. Mebendazole is a relatively safe drug, although some mild, transient gastrointestinal problems may occur.

Niclosamide

Niclosamide (Niclocide) is effective against several types of tapeworm. This drug inhibits certain mitochondrial enzymes in these parasites, which ultimately results in the breakdown of the protective integument of the worm, thus allowing the digestive enzymes in the host (human) intestine to attack the parasite. Ultimately, the worm is digested and expelled from the gastrointestinal tract. There are relatively few adverse effects of niclosamide treatment, probably because the drug is not absorbed to any great extent from the human intestine. Thus, this drug remains in the intestinal lumen, where it can act directly on the tapeworm.

Oxamniquine

Oxamniquine (Vansil) is effective against a genus of parasitic worms known as blood flukes (schistosomes). These parasites typically adhere to the wall of blood vessels such as the hepatic portal vein. Oxamniquine inhibits muscular contraction of the sucker that holds the fluke to the vessel wall, thus allowing the worm to dislodge and travel to the liver. In the liver, the parasite is engulfed and destroyed by hepatic phagocytes. Common side effects associated with this drug include headache, dizziness, and drowsiness. However, these adverse effects are generally mild and transient.

Piperazine Citrate

Piperazine citrate is typically used as a secondary agent in ascariasis (roundworm) and enterobiasis (pin-worm) infections. This drug appears to paralyze the worm by blocking the effect of acetylcholine at the parasite's neuromuscular junction. The paralyzed worm can then be dislodged and expelled from the host (human) intestine during normal bowel movements. Side effects such as headache, dizziness, and gastrointestinal disturbance may occur during piperazine citrate administration, but these effects are generally mild and transient.

Praziquantel

Praziquantel (Biltricide) is one of the most versatile and important anthelmintic agents, and is the drug of choice in treating all major trematode (fluke) infections and several common types of tapeworm infections. This drug's exact mechanism of action is unknown. Praziquantel may stimulate muscular contraction of the parasite, resulting in a type of spastic paralysis, which causes the worm to lose its hold on intestinal or vascular tissue. At higher concentrations, this drug may initiate destructive changes in the integument of the worm, allowing the host defense mechanisms (e.g., enzymes, phagocytes) to destroy the parasite. Praziquantel is associated with a number of frequent side effects, including gastrointestinal problems (abdominal pain, nausea, vomiting), CNS effects (headache, dizziness), and mild hepatotoxicity. These effects can usually be tolerated, however, for the relatively short time that the drug is in effect.

Pyrantel Pamoate

Pyrantel pamoate (Antiminth, other names) is one of the primary agents used in several types of roundworm and pinworm infections. This drug stimulates acetylcholine release and inhibits acetylcholine breakdown at the neuromuscular junction, thus producing a prolonged state of excitation and muscular contraction that causes spastic paralysis of the worm. The worm is unable to retain its hold on the intestinal tissue and can be expelled from the digestive tract by normal bowel movements. This drug is generally well tolerated, with only occasional problems of mild gastrointestinal disturbances.

Thiabendazole

Thiabendazole (Mintezol) is often used in trichinosis and several other types of roundworm infections. The anthelmintic mechanism of this drug is not fully understood, but selective inhibition of certain key metabolic enzymes in susceptible parasites is probable. Although thiabendazole is quite effective, the use of this drug has declined somewhat in favor of less toxic agents such as mebendazole. The most common side effects associated with this drug involve gastrointestinal distress (nausea, vomiting, loss of appetite). Allergic reactions (skin rash, itching, chills) may also occur in some individuals.

11

ANTIBACTERIAL DRUGS

This chapter address drugs used to treat infections caused by pathogenic microorganisms and parasites. Microorganisms such as bacteria, viruses, and protozoa, as well as larger multicellular parasites, frequently invade human tissues and are responsible for various afflictions ranging from mild and annoying symptoms to life-threatening diseases. Often, the body's natural defense mechanisms are unable to deal with these pathogenic invaders, and pharmacologic treatment is essential in resolving infections and promoting recovery. Drugs used to treat infection represent one of the most significant advances in medical history, and these agents are among the most important and widely used pharmacologic agents throughout the world.

Drugs used to treat infectious diseases share a common goal of *selective toxicity*, meaning they must selectively kill or attenuate the growth of the pathogenic organism without causing excessive damage to the host (human) cells. In some cases, the pathogenic organism may have some distinctive structural or biochemical feature that allows the drug to selectively attack the invading cell. For instance, drugs that capitalize on certain differences in membrane structure, protein synthesis, or other unique aspects of cellular metabolism in the pathogenic organism will be effective and safe anti-infectious agents. Of course, selective toxicity is a relative term, because all of the drugs discussed in the following chapters exert some adverse effects on human tissues. However, drugs used to treat various infections generally impair function much more in the pathogenic organism than in human tissues.

Several other general terms are also used to describe the drugs used to treat infectious disease. Agents used specifically against small, unicellular organisms (e.g., bacteria, viruses) are often referred to as *antimicrobial drugs*. Antimicrobial agents are also commonly referred to as *antibiotics*, indicating that these substances are used to kill other living organisms (i.e., anti- "bios," or life). To avoid confusion, drugs in this text are classified and identified according to the primary type of infectious organism they are used to treat--that is, whether they are antibacterial, antiviral, antifungal, and so on.

This chapter discusses drugs used to treat bacterial infections. Drugs used to treat and prevent viral infections followed by the pharmacologic management of other parasitic infections (antifungal, antiprotozoal, and anthelmintic drugs). Because infectious disease represents one of the most common forms of illness, many patients undergoing therapists physical rehabilitation take one or more of these drugs. Physical therapists and occupational therapists will undoubtedly deal with patients undergoing chemotherapy for infectious disease on a routine basis. The pharmacotherapeutic management of infectious disease should be of interest to all rehabilitation specialists.

Bacteria: Basic Concepts

Bacterial Structure and Function

Bacteria are unicellular microorganisms, ranging in size from 0.8 to 15.0 μm in diameter. Bacteria are distinguished from other microorganisms by several features, including a rigid cell wall that surrounds the bacterial cell and the lack of a true nuclear membrane (i.e., the genetic material within the bacterial cell is not confined by a distinct membrane). Bacteria usually contain the basic subcellular organelles needed to synthesize proteins and maintain cellular metabolism, including ribosomes, enzymes, and cytoplasmic storage granules. Bacteria, however, must depend on some kind of nourishing medium to provide metabolic substrates to maintain function. Hence, these microorganisms often invade human tissues to gain access to a supply of amino acids, sugars, and other substances.

Pathogenic Effects of Bacteria

Bacterial infections can be harmful to host organisms in several ways. First, bacteria multiply, competing with host (human) cells for essential nutrients. Bacteria also may directly harm human cells by releasing toxic substances. Moreover, bacteria may cause an immune response that will ultimately damage human tissues and the invading bacteria. Of course, not all bacteria in the human body are harmful. For example, certain bacteria in the gastrointestinal system inhibit the growth of other microorganisms and assist in the digestion of food and synthesis of certain nutrients. In addition, many bacteria that enter the body are adequately dealt with by normal immunologic responses. However, the invasion of pathogenic bacteria can lead to severe infections and death, especially if the patient's immune system is compromised or the body's endogenous defense mechanisms are unable to combat the infection. In some cases, bacteria may establish growth areas or colonies that remain innocuous for extended periods. However, this colonization may begin to proliferate and become a health threat when the patient succumbs to some other disorder or illness. Consequently, the chance of severe, life-threatening infections is especially high in individuals who are debilitated or have some immune system defect.

Bacterial Nomenclature and Classification

Bacteria are usually named according to their genus and species; these names are identified in italic typeface. For instance, *Escherichia coli* refers to bacteria from the *Escherichia* genus, *coli* species. According to this nomenclature, the genus is capitalized and refers to bacteria with common genetic, morphologic, and biochemical characteristics. The species name is not capitalized and often refers to some physical, pathogenic, or other characteristic of the species. For example, *Streptococcus pyogenes* refers to bacteria from the *Streptococcus* genus, which are commonly associated with pyogenic or pus-producing characteristics.

Because of diverse bacterial genera, bacteria are often categorized according to common characteristics, such as the shape and histologic staining of the bacterial cell. For example, *gram-positive cocci* refers to spherical bacteria (cocci) that retain the discoloration of a particular staining technique (Gram's method of staining). However, development of a comprehensive taxonomy that neatly categorizes all bacteria is difficult because of the diverse morphologic and biochemical characteristics of the various bacterial families and genera. This classification scheme does not fully identify all of the various characteristics of the many bacterial families. The classifications are used here only to categorize bacteria according to the use of antibacterial agents.

Treatment of Bacterial Infections: Basic Principles

Spectrum of Antibacterial Activity

Some drugs are effective against a variety of bacteria; these are usually referred to as *broad-spectrum agents*. For example, a drug such as tetracycline is considered to have a broad spectrum of activity because this drug is effective against many gram-negative, gram-positive, and other types of bacteria. In contrast, a drug such as isoniazid is specific for the bacillus that causes tuberculosis (i.e., *Mycobacterium tuberculosis*), and its spectrum of activity is relatively narrow. Hence, the antibacterial spectrum is one property of an antibacterial drug that determines the clinical applications of that agent. Other factors, including patient tolerance, bacterial resistance, and physician preference, also influence the selection of a particular drug for a particular condition. The clinical use of antibacterial drugs relative to specific bacterial pathogens is discussed in "Clinical Use of Antibacterial Drugs: Relationship to Specific Bacterial Infections."

Bactericidal versus Bacteriostatic Activity

The term bactericidal refers to drugs that typically kill or destroy bacteria. In contrast, drugs that do not actually kill bacteria but limit the growth and proliferation of bacterial invaders are referred to as bacteriostatic. Antibacterial drugs are usually classified as either bactericidal or bacteriostatic, depending on their mechanism of action. In addition, the classification of whether a drug is bactericidal or bacteriostatic may depend on the drug dosage. For instance, drugs such as erythromycin exhibit bacteriostatic activity at lower doses but are bactericidal at higher doses.

Basic Mechanisms of Antibacterial Drugs

As mentioned previously, antibacterial and other antimicrobial drugs must be selectively toxic to the infectious microorganism, without causing excessive damage to human cells. These mechanisms include (1) inhibition of bacterial cell wall synthesis and function, (2) inhibition of bacterial protein synthesis, and (3) inhibition of bacterial DNA/RNA function.

Inhibition of Bacterial Cell Wall Synthesis and Function

Penicillin, cephalosporins, and several other commonly used drugs exert antibacterial effects by inhibiting the synthesis of bacterial cell walls. These drugs are selectively toxic because the bacterial cell walls differ considerably from those of their mammalian counterparts. The membrane surrounding most bacterial cells (with the exception of the *Mycoplasma* genus) is a relatively rigid, firm structure. This rigidity appears to be essential in constraining the high osmotic pressure within the bacterial cell. This behavior contrasts with the relatively supple, flexible membrane encompassing the mammalian cell.

The increased rigidity of bacterial cell walls is caused by the presence of protein-polysaccharide structures known as *peptidoglycans*. Peptidoglycan units (also known as mureins) are cross-linked to one another within the cell wall in such a way as to provide a remarkable amount of rigidity and firmness to the cell. If these peptidoglycans are not present, the bacterial membrane will lack integrity and will cause altered function and impaired homeostasis within the bacterial cell. Also, the lack of adequate membrane cytoarchitecture appears to initiate a suicidal autolysis, whereby bacterial hydrolases released from lysosomes begin to break down the cell wall, thus further contributing to destruction of the microorganism.

Consequently, drugs that cause inadequate production of peptidoglycans or other structural components within the cell wall may produce a selective bactericidal effect. Also, a limited number of antibacterial agents directly punch holes in the bacterial cell membrane, destroying the selective permeability and separation of internal from external environment, which is crucial for the life of the microorganism. These agents include the polymyxin antibiotics (polymyxin B, colistin). These drugs are cationic compounds that are attracted to negatively charged phospholipids in the bacterial cell membrane. The selectivity of these agents for bacterial cell membranes may be due to a greater attraction to certain bacterial phospholipids, as opposed to human cell membrane phospholipids. In any event, these drugs penetrate and disrupt the architecture and integrity of the surface membrane. In essence, these drugs act as detergents that break apart the phospholipid bilayer, creating gaps and leaks in the bacterial cell membrane. The loss of cell membrane integrity leads to rapid death of the bacteria.

Inhibition of Bacterial Protein Synthesis

Bacteria, like most living organisms, must continually synthesize specific proteins to carry out various cellular functions, including enzymatic reactions and membrane transport. A fairly large and well-known group of antibacterial agents works by inhibiting or impairing the synthesis of these bacterial proteins. Drugs that exert their antibacterial effects in this manner include the aminoglycosides (e.g., gentamicin, streptomycin), erythromycin, the tetracyclines, and several other agents. Generally, drugs that inhibit bacterial protein synthesis enter the bacterial cell and bind to specific ribosomal subunits. Antibacterial drugs that work by this mechanism have a much greater affinity for bacterial ribosomes than for human ribosomes, hence their relative specificity in treating bacterial infections. Binding of the drug to the ribosome either blocks protein synthesis or causes the ribosome to misread the messenger RNA (mRNA) code, resulting in the production of meaningless or nonsense proteins. The lack of appropriate protein production impairs bacterial cell membrane transport and metabolic function, resulting in retarded growth or death of the bacteria.

Inhibition of Bacterial DNA/RNA Synthesis and Function

As in any cell, bacteria must be able to replicate their genetic material to reproduce and function normally. An inability to produce normal DNA and RNA will prohibit the bacteria from mediating continued growth and reproduction. Drugs that exert their antibacterial activity by directly or indirectly interfering with the structure, synthesis, and function of DNA and RNA in susceptible bacteria include the fluoroquinolones, sulfonamides, and several other agents. Apparently, these drugs are able to selectively impair bacterial DNA/RNA function because they have a greater affinity for bacterial genetic material and enzymes related to bacterial DNA/RNA synthesis.

Several antibacterial drugs inhibit bacterial nucleic acid synthesis by inhibiting the production of folic acid. Folic acid serves as an enzymatic cofactor in a number of reactions, including synthesis of bacterial nucleic acids and certain essential amino acids. Certain antibacterial drugs block specific steps in the folate pathway, thus impairing the production of this enzymatic cofactor and ultimately impairing the production of nucleic acids and other essential metabolites. Examples of drugs that exert antibacterial effects by this mechanism are trimethoprim and the sulfonamide drugs (e.g., sulfadiazine, sulfamethoxazole).

Specific Antibacterial Agents

Considering the vast number of antibacterial drugs, we cannot explore the pharmacokinetic and pharmacologic details of each individual agent. For the purposes of this chapter, the major groups of antibacterial drugs are categorized according to the basic modes of antibacterial action that were previously discussed (inhibition of cell wall synthesis, etc.). Pertinent aspects of each group's actions, uses, and potential side effects are briefly discussed. For a more detailed description of any specific agent, the reader is referred to one of the current drug indexes, such as the *Physician's Desk Reference (PDR)*.

Antibacterial Drugs That Inhibit Bacterial Cell Wall Synthesis and Function

Clinical use and specific aspects of these drugs are presented below.

Penicillins

Penicillin, the first antibiotic, was originally derived from mold colonies of the *Penicillium* fungus during the early 1940s. Currently, there are several forms of natural and semisynthetic penicillins. These agents have a chemical structure and mode of action similar to the cephalosporin drugs and several other agents. Collectively, the penicillins and these other drugs are known as ***beta-lactam antibiotics*** because they share a common structure known as a *beta-lactam ring*.

Penicillin and other beta-lactam agents exert their effects by binding to specific enzymatic proteins within the bacterial cell wall. These enzymatic proteins, known as penicillin-binding proteins (PBPs), are responsible for the normal synthesis and organization of the bacterial cell wall. In particular, PBPs help manufacture the peptidoglycans, which are essential for normal membrane structure and function. Penicillins and other beta-lactam drugs attach to the PBPs and inhibit their function. Thus, construction of the bacterial cell wall is impaired, and the cell dies from the membrane's inability to serve as a selective barrier and to contain the high internal osmotic pressure of the bacterial cell.

Classification and use of penicillins

Penicillins can be classified according to their chemical background, spectrum of antibacterial activity, or pharmacokinetic features. The naturally occurring penicillins (penicillin G and V) can be administered orally but have a relatively narrow antibacterial spectrum. Some semisynthetic penicillins (amoxicillin, ampicillin) have a broader antibacterial spectrum and may be administered either orally or parenterally, depending on the specific agent.

Penicillinase-resistant forms of penicillin were developed to overcome strains of bacteria that contain an enzyme known as a penicillinase or beta-lactamase. This enzyme destroys natural and some semisynthetic penicillins, rendering these drugs ineffective in bacteria containing this enzyme. For penicillinase-containing bacteria, the semisynthetic forms of penicillin that are resistant to destruction by the penicillinase must be used.

Discussing all the clinical applications of the penicillins goes well beyond the scope of this chapter. These agents are a mainstay in the treatment of infection and remain the drugs of choice in a diverse array of clinical disorders. Clearly, these agents continue to be one of the most important and effective antibacterial regimens currently available.

Adverse effects

One of the primary problems with penicillin drugs is the potential for allergic reactions. Hypersensitivity to penicillin is exhibited by skin rashes, hives, itching, and difficult breathing. In some individuals, these reactions may be minor and can often be resolved by changing the type of penicillin or the method of administration. In others, however, penicillin hypersensitivity may be severe and lead to an anaphylactic reaction (severe bronchoconstriction and cardiovascular collapse).

During prolonged administration, penicillin drugs may also cause central nervous system (CNS) problems (e.g., confusion, hallucinations), as well as certain blood disorders, such as hemolytic anemia and thrombocytopenia. Other relatively minor side effects of penicillin drugs include gastrointestinal problems such as nausea, vomiting, and diarrhea.

Cephalosporins

The cephalosporin drugs, which are also classified as beta-lactam antibiotics, exert their bactericidal effects in a manner similar to that of the penicillins (inhibition of PBPs, resulting in inadequate peptidoglycan production). Generally, the cephalosporins serve as alternative agents to penicillins if the penicillin drugs are ineffective or poorly tolerated by the patient. Cephalosporins may also be the drugs of choice in certain types of urinary tract infections.

Cephalosporins can be subdivided into first-, second-, third-, and fourth-generation groups, according to their spectrum of antibacterial activity. First-generation cephalosporins, which are generally effective against gram-positive cocci, may also be used against some gram-negative bacteria. Second-generation cephalosporins are also effective against gram-positive cocci, but they are somewhat more effective than first-generation agents against gram-negative bacteria. Third-generation cephalosporins have the broadest spectrum of effectiveness against gram-negative bacteria, but they have limited effects on gram-positive cocci. Fourth-generation agents have the broadest antibacterial spectrum of the cephalosporins, and they are effective against gram-positive and gram-negative organisms.

Adverse effects

In some patients, cephalosporins may cause an allergic reaction similar to the penicillin hypersensitivity described previously. A cross-sensitivity often exists: a patient who is allergic to penicillin drugs will also display hypersensitivity to cephalosporin agents. Other principal adverse effects of cephalosporins include gastrointestinal problems such as stomach cramps, diarrhea, nausea, and vomiting.

Other Agents that Inhibit Bacterial Cell Wall Synthesis

Aztreonam

Aztreonam (Azactam) is another type of beta-lactam antibiotic, but this drug is classified as a carbapenam agent rather than a penicillin or cephalosporin. Nonetheless, aztreonam acts like the other beta-lactam agents and inhibits the synthesis and structure of the cell membrane in susceptible bacteria. Aztreonam has a limited spectrum, but it may be useful against serious infections caused by certain gram-negative bacilli (*Enterobacter aerogenes* and *Pseudomonas aeruginosa*). The principal problems associated with aztreonam include skin rashes, redness, and itching due to hypersensitivity in susceptible individuals.

Bacitracin

Bacitracin refers to a group of polypeptide antibiotics that have similar chemical and pharmacologic properties. These compounds inhibit bacterial cell wall synthesis by inhibiting the incorporation of amino acids and nucleic acid precursors into the bacterial cell wall. Bacitracin compounds, which have a broad range of antibacterial activity, are effective against many gram-positive bacilli and gram-positive cocci, as well as several other microorganisms. Bacitracin is usually applied topically to prevent and treat infection in superficial skin wounds and certain ophthalmic infections. Commercial preparations containing bacitracin may also contain other antibiotics, such as neomycin and polymyxin B. The primary problem associated with bacitracin is local hypersensitivity, as indicated by skin rashes and itching.

Colistin

Colistin (also known as *colistimethate* or *polymyxin E*) is similar to polymyxin B in terms of pharmacologic mechanism and antibacterial effects. Colistin is used primarily in combination with other agents (neomycin and hydrocortisone) to treat local infections of the external auditory canal. Adverse effects are relatively rare during the local and topical use of this drug.

Cycloserine

Cycloserine inhibits bacterial wall synthesis by interfering with the final stage of peptidoglycan synthesis. Adding two units of the amino acid D-alanine completes the synthesis of peptidoglycans. Cycloserine, which is similar in structure to D-alanine, competitively inhibits the enzyme that adds the final D-alanine units onto the peptidoglycan structures. Cycloserine is considered a broad-spectrum antibiotic but is used primarily as an adjunct in the treatment of tuberculosis. The primary adverse effect of this drug is CNS toxicity, which may occur during prolonged use at relatively high dosages.

Ertapenem

Ertapenem (Invanz) is another carbapenam antibacterial agent that is similar to meropenem. Ertapenem is effective against gram-positive and gram-negative aerobic and anaerobic bacteria, and is often used to treat intra-abdominal and pelvic infections, as well as infections in the skin, urinary tract, and respiratory tract. Side effects include chest pain, gastrointestinal problems (nausea, diarrhea), headache, and fever.

Imipenem and cilastatin

Imipenem is a betalactam drug that is classified as a carbapenam antibiotic. Imipenem exerts bactericidal effects similar to the other beta-lactam agents (penicillins and cephalosporins); that is, imipenem inhibits PBP function and peptidoglycan synthesis. This drug is typically administered along with a second agent, cilastatin. Cilastatin enhances the bactericidal effects of imipenem by inhibiting metabolic inactivation of imipenem within the kidneys, even though cilastin does not exhibit any antibacterial activities by itself. Imipenem has one of the broadest antibacterial spectrums of the beta-lactam drugs and may be useful against a variety of aerobic gram-positive or gram-negative bacteria, as well as some anaerobic bacterial strains. Side effects associated with imipenem include nausea, hypotension, and hypersensitivity (skin rashes, redness, itching). CNS abnormalities such as confusion, tremors, and seizures have also been reported in certain patients. The risk of imipenem-induced seizure is increased in patients who have a preexisting seizure disorder or if the drug dosage is too high, based on the patient's body weight.

Meropenem

Meropenem is a carbapenam antibacterial with effects and spectrum similar to imipenem. Meropenem, however, does not need to be administered with cilastatin. This agent may likewise be effective against certain forms of gram-positive and gram-negative bacteria that are resistant to other betalactam drugs. Meropenem may cause CNS problems—including seizures—but the risk is relatively low when compared with the risk of seizures with imipenem.

Polymyxin B

Polymyxin antibiotics are cationic compounds that are attracted to negatively charged phospholipids in the bacterial cell membrane. These drugs penetrate and disrupt the architecture and integrity of the surface membrane. Essentially, polymyxins act as detergents that break apart the phospholipid bilayer, which creates gaps in the bacterial cell wall, leading to the subsequent destruction of the bacteria.

Polymyxin B is effective against many gram-negative bacteria, including *E. coli*, *Klebsiella*, and *Salmonella*. Systemic administration of this drug, however, is often associated with extreme nephrotoxicity. Hence, this agent is used primarily for the treatment of local, superficial infections of the skin, eyes, and mucous membranes. When applied topically for these conditions, adverse reactions are relatively rare. Polymyxin B is often combined with other antibiotics such as bacitracin and neomycin in commercial topical preparations.

Vancomycin

Vancomycin appears to bind directly to bacterial cell wall precursors such as D-alanine and to impair the incorporation of these precursors into the cell wall. Vancomycin is effective against gram-positive bacilli and cocci and primarily serves as an alternative to the penicillins in a variety of infections. The emergence of bacteria that are resistant to vancomycin, however, has generated concern about the continued use of this drug. The primary adverse effects associated with vancomycin include hypersensitivity (e.g., skin rashes), a bitter or unpleasant taste in the mouth, and gastrointestinal disturbances (nausea and vomiting). Vancomycin also has the potential to cause nephrotoxicity and ototoxicity.

Use of Beta-Lactamase Inhibitors

A primary problem in using penicillins, cephalosporins, and other beta-lactam antibiotics is that certain bacteria produce enzymes known as beta-lactamases. These beta-lactamase enzymes bind to the beta-lactam drug and destroy it before it can exert an antibacterial effect. Bacteria that produce these beta-lactamase enzymes are therefore resistant to penicillin and other beta-lactam antibacterial drugs. Fortunately, several drugs are available that inhibit these beta-lactamase enzymes. These drugs include clavulanate, sulbactam, and tazobactam. These betalactamase inhibitors are typically combined with a specific type of penicillin in order to treat infections caused by bacteria that produce beta-lactamase enzymes. The beta-lactamase inhibitor prevents the beta-lactamase enzyme from destroying the penicillin, thus allowing the penicillin to remain intact and effective against the bacterial infection.

Administration of these drug combinations may produce side effects that are caused primarily by the penicillin component; that is, penicillin-related side effects such as headache, gastrointestinal problems, and allergic reactions. Nonetheless, combining a beta-lactamase inhibitor with a penicillin can be an effective way of treating bacterial infections that might otherwise be resistant to traditional antibacterial therapy.

Drugs that Inhibit Bacterial Protein Synthesis

Aminoglycosides

The aminoglycosides are a group of antibacterial agents including streptomycin, gentamicin, neomycin, and similar agents. These agents bind irreversibly to certain parts of bacterial ribosomes and cause several changes in protein synthesis, including alterations in the ribosome's ability to read the mRNA genetic code. This misreading results in the improper synthesis of proteins that control specific aspects of cell function, such as membrane structure and permeability. The lack of normal cell proteins leads to the bacterial cell's death.

Antibacterial spectrum and general indications

Aminoglycosides have a very broad spectrum of antibacterial activity and are effective against many aerobic gram-negative bacteria, including *E. coli*, *Pseudomonas*, and *Salmonella*. Aminoglycosides are active against some aerobic gram-positive bacteria, such as certain species of *Staphylococcus*, and many anaerobic bacteria. Consequently, aminoglycosides are used to treat a variety of tissue and wound infections.

Adverse effects

Aminoglycoside use is limited somewhat by problems with toxicity. Nephrotoxicity, as indicated by bloody urine, acute renal tubular necrosis, and so on, is one of the more common and serious adverse effects. Ototoxicity, as indicated by dizziness and ringing or fullness in the ears, may also occur. This effect can be irreversible in severe cases. Toxicity may occur more frequently in certain individuals, such as patients with liver or kidney failure, or in elderly patients. To reduce the risk of toxicity, drug levels in the bloodstream must be periodically monitored so dosages can be adjusted for individual patients. Other adverse effects include hypersensitivity (e.g., skin rashes, itching) in susceptible individuals.

Erythromycin and Other Macrolides

Erythromycin and its chemical derivatives (azithromycin, clarithromycin, dirithromycin) comprise a group of agents known as macrolide antibiotics. These drugs inhibit bacterial protein synthesis by binding to specific parts of the ribosomes in susceptible bacteria. This binding impairs protein synthesis primarily by inhibiting the formation of peptide bonds between adjacent amino acids. In particular, erythromycin seems to encourage the dissociation of transfer RNA (tRNA) units from their binding site on the ribosome. Normally, the tRNAs bring amino acids to the ribosome, where the amino acids are linked together to form proteins. By stimulating the detachment of tRNA, peptide bond formation is averted.

Antibacterial spectrum and general indications

Erythromycin and the other macrolides exhibit a very broad spectrum of antibacterial activities and are active against many gram-positive bacteria, as well as some gram-negative bacteria. These agents are often used as the primary or alternative drug in a variety of clinical conditions. Macrolides may be especially useful in patients who are allergic to penicillin. Macrolides may produce other beneficial effects that compliment their antibacterial properties. These drugs, for example, seem to have anti-inflammatory effects, especially in diseases associated with airway inflammation. Hence, these drugs may be particularly useful in treating certain airway infections in people with cystic fibrosis or other respiratory disorders associated with infection and inflammation in airway tissues.

Adverse effects

When given in high (bactericidal) dosages, gastrointestinal distress is a common problem with erythromycin administration; for example, stomach cramps, nausea, vomiting, and diarrhea may occur. Hence, erythromycin is usually given in doses that only impair the growth of bacteria (bacteriostatic doses). Some of the newer macrolides (clarithromycin, dirithromycin) may be somewhat safer and produce fewer side effects than erythromycin. However, various degrees of allergic reactions—ranging from mild skin rashes to acute anaphylaxis—may occur when these drugs are used in susceptible individuals.

Tetracyclines

Tetracycline and tetracycline derivatives inhibit protein synthesis by binding to several components of the ribosomal apparatus in susceptible bacteria. Hence, these drugs may cause misreading of the mRNA code, as well as impair the formation of peptide bonds at the bacterial ribosome. Thus, tetracyclines are very effective in preventing bacterial protein synthesis.

Antibacterial spectrum and General Indications

Tetracyclines are active against a variety of bacteria, including many gram-positive and gram-negative bacteria, as well as other bacterial microorganisms (*Rickettsia*, spirochetes). Their use as a broad-spectrum antibiotic has diminished somewhat, however, because of the development of tetracycline-resistant bacterial strains. Some of the newer tetracycline derivatives such as doxycycline may be used to overcome bacterial strains that are resistant to the traditional drugs. Currently, tetracyclines are used to treat specific infections relating to such bacilli as *Chlamydia*, *Rickettsia*, and certain spirochetes. Tetracyclines may also be used as alternative agents in treating bacterial strains that are resistant to other drugs, such as chloramphenicol, streptomycin, and various penicillins. Tetracyclines also seem to have anti-inflammatory and immunomodulating effects. Although the exact reasons for these effects are unclear, tetracyclines have been used in a variety of noninfectious diseases with an inflammatory or autoimmune basis, including scleroderma and rheumatoid arthritis. Clinical studies will continue to investigate how these drugs can be used effectively in the long-term management of chronic disease.

Adverse effects

Gastrointestinal distress (nausea, vomiting, diarrhea) may be a problem with tetracycline use. Hypersensitivity reactions (such as rashes) may also occur, as well as an increase in skin sensitivity to ultraviolet light (photosensitivity). Tetracyclines form chemical complexes with calcium that may impair the growth and development of calcified tissues such as bone and teeth, especially in children. Tetracyclines also cause discoloration of teeth in children and pregnant women, apparently because of the tetracycline-calcium interaction. As mentioned previously, development of tetracycline-resistant strains and resulting superinfections may be a serious problem during tetracycline therapy.

Other Agents that Inhibit Bacterial Protein Synthesis

Chloramphenicol

Chloramphenicol (Chloromycetin) is a synthetically produced agent that exerts antibacterial effects similar to those of erythromycin; that is, it binds to the 50S subunit of bacterial ribosomes and inhibits peptide bond formation. Chloramphenicol is a broad-spectrum antibiotic that is active against many gram-negative and gram-positive bacteria. This drug is administered systemically to treat serious infections such as typhoid fever, *Haemophilus* infections such as osteomyelitis, rickettsial infections such as Rocky Mountain spotted fever, and certain forms of meningitis. Chloramphenicol may also be administered topically to treat various skin, eye, and ear infections.

The most serious problem associated with chloramphenicol is the potential for bone marrow aplasia, which can lead to aplastic anemia and possibly death. Chloramphenicol is also associated with other blood dyscrasias such as agranulocytosis and thrombocytopenia. Because of these risks, chloramphenicol is not typically used as a first-choice drug, but is reserved for severe infections that do not respond to other antibacterials, or situations where safer drugs are contraindicated (e.g., patients are allergic to other medications).

Clindamycin

Clindamycin (Cleocin) is derived from lincomycin. Both drugs are similar in structure and function to erythromycin and inhibit protein synthesis by binding to the 50S ribosomal subunit of susceptible bacteria. These agents are effective against most gram-positive bacteria and some gram-negative microorganisms. Typically, clindamycin and lincomycin are reserved as alternative drugs (rather than primary agents) in the treatment of local and systemic infections; these agents may be especially useful if patients are unable to tolerate either penicillin or erythromycin. The principal adverse effects associated with these drugs include gastrointestinal distress (nausea, diarrhea, colitis) and various allergic reactions, ranging from mild skin rashes to anaphylactic shock.

Ethionamide

Ethionamide (Trecator-SC) appears to inhibit bacterial protein synthesis, but the exact mechanism of action is unknown. This drug may act in a manner similar to that of some of the other drugs discussed previously in this section (binding to bacterial ribosomes), or it may mediate its effect by some other means. Ethionamide is effective against *M. tuberculosis* and is used primarily in the treatment of tuberculosis. This drug is usually used as a secondary agent when primary antituberculosis drugs are ineffective. Gastrointestinal distress (nausea, vomiting) is the most frequent problem encountered with ethionamide use. CNS disorders (drowsiness, mental depression, etc.), as well as severe postural hypotension, may also occur.

Lincomycin

Lincomycin (Lincocin, Lincorex) is similar in mechanism of action, clinical indications, and adverse side effects to clindamycin.

Linezolid

Linezolid (Zyvox) binds to a specific site on the bacterial ribosome and inhibits protein synthesis in many gram-positive bacteria including staphlocci, streptococci, and enterococci. Hence, this drug is commonly used to treat pneumonia caused by *S. aureus* or *S. pneumoniae*, and other susceptible skin and soft tissue infections. Common side effects include gastrointestinal problems (nausea, diarrhea), with more serious blood dyscrasias (anemia, leukopenia, thrombocytopenia) occurring in some patients during prolonged drug administration.

Quinupristin and dalfopristin

Quinupristin and dalfopristin are combined in the same product (Synercid), which is used to treat certain gram-positive bacteria such as staphylococci and some enterococcal strains. These agents bind to the bacterial ribosome at slightly different sites, and work together to prevent the formation of bacterial polypeptide chains. Treatments are administered via intravenous infusion; primary side effects involve pain, irritation, and thrombophlebitis at the infusion site. Other side effects include muscle and joint pain and gastrointestinal disturbances (nausea, vomiting, diarrhea).

Telithromycin

Telithromycin (Ketek) is the first agent from a new class of drugs known as ketolide antibacterials. This drug is derived from erthythromycin, but is altered structurally so that it is able to overcome certain forms of bacterial resistance. Telithromycin acts by binding to the bacterial ribosome and inhibiting protein synthesis. It has an antibacterial spectrum similar to erthythromycin, but is typically reserved for gram-negative strains that are resistant to other agents. Primary side effects include gastrointestinal disturbances (nausea, vomiting, diarrhea), liver toxicity, and cardiac arrhythmias in susceptible patients.

Tigecycline

Tigecycline (Tygacil) is a relatively new antibacterial drug that is classified chemically as a glycycline agent. This drug is similar to tetracycline in structure and antibacterial spectrum, but tigecycline may be somewhat more effective in treating certain infections that are tetracycline-resistant. This drug may also be useful against other resistant strains including methicillin-resistant *S. aureus*, and vancomycin-resistant *E. faecalis* and *E. faecium*. The primary side effects of tigecycline include nausea, vomiting, headache, and dizziness.

Drugs that Inhibit Bacterial DNA/RNA Synthesis and Function

Aminosalicylic Acid

Aminosalicylic acid (Paser, PAS) exerts its effects in a manner similar to the sulfonamide drugs; that is, aminosalicylic acid is structurally similar to paraaminobenzoic acid (PABA) and inhibits folic acid synthesis by competing with PABA in tuberculosis bacteria. This drug is used as an adjunct to the primary antitubercular agents, isoniazid and rifampin. Adverse effects are fairly common with aminosalicylic acid use and include gastrointestinal problems, hypersensitivity reactions, and blood dyscrasias (e.g., agranulocytosis, thrombocytopenia).

Clofazimine

Although the exact mechanism of clofazimine (Lamprene) is unclear, this drug appears to bind directly to bacterial DNA in susceptible microorganisms. Drug binding may prevent the double-stranded DNA helix from unraveling to allow replication of the DNA genetic code. An inability to replicate its genetic material will prevent the bacteria from undergoing mitosis.

Clofazimine is effective against *Mycobacterium leprae* and is used primarily as an adjunct in the treatment of leprosy. During clofazimine therapy, many patients experience problems with red to brownish-black discoloration of the skin. Although this discoloration is reversible, it may take several months to years before skin color returns to normal. Other adverse effects include abdominal pain, nausea, vomiting, and rough, scaly skin.

Dapsone

Dapsone (Avlosulfon) is a member of a class of chemical agents known as the sulfones. Dapsone is especially effective against *M. leprae* and is used with rifampin as the primary method of treating leprosy. Dapsone appears to exert its antibacterial effects in a manner similar to that of the sulfonamide drugs; that is, dapsone impairs folic acid synthesis by competing with PABA in bacterial cells. Primary adverse effects associated with dapsone include peripheral motor weakness, hypersensitivity reactions (skin rashes, itching), fever, and blood dyscrasias, such as hemolytic anemia.

Ethambutol

The mechanism of ethambutol (Myambutol) is not fully understood. This drug apparently suppresses RNA synthesis in susceptible bacteria, but it is not known how this occurs. Ethambutol is primarily effective against *M. tuberculosis* infections and is a secondary agent in the treatment of tuberculosis. Adverse effects associated with this drug include joint pain, nausea, skin rash and itching, and CNS abnormalities (dizziness, confusion, hallucinations).

Fluoroquinolones

The fluoroquinolone antibiotics include ciprofloxacin (Cipro), enoxacin (Penetrex), gatifloxacin (Tequin), levofloxacin (Levaquin), lomefloxacin (Maxaquin), moxifloxacin (Avelox), norfloxacin (Noroxin), ofloxacin (Floxin), and sparfloxacin (Zagam). These drugs inhibit two specific enzymes—DNA-gyrase and topoisomerase IV—that affect DNA function in certain bacteria. DNA-gyrase is responsible for controlling the amount of DNA winding (supercoiling) in bacterial cells. Topoisomerase IV enzymatically separates two new DNA strands that are formed during bacterial cell division. Fluoroquinolones inhibit these enzymes, thereby impairing the normal DNA structure and function that is needed for cell growth and replication.

Fluoroquinolones are effective against a wide range of gram-positive and gram-negative aerobic bacteria and are especially useful in urinary tract infections caused by *E. coli*, *Klebsiella*, *Proteus*, and *Enterobacter aerogenes*. Other indications include the treatment of gastrointestinal infections, respiratory infections, osteomyelitis, and certain sexually transmitted diseases (gonorrhea). A specific agent, ciprofloxacin (Cipro), is particularly effective against anthrax infections, and this drug received considerable attention as an intervention against bioterrorist activities that use anthrax. Primary adverse effects include CNS toxicity, manifested by visual disturbances, headache, and dizziness. Gastrointestinal distress (nausea, vomiting, diarrhea) and allergic reactions (skin rashes, itching) may also occur. These drugs produce photosensitivity and increase the skin's sensitivity to ultraviolet light. Rare but potentially serious cases of nephrotoxicity may occur in certain patients.

Finally, these drugs may cause tendon pain and inflammation (tendinopathy) that can be severe and can ultimately lead to tendon rupture in some patients. Tendinopathy seems to occur most commonly in the Achilles tendon, but other tendons such as the patellar tendon and supraspinatus tendon may also be affected. Although the overall incidence of tendinopathy is fairly low, patients may be more susceptible if they are older, have renal failure, are taking glucocorticoids, or have a history of fluoroquinolone-induced tendinopathy. Although all of the fluoroquinolones can potentially cause tendinopathy, the risk of tendon damage seems highest with ofloxacin. Hence, complaints of pain in any tendon should be carefully evaluated in patients taking fluoroquinolones, and the affected tendon(s) should not be exercised until the cause of tendinopathy can be determined. If it seems that fluoroquinolones are causing tendinopathy, these drugs should be discontinued, and efforts should be made to protect the tendon from excessive stress until the tendinopathy is resolved.

Metronidazole

The exact mechanism of metronidazole (Flagyl, Protostat, others) is not fully understood. This drug appears to be incorporated into bacterial cells, where it undergoes chemical reduction. Apparently, the reduced metabolite of metronidazole interacts with bacterial DNA and causes it to lose its characteristic double-helix structure. This leads to the disintegration of DNA molecules and loss of the ability to replicate and carry out normal genetic functions. Further details of this bactericidal effect remain to be determined.

Metronidazole is effective against most anaerobic bacteria and is useful in treating serious infections caused by *Bacteroides*, *Fusobacterium*, and other anaerobic bacteria. Metronidazole, is also effective against certain protozoa with regard to its antiprotozoal effects. Common side effects associated with metronidazole include gastrointestinal distress (nausea, diarrhea), allergic reactions (such as rashes), and CNS symptoms (confusion, dizziness, mood changes). This drug may also cause peripheral neuropathies as indicated by numbness and tingling in the hands and feet.

Mupirocin

Mupirocin (Bactroban) inhibits a specific enzyme responsible for tRNA synthesis in susceptible bacteria. This drug is used topically to treat skin infections caused by *Staphylococcus aureus* or *Streptococcus pyogenes*. Likewise, mupirocin can be administered by nasal spray to treat local colonization of *S. aureus* in the nasal mucosa. This idea may be especially helpful in preventing systemic infection in individuals such as health care workers who are exposed to an outbreak of resistant strains of *S. aureus*. Local/topical administration of this drug is well tolerated, although some irritation of the skin may occur during topical use, and cough and respiratory irritation can occur when mupirocin is administered by nasal spray.

Rifampin

Rifampin (Rifadin, Rimactane), and similar agents such as rifabutin (Mycobutin) and rifapentine (Priftin), directly impair DNA replication by binding to and inhibiting the DNA-dependent RNA polymerase enzyme in susceptible bacteria. This enzyme initiates the replication of genetic material by generating the formation of RNA strands from the DNA template. By inhibiting this enzyme, rifampin blocks RNA chain synthesis and subsequent replication of the nucleic acid code in bacterial cells.

Rifampin is effective against many gram-negative and gram-positive bacteria and is one of the principal agents used to treat tuberculosis and leprosy. Typically, this drug is combined with another agent—for example, rifampin plus dapsone for leprosy, or rifampin plus isoniazid for tuberculosis—to increase effectiveness and to prevent the development of resistance to rifampin. Rifampin is also used in combination with erythromycin to treat Legionnaire disease and certain forms of meningitis.

Common adverse effects include gastrointestinal distress (nausea, vomiting, stomach cramps) and various hypersensitivity reactions (rashes and fever). Disturbances in liver function have also been noted, and serious hepatic abnormalities may occur in patients with preexisting liver disease.

Sulfonamides

The sulfonamides include sulfadiazine, sulfamethizole, and similar agents. Sulfonamides interfere with bacterial nucleic acid production by disrupting folic acid synthesis in susceptible bacteria. Sulfonamide drugs are structurally similar to PABA, which is the substance used in the first step of folic acid synthesis in certain types of bacteria. Sulfonamides either directly inhibit the enzyme responsible for PABA utilization or become a substitute for PABA, which results in the abnormal synthesis of folic acid. In either case, folic acid synthesis is reduced, and bacterial nucleic acid synthesis is impaired.

Sulfonamides have the potential to be used against a wide variety of bacteria, including gram-negative and gram-positive bacilli and cocci. The development of resistance in various bacteria, however, has limited the use of these drugs. Currently, sulfonamides are used systemically to treat certain urinary tract infections and infections caused by *Nocardia* bacteria. Sulfonamides may also be applied topically to treat vaginal infections, ophthalmic conditions, and other local infections. A specific agent, sulfadiazine, can also be combined with silver nitrate to form silver sulfadiazine, which is often applied topically to control bacterial infection in burns. The problems encountered most frequently with sulfonamide drugs include gastrointestinal distress, increased skin sensitivity to ultraviolet light, and allergic reactions. Serious disturbances in the formed blood elements, including blood dyscrasias such as agranulocytosis and hemolytic anemia, may also occur during systemic sulfonamide therapy.

Trimethoprim

Trimethoprim (Proloprim, Trimpex) interferes with the bacterial folic acid pathway by inhibiting the dihydrofolate reductase enzyme in susceptible bacteria. This enzyme converts dihydrofolic acid to tetrahydrofolic acid during the biosynthesis of folic acid cofactors. By inhibiting this enzyme, trimethoprim directly interferes with the production of folic acid cofactors, and subsequent production of vital bacterial nucleic acids is impaired. Trimethoprim is effective against several gram-negative bacilli, including *E. coli*, *Enterobacter*, *Proteus mirabilis*, and *Klebsiella*. Trimethoprim is used primarily in the treatment of urinary tract infections caused by these and other susceptible bacteria. Trimethoprim is frequently used in combination with the sulfonamide drug sulfamethoxazole. Primary adverse effects associated with trimethoprim include headache, skin rashes and itching, decreased appetite, an unusual taste in the mouth, and gastrointestinal problems (nausea, vomiting, diarrhea). Trimethoprim may also cause excessively high levels of potassium in the blood (hyperkalemia), especially in older adults.

OTHER ANTIBACTERIAL DRUGS

Several other antibacterial drugs work by mechanisms that are either unknown or are different from the classical antibacterial mechanisms described previously. These drugs are discussed individually here.

Capreomycin

Capreomycin (Capastat) is used as an adjunct or alternative drug for the treatment of tuberculosis. The drug's mechanism of action is unknown. The primary problems associated with this drug include ototoxicity and nephrotoxicity.

Daptomycin

Daptomycin (Cubicin) is unique in that this drug binds to the cell membrane of susceptible bacteria and depolarizes the cell. Loss of membrane polarity results in a general inhibition of cell function and subsequent death of the bacterium. This drug is used primarily to treat skin infections caused by certain staphylococcal, streptococcal, and enterococcal bacteria. Because of its unique mechanism of action, daptomycin may also be helpful in treating strains that are resistant to more traditional antibacterial drugs. Primary side effects of this drug include gastrointestinal problems (nausea, constipation, diarrhea), and higher doses may cause myopathy and neuropathy in some patients.

Isoniazid

Isoniazid (INH, Laniazid, Nydrazid, other names) is one of the primary drugs used to treat tuberculosis. Although the exact mechanism of action is unknown, this drug appears to interfere with several enzymatic pathways involving protein, lipid, carbohydrate, and nucleic acid metabolism in susceptible bacteria. Adverse reactions to isoniazid are common, and patients may develop disorders such as hepatitis and peripheral neuropathies.

Methenamine

Methenamine (Hiprex, Mandelamine, Urex) exerts antibacterial properties in a unique fashion. In an acidic environment, this drug decomposes into formaldehyde and ammonia. Formaldehyde is bactericidal to almost all bacteria, and bacteria do not develop resistance to this toxin. This mechanism enables methenamine to be especially useful in treating urinary tract infections, because the presence of this drug in acidic urine facilitates the release of formaldehyde at the site of infection (i.e., within the urinary tract). Use of methenamine is safe, although high doses are associated with gastrointestinal upset and problems with urination (bloody urine, pain while urinating).

Nitrofurantoin

Bacterial enzymes reduce nitrofurantoin (Macrobid, Macrodantin, others) into a metabolite that is toxic to the bacterial cell. This toxic metabolite inhibits bacterial metabolic function by interfering with ribosomal function and other molecules involved in energy production and utilization in the bacterial cell. Nitrofurantoin is primarily used to treat urinary tract infections caused by a number of gram-negative and some gram-positive bacteria. Adverse effects associated with this drug include gastrointestinal distress (nausea, vomiting, and diarrhea) and neurotoxicity (as indicated by headache, numbness, and excessive fatigue). Acute pneumonitis (as indicated by coughing, chills, fever, and difficulty in breathing) may also occur soon after nitrofurantoin is initiated. This pneumonitis appears to be a direct chemical effect of the drug and usually disappears within hours after the drug is withdrawn.

Pyrazinamide

Pyrazinamide (generic) is used primarily as an adjunct to other drugs in treating tuberculosis. This drug's mechanism of action against *M. tuberculosis* is unknown. Problems associated with pyrazinamide include hepatotoxicity and lower-extremity joint pain.

Clinical Use of Antibacterial Drugs: Relationship to Specific Bacterial Infections

An incredible array of antibacterial agents is currently being used clinically. As mentioned previously, selection of a particular agent is based on the effectiveness of the drug against a range or spectrum of different bacteria. Various antibacterial drugs can serve as either the primary or the alternative agents against specific bacterial infections. The actual selection of an antibacterial agent is often highly variable, depending on the particular patient, the type and location of the infection, the experience of the physician, and many other factors.

Resistance to Antibacterial Drugs

One of the most serious problems of antibacterial therapy is the potential for development of strains of bacteria that are resistant to one or more antibacterial agents. Certain bacterial strains have a natural or acquired defense mechanism against specific antibacterial drugs. This enables the strain to survive the effects of the drug and continue to grow and reproduce similar resistant strains, thus representing a genetic selection process in which only the resistant strains survive the drug. As a result, bacteria that are invulnerable to the drug can breed. If other drugs are not effective against the resistant strain, or if cross-resistance to several antibacterial drugs occurs, the resistant bacteria become especially dangerous because of their immunity from antibacterial chemotherapy.

Bacterial resistance can occur because of several mechanisms. Certain bacterial strains may be able to enzymatically destroy the antibacterial drug. The best example is the beta-lactamase enzyme that is found in bacteria that are resistant to beta-lactam drugs (penicillins and cephalosporins). As previously discussed, bacteria containing this enzyme can destroy certain penicillin and cephalosporin drugs, thus rendering the drug ineffective against these strains.

Resistance may also occur because the bacterial cell modifies or masks the site where the antibacterial drug typically binds on or within the cell. For instance, penicillins, aminoglycosides, vancomycin, and other drugs must bind to membrane proteins, intracellular proteins, ribosomes, and the like to exert their effect. Differences in the affinity of these binding sites may be acquired by bacterial mutation, thus decreasing the drug's effectiveness. Bacteria may also develop resistance through genetic mutations that change the enzymes targeted by certain drugs. For example, fluoroquinolones, rifampin, and other drugs that normally inhibit enzymes responsible for bacterial DNA/RNA function will be ineffective if enzymes are modified within resistant bacteria.

Resistance can likewise occur if the drug's ability to penetrate the bacterial cell is reduced. Most drugs must first penetrate the cell membrane and then enter the bacterial cell to exert their bactericidal effects. Specific bacteria that have a natural or acquired opposition to drug penetration render the drug useless, thus leading to the development of strains that are resistant to aminoglycosides and other agents. Certain bacteria also develop drug efflux pumps that expel the drug from the bacterial cell, thus rendering the drug ineffective. These pumps are a common way that bacteria develop resistance to tetracyclines and a number of other antimicrobial agents.

Consequently, a number of factors may be responsible for mediating the formation of bacterial resistance to penicillins, cephalosporins, aminoglycosides, tetracyclines, and other antibacterial agents.

Antibacterial resistance is typically categorized according to the name of the drug and the associated resistant bacterial strain. For example, some of the best known and most important types of resistance include vancomycin-resistant *Staphylococcus aureus* (*VRSA*), methicillin-resistant *S. aureus* (*MRSA*), vancomycinresistant *Enterococcus* (*VRE*), and penicillin-resistant *Streptococcus pneumoniae* (*PRSP*). Even though a resistant organism may be linked to a specific drug by name, the organism is typically resistant to other drugs as well (multidrug resistance).

Development of resistant bacteria is understandably a very serious problem in contemporary drug therapy. In addition, the number of resistant bacterial strains continues to progressively increase in certain institutions and in the community. To limit the development of resistant strains, antibacterial drugs should be used judiciously and not overused. For instance, it is often worthwhile to perform culture and sensitivity tests on sputum, blood, and other body fluids so that the pathogenic bacteria can be identified, leading to the use of more selective agents. Administering selective agents as opposed to broad-spectrum antibiotics may help attenuate and kill resistant strains more effectively, thus limiting the spread of bacterial resistance. The selective use of current antibacterial drugs and the development of new bactericidal agents are needed to help control the problem of bacterial resistance.

Antibacterial drugs are used to prevent and treat infection in a variety of clinical situations. Some drugs are effective against a limited number of bacteria (narrow-spectrum), whereas other agents may be used against a relatively wide variety of bacterial pathogens (broad-spectrum). Specific agents may exert their antibacterial effects by preventing bacterial cell wall synthesis and function, or by inhibiting either bacterial protein synthesis or bacterial DNA/RNA synthesis and function. Although most bacterial infections can be effectively treated with one or more agents, the development of bacterial strains that are resistant to drug therapy continues to be a serious problem. Rehabilitation specialists will routinely treat patients receiving antibacterial drugs for conditions that are directly or indirectly related to the need for physical therapy and occupational therapy. Therapists should be cognizant of the potential side effects of these drugs and should know how these drugs may interfere with specific physical therapy and occupational therapy procedures.

12

ANTIVIRAL DRUGS

A virus is one of the smallest microorganisms, consisting of only a nucleic acid core that is surrounded by a protein shell. Several types of viruses commonly infect human cells and are responsible for a diverse range of pathologies. Viral infections extend from relatively mild disorders such as the common cold to serious, life- threatening conditions such as acquired immunodeficiency syndrome (AIDS). Viruses are somewhat unique in that they must rely totally on the metabolic processes of the host (human) cell to function. Hence, the pharmacologic treatment of viral infections is complex, because it is often difficult to selectively destroy the virus without also destroying human cells.

This chapter describes the basic characteristics of viruses and the relatively limited number of drugs that can act selectively as antiviral agents. Methods of preventing viral infections (antiviral vaccines) are also briefly discussed. Finally, the current methods of treating a specific viral-induced disease—AIDS—are presented. Rehabilitation specialists often treat patients who are in the active stages of a viral infection, as well as those suffering from the sequelae of viral disorders, such as gastroenteritis, encephalitis, and influenza. Hence, the pharmacotherapeutic treatment and prophylaxis of viral infections should concern physical therapists and occupational therapists.

VIRAL STRUCTURE AND FUNCTION

Classification of Viruses

Viruses are classified according to several criteria, including physical, biochemical, and pathogenic characteristics. The viruses can be divided into two categories, depending on the type of genetic material contained in the virus (DNA or RNA viruses). Families within each major subdivision are classified according to physical characteristics (configuration of the genetic material, shape of the virus capsule) and other functional criteria.

Characteristics of Viruses

Viruses are somewhat unique in structure and function as compared with other microorganisms. A virus essentially consists of a core of viral DNA or RNA. The genetic core is surrounded by a protein shell, or *capsid*. This structure—the capsid enclosing the nucleic acid core—is referred to as the *nucleocapsid*. In some viruses, the nucleocapsid is also surrounded by a viral membrane, or envelope, which is composed of glycoproteins extending outward from a lipid bilayer.

The virus, however, does not contain any of the cellular components necessary to replicate itself or synthesize proteins and other macromolecules; that is, the virus lacks ribosomes, endoplasmic reticulum, and so on. The virus contains only the genetic code (viral genome) that will produce additional viruses. To replicate itself, the virus must rely on the biochemical machinery of the host cell. In

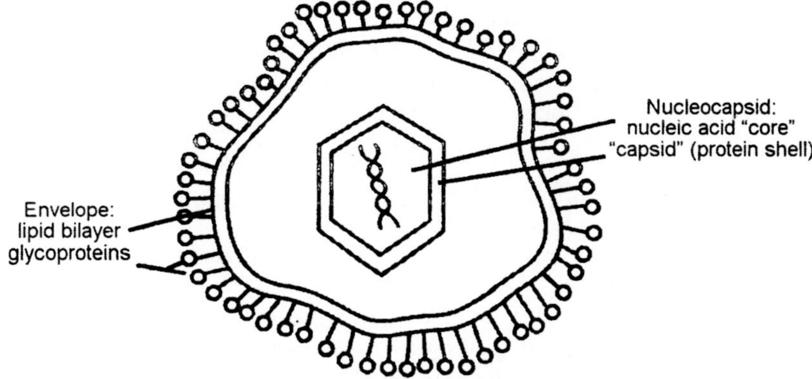

Fig. 12.1. Basic components of a virus.

essence, the virus invades the host cell, takes control of the cell's metabolic function, and uses the host cell's macromolecular-synthesizing apparatus to crank out new viruses.

Viral Replication

Self-replication of a virus occurs in several distinct steps: (1) adsorption, (2) penetration and uncoating, (3) biosynthesis, and (4) maturation and release.

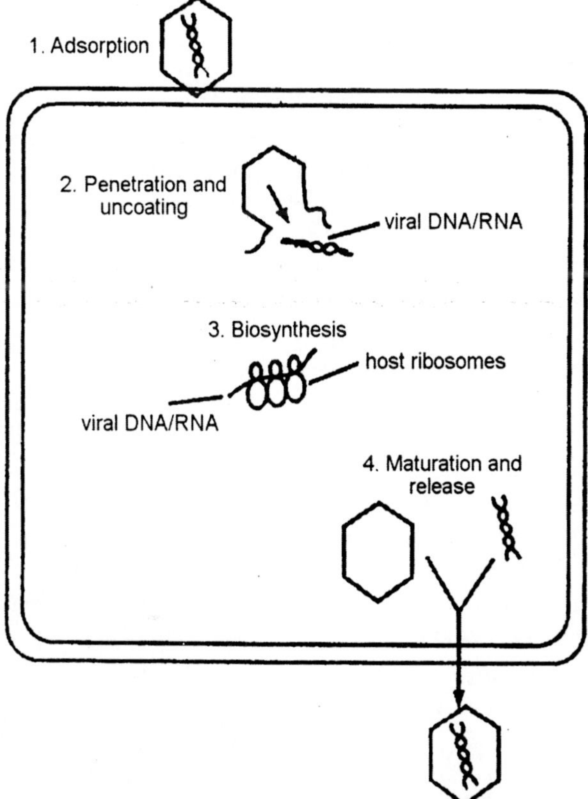

Fig. 12.2. Basic sequence of viral replication.

Adsorption

Initially, the virus attaches or adsorbs to the surface of the host cell. Most viruses are attracted to the host cell because of the interaction between proteins on the outer surface of the virus and receptorlike proteins on the host-cell membrane. The interaction of the virus with these surface proteins causes the virus to adhere to the outer surface of the host-cell membrane.

Penetration and uncoating

The virus enters the host cell either by passing directly through the cell membrane or by fusing with the host-cell membrane and releasing the viral genetic material into the host cell. Once inside the host cell, its proteolytic enzymes usually remove any coating that remains on the virus.

Biosynthesis

When viral genetic material is released within the host cell, the virus takes control of the cell's molecular synthesizing machinery to initiate the biosynthesis of new viral enzymes and proteins. Different viruses exert their effects on the host cell in different ways, but many viruses control the host cell through a direct effect on the cell's nucleus. Some viruses, including the virus that causes AIDS, actually insert their genetic material directly into the host cell's DNA, thereby becoming integrated within the genetic control of the infected cell.

Regardless of the exact mechanism of infection, the virus essentially commands the cell to synthesize the enzymes that produce more copies of viral DNA or RNA and to synthesize structural proteins that will ultimately be used to form new viral shells or capsids. Thus, the virus uses the biosynthetic machinery as well as the structural components and nutrients of the cell (amino acids, nucleic acids, etc.) to replicate itself. Likewise, the virus often incapacitates the infected cell so that the infected cell cannot carry out its normal physiologic activities.

Maturation and release

The component parts of the virus (the genetic core and surrounding shell) are assembled into mature viruses and released from the host cell. In some cases, the virus is released by a process of exocytosis, leaving the host cell relatively intact (although still infected with the original virus). Alternatively, the host cell may simply be destroyed (undergo lysis), thus releasing the viral offspring. Lysis of the host cell not only results in the release of the virus and the death of the cell, but also may stimulate the production of inflammatory mediators (prostaglandins, kinins, etc.), which create a hypersensitivity response. The steps involved in viral replication are important pharmacologically because antiviral drugs may interrupt this process at one or more of the steps.

Specific Antiviral Drugs

Acyclovir and Valacyclovir

Antiviral efficacy and clinical use

Acyclovir (Zovirax) is effective against herpesvirus infections, especially those involving herpes simplex types I and II. Acyclovir is the principal drug used to treat genital herpes and herpes simplex–related infections in other mucosal and cutaneous areas (lips and face). Acyclovir is also effective against other members of the herpesvirus family, including the varicella-zoster and Epstein-Barr virus. This agent may be used to treat varicella-zoster–related infections such as herpes zoster and chickenpox. Epstein-Barr virus infections, including infectious mononucleosis, may also respond to acyclovir. This drug can also help decrease the risk of cytomegalovirus (CMV) infection in people receiving kidney transplants and transplants of other solid organs.

Acyclovir can be applied topically as a cream to treat cutaneous and mucosal infections. This drug can also be administered systemically, either orally or intravenously in severe, acute infections.

Valacyclovir (Valtrex) is the precursor or "*prodrug*" of acyclovir. When administered orally, valacyclovir is converted to acyclovir in the intestinal tract and liver. This conversion typically results in the eventual appearance of higher levels of acyclovir in the bloodstream, because valacyclovir is absorbed more readily from the gastrointestinal tract than acyclovir. Thus, administration of valacyclovir is a more effective way to achieve the therapeutic effects of acyclovir when these drugs are orally administered.

Mechanism of action

Acyclovir inhibits viral DNA replication by inhibiting the function of the DNA polymerase enzyme. This drug is taken into virus-infected cells and converted to acyclovir triphosphate by an enzyme known as viral thymidine kinase. The phosphorylated drug directly inhibits the function of the viral DNA polymerase, thus impairing the replication of viral genetic material. The virus also incorporates the drug into viral DNA strands, which halts further production of DNA because of the presence of a false nucleic acid.

The antiviral specificity of acyclovir is due to the drug's higher affinity for viral DNA polymerase rather than the analogous enzyme in human cells. Also, the first step in the phosphorylation of acyclovir is greatly accelerated in virus-infected cells versus healthy cells. Hence, the amount of the activated (phosphorylated) form of acyclovir is much greater in the cells that really need it—that is, cells infected with the virus.

Adverse effects

Topical application of acyclovir may produce local irritation of cutaneous and mucosal tissues. Prolonged systemic administration of acyclovir or valacyclovir may cause headaches, dizziness, skin rashes, and gastrointestinal problems (nausea, vomiting, diarrhea).

Amantadine and Rimantadine

Antiviral efficacy and clinical use

Amantadine (Symmetrel) and rimantadine (Flumadine) are used in the prevention and treatment of infections caused by the influenza A virus. When administered prophylactically, these drugs appear to be approximately 70 to 90 percent effective in preventing influenza A infections. Also, these drugs usually decrease the severity and duration of flu symptoms in people infected with influenza A if drug therapy is initiated when symptoms first appear. Amantadine is also effective in alleviating some of the motor abnormalities of Parkinson disease. As an anti- Parkinson drug, amantadine may block the effects of excitatory neurotransmitters in the basal ganglia, thus exerting effects that are quite different from its antiviral effects. Amantadine and rimantadine are administered to individuals already infected with influenza A to lessen the extent of the illness associated with the virus. These drugs are also given prophylactically to individuals who may have been exposed to influenza A and to high-risk patients such as the elderly or those with cardiopulmonary and other diseases. Amantadine may also be somewhat effective in treating certain cases of hepatitis C infection. These drugs are typically administered orally, either in capsule form or in a syrup preparation.

Mechanism of action

Amantadine and rimantadine appear to inhibit one of the early steps in influenza A replication by blocking the uncoating of the virus and preventing the release of viral nucleic acid within the host cell. These drugs may also interfere with the assembly of viral components, thus inhibiting one of the final steps in the replication process. This dual inhibitory effect on the early and late steps of viral replication accounts for these drugs' antiviral effectiveness.

Adverse effects

These drugs may produce central nervous system (CNS) symptoms such as confusion, loss of concentration, mood changes, nervousness, dizziness, and light-headedness. These symptoms may be especially problematic in elderly patients. Excessive doses of amantadine and rimantadine may increase the severity of these CNS symptoms, and overdose may cause seizures.

Cidofovir

Antiviral efficacy and clinical use

Cidofovir (Vistide) is used primarily to treat CMV retinitis in people with AIDS. When used clinically, this drug is often combined with probenecid, an agent that inhibits renal excretion of cidofovir, thereby providing higher plasma levels of this antiviral agent.

Mechanism of action

Cidofovir works like acyclovir and ganciclovir; these drugs inhibit viral DNA replication by inhibiting DNA polymerase activity and by halting elongation of viral DNA chains.

Adverse effects

Cidofovir may cause nephrotoxicity, especially at higher doses. This drug may also decrease the number of neutrophilic leukocytes, resulting in neutropenia and related symptoms such as fever, chills, and sore throat. Other side effects include headache and gastrointestinal disturbances (anorexia, nausea, diarrhea).

Docosanol

Antiviral efficacy and clinical use

Docosanol (Abreva) is applied topically to treat blisters and cold sores caused by herpes virus simplex. This drug is available as an over-the-counter product, and is used primarily to treat recurrent outbreaks of orofacial herpes lesions.

Mechanism of action

Docosanol does not inactivate the herpes virus, but appears to act on the host (human) cells so that the virus cannot adsorb to the surface of the cell. As such, it must be applied early in the course of outbreaks before the virus has a chance to cause substantial lesions.

Adverse effects

Patients may experience headache and some local skin irritation during topical use of this drug.

Enfuvirtide

Antiviral efficacy and clinical use

Enfuvirtide (Fuzeon) is the first approved drug that limits the ability of human immunodeficiency virus (HIV) to enter host cells. As such, this drug is used as part of the antiviral regimen against HIV infection. Enfuvirtide is typically added to other agents (reverse transcriptase inhibitors, protease inhibitors) in patients who do not respond adequately to traditional anti-HIV treatment. This drug is effective against HIV type 1, but not against HIV type 2. Enfuvirtide must be administered parenterally; it is associated with frequent and potentially serious side effects. At the time of this writing, enfuvirtide is the only drug of its type, but other HIV entry inhibitors are currently in development, and the use of these drugs may be expanded in the future if newer, safer agents reach the market.

Mechanism of action

As indicated, enfuvirtide inhibits the ability of HIV to bind to, and enter, susceptible host cells such as CD4 lymphocytes. The drug actually binds to specific components on the outer glycoprotein envelop of the virus, thereby retarding the ability of the virus to change its shape in preparation for adsorbing to the surface of the host cell. If the virus cannot attach to host cells, the risk of infection is reduced.

Adverse effects

Enfuvirtide must be administered by subcutaneous injection, and local pain and irritation occurs at the injection site in most patients. Other common side effects include peripheral neuropathy and immune complex reactions that can lead to serious problems including respiratory distress syndrome, kidney dysfunction, and possibly GuillainBarre syndrome.

Famciclovir and Penciclovir

Antiviral efficacy and clinical use

Penciclovir (Denavir) is similar to acyclovir in terms of its antiviral effects and clinical indications. However, penciclovir is absorbed poorly from the gastrointestinal tract. This drug is primarily administered topically to treat recurrent herpes simplex infections of the lips and face (cold sores).

Famciclovir (Famvir) is the precursor (prodrug) to penciclovir; the drug is converted to penciclovir following oral administration. This situation is analogous to the relationship between acyclovir and valacyclovir, where it is advantageous to administer the prodrug because it will be absorbed more completely and will ultimately result in higher plasma levels of the drug's active form. Hence, famciclovir is administered orally to treat infections related to herpes simplex (e.g., genital herpes) and varicella zoster (e.g., herpes zoster). However, the actual antiviral effects of famciclovir occur because this drug is converted to penciclovir within the body.

Mechanism of action

Penciclovir acts like acyclovir; that is, the drug is activated (phosphorylated) within virus-infected cells, where it subsequently inhibits viral DNA synthesis and viral replication. As indicated, famciclovir exerts its antiviral effects after being converted to penciclovir in vivo.

Adverse effects

Topical application of penciclovir may cause some skin reactions (rashes, irritation) at the application site, but the incidence of these reactions is fairly low. Systemic (oral) administration of famciclovir is generally well tolerated, with only minor side effects such as headache, dizziness, and gastrointestinal disturbances (nausea, diarrhea).

Fomivirsen

Antiviral efficacy and clinical use

Fomivirsen (Vitravene) is injected into the vitreous humour to treat CMV infection in the eye. This drug is often used to treat ocular CMV infections that are resistant to more traditional agents such as ganciclovir or foscarnet.

Mechanism of action

Fomivirsen has a unique mechanism of antiviral action. This drug contains an amino acid sequence that is opposite or complimentary to the messenger RNA sequence controlling CMV replication. Because of this opposing or "*antisense*" sequence, fomivirsen inhibits several aspects of CMV replication, and also inhibits the viruses' ability to adsorb to the surface of host cells.

Adverse effects

Injecting fomivirsen into the eye may cause localized pain, redness, or swelling, but serious side effects or vision disturbances are rare.

Foscarnet

Antiviral efficacy and clinical use

Foscarnet (Foscavir) is primarily given to treat CMV retinitis in patients with AIDS. This agent may also help control other infections in patients with a compromised immune system, including serious cytomegaloviral infections (pneumonia, gastrointestinal infections) and some herpesvirus infections (herpes simplex, varicellazoster).

Mechanism of action

Foscarnet works somewhat like acyclovir and ganciclovir; that is, foscarnet inhibits the DNA polymerase enzyme necessary for viral DNA replication. Foscarnet differs from these other antiviral drugs, however, in that it does not require phosphorylation (activation) by enzymes such as viral thymidine kinase. Certain strains of viruses are thymidine-kinase deficient, meaning that these viruses lack the enzyme needed to activate antiviral agents such as acyclovir and ganciclovir. Hence, foscarnet is often used in patients with thymidine-kinase-resistant viruses who do not respond to acyclovir or ganciclovir.

Adverse effects

The primary problem associated with foscarnet is impaired renal function, including acute tubular necrosis. Hematologic disorders (anemia, granulocytopenia, leukopenia), gastrointestinal disturbances (cramps, nausea, vomiting), and CNS toxicity may also occur during foscarnet treatment.

Ganciclovir and Valganciclovir

Antiviral efficacy and clinical use

Ganciclovir (Cytovene) is given primarily to patients with AIDS to treat problems related to CMV infection, including CMV retinitis, polyradiculopathy, and other systemic CMV infections. Valganciclovir (Valcyte) is the precursor (prodrug) form that is converted to ganciclovir within the body. Ganciclovir and similar agents can also help reduce the risk of CMV infection in people receiving solid organ transplants such as kidney transplants.

Mechanism of action

Ganciclovir, like acyclovir, inhibits viral DNA replication by inhibiting DNA polymerase activity and by halting elongation of viral DNA chains.

Adverse effects

The most serious problems associated with ganciclovir include anemia, granulocytopenia, thrombocytopenia, and related hematologic disorders. Ganciclovir may also cause gastrointestinal disturbances (nausea, loss of appetite) and CNS disturbances (mood changes, nervousness, tremor).

Imiquimod

Antiviral efficacy and clinical use

Imiquimod (Aldara) is applied topically to treat condylomata acuminate infections that cause genital and perianal warts. It can also be used to treat certain skin conditions such as actinic keratoses of the face and scalp.

Mechanism of action

Although the details are unclear, imiquimod enhances the local production of interferons, tumour necrosis factor-alpha, and possibly other cytokines that produce antiviral responses. Hence, this drug does not act directly on the virus, but instead modulates the host (human) immune responses that have antiviral effects.

Adverse effects

Some local skin irritation and blistering can occur when imiquimod is applied topically.

Trifluridine

Antiviral efficacy and clinical use

Trifluridine (Viroptic) is administered by eye drops to treat local eye infections associated with herpes simplex virus; that is, herpes virus-related keratitis and keratoconjunctivitis.

Mechanism of action

This drug impairs viral DNA synthesis by inhibiting the enzymes that incorporate a specific nucleotide (thymidine) into viral DNA. The drug also substitutes itself for thymidine in the viral DNA sequence, thus creating a false DNA code that is ineffective in promoting viral replication.

Adverse effects

Some local redness and irritation of the eye may develop during local/topical application of trifluridine, but serious adverse effects are rare.

Oseltamivir and Zanamivir

Antiviral efficacy and clinical use

Oseltamivir (Tamiflu) and Zanamivir (Relenza) are effective against influenza virus types A and B. These drugs can reduce the duration and severity of flu symptoms if the drug is administered within 48 hours after symptoms first appear. These drugs can also be taken prophylactically to reduce the risk of getting the flu, especially in people who are at high risk (older adults, people with respiratory disorders), or in cases where an individual is exposed to a family member or someone else with the flu.

Mechanism of action

Oseltamivir and zanamivir inhibit a specific enzyme (neuraminidase) that the influenza virus uses to complete its biosynthesis and release. By inhibiting this enzyme, these drugs impair a key step in viral replication, and reduce the ability of the virus to infect other respiratory cells.

Adverse effects

Oral administration of oseltamivir can cause gastrointestinal disturbances such as nausea, vomiting, diarrhea, and abdominal cramps. Zanamivir, which is administered by inhalation, is associated with bronchospasm and reduced opening of the airway. The adverse effects of zanamivir can be quite severe in people with bronconstrictive disease (asthma, chronic obstructive pulmonary disease), and this drug should probably be avoided in these individuals.

Protease Inhibitors

Antiviral efficacy and clinical use

These drugs inhibit an enzyme known as HIV protease. This enzyme is needed to manufacture specific HIV proteins, including enzymes such as the HIV reverse transcriptase enzyme and structural proteins that comprise the HIV molecule. By inhibiting this enzyme, protease inhibitors prevent the synthesis and maturation of HIV, thus helping to prevent HIV replication and progression of HIV-related disease. The protease inhibitors currently available include amprenavir (Agenerase), atazanavir (Reyataz), fosamprenavir (Lexiva), indinavir (Crixivan), lopinavir (Kaltetra; the trade name for lopinavir combined with ritonavir), nelfinavir (Viracept), ritonavir (Norvir), and saquinavir (Fortovase, Invirase).

Protease inhibitors are often incorporated into the comprehensive treatment of people with HIV infection. In addition, a specific protease inhibitor can be combined with a low dose of ritonavir—a process known as protease-inhibitor "*boosting*." Ritonavir inhibits the hepatic breakdown of the other (primary) protease drug, thereby enabling the primary drug to exert better therapeutic effects at a lower dose.

Mechanism of action

Protease inhibitors bind to the HIV protease and prevent this enzyme from acting on HIV substrates. This effect negates the ability of the protease enzyme to cleave polypeptide precursors from larger, polypeptide chains. If these precursors are not available for the manufacture of HIV proteins, the virus cannot fully develop. Treatment with protease inhibitors therefore results in the manufacture of incomplete and noninfectious fragments of HIV rather than the mature virus.

Adverse effects

Protease inhibitors may cause alterations in fat deposition in the body (lipodystrophy)—fat deposits atrophy in the limbs, but excess fat is deposited in the abdomen. Blood lipids may also be adversely affected, resulting in increased plasma cholesterol, increased triglycerides, and decreased high-density lipoproteins. These drugs may also cause other metabolic disturbances, including insulin resistance. These drug-induced problems create a metabolic syndrome that can increase the risk of cardiovascular disease in people receiving protease inhibitors. The extent of these metabolic problems depends on several factors, including the specific protease inhibitor, other anti-HIV medications that are also being administered, and the characteristics of each patient. Other side effects include diarrhea, headache, and fatigue.

Reverse Transcriptase Inhibitors

Antiviral efficacy and clinical use

Reverse transcriptase inhibitors (RTIs) are used to inhibit the replication and proliferation of HIV type I (HIV-1). These agents act on a specific enzyme and inhibit a key step in HIV replication. Although these drugs do not eliminate the virus from infected cells, they are often effective in reducing HIV proliferation and the spread of HIV to noninfected cells. These drugs are therefore beneficial in preventing or delaying the progression of HIV and AIDS.

Zidovudine (Retrovir), also known generically as azidothymidine or AZT, was the first RTI approved for treating people who are infected with HIV. Other zidovudine-like drugs have also been developed; currently available agents include abacavir (Ziagen), didanosine (Videx), lamivudine (Epivir), stavudine (Zerit), tenofovir (Viread), and zalcitabine (HIVID). These RTIs can also be subclassified as nucleoside reverse transcriptase inhibitors (NRTIs) because they share a common chemical background.

More recently, RTIs that are chemically distinct from zidovudine and other NRTIs have also been developed. These agents are known as nonnucleoside reverse transcriptase inhibitors (NNR-TIs), and include drugs such as delavirdine (Rescriptor), efavirenz (Sustiva), and nevirapine (Viramune). These drugs also inhibit the reverse transcriptase enzyme, but act at a different site on the enzyme than do their NRTI counterparts.

Therefore, several types of RTIs are available that can help prevent HIV replication and inhibit the proliferation and spread of this virus to noninfected cells. Although these drugs do not kill HIV, RTIs are the cornerstone of treatment for preventing the progression of HIV disease.

Mechanism of action

RTIs impair HIV replication by inhibiting the reverse transcriptase enzyme that is needed to convert viral RNA to viral DNA. With regard to zidovudine and the other NRTIs, these agents enter viral-infected cells, where they are progressively phosphorylated (activated) by various intracellular enzymes. The phosphorylated version of the drug then acts as a false nucleic acid, competing with the real nucleic acid (thymidine) for incorporation into growing viral DNA strands. This competition slows down the reverse transcriptase enzyme because the enzyme cannot handle the false nucleic acid (the drug) as easily as the real nucleic acid (thymidine). Even if the reverse transcriptase is successful in incorporating the drug into viral DNA strands, this action prematurely terminates DNA strand synthesis because a false nucleic acid has been added to the viral DNA instead of the real nucleic acid.

The newer agents (NNRTIs) such as delaviridine, efavirenz, and nevirapine directly inhibit the reverse transcriptase enzyme by binding to the enzyme's active (catalytic) site and preventing this enzyme from converting viral RNA to viral DNA. Thus, these agents offer an alternative way to impair reverse transcriptase function and prevent viral replication.

Adverse effects

RTIs are associated with a number of bothersome side effects, and certain agents can also cause potentially serious problems. The most common problems associated with zidovudine are blood dyscrasias, such as anemia and granulocytopenia. Other symptoms occurring during zidovudine administration may include fever, chills, nausea, diarrhea, dizziness, headache, and excessive fatigue. NRTI drugs may also cause myopathy, as indicated by skeletal muscle tenderness, weakness, and atrophy. Likewise, peripheral neuropathies are common, especially when NRTIs such as didanosine, stavudine, and zacitabine are administered in higher doses. These adverse neuromuscular effects are probably due to the toxic effects of these drugs on mitochondrial function in muscle and nerve tissues. However, considering that these drugs are often used in severely immunocompromised patients (such as patients with AIDS), adverse neuromuscular effects may be also be caused by other sequelae of AIDS in addition to the drug's effects. Hence, neuromuscular problems are seen frequently in patients with advanced cases of HIV infection and AIDS. Other effects associated with NRTIs include pancreatitis, CNS toxicity (headache, irritability, insomnia), and gastrointestinal disturbances (nausea, diarrhea). Abacavir can cause an allergic (hypersensitivity) reaction that produces symptoms such as fever, joint and muscle pain, skin rashes, abdominal pain, nausea, diarrhea, and vomiting. In severe cases, this reaction can progress to anaphylactic shock and possibly death. Skin rashes are the most common side effect of the NNRTIs, and efavirenz may cause nervous system symptoms such as headache, dizziness, and insomnia.

Ribavirin

Antiviral efficacy and clinical use

Ribavirin (Virazole) is active against several RNA and DNA viruses, including respiratory syncytial virus (RSV). Clinically, this drug is used to treat severe RSV pneumonia in infants and young children, and RSV in certain adult populations, including the elderly, people with cardiopulmonary problems, and people with a compromised immune system. Ribavirin may also be useful as a secondary agent in the treatment of influenza A and B in young adults. The combination of ribavirin and interferons is often the treatment of choice in chronic hepatitis C infection. Ribavirin is administered through oral inhalation. This drug is suspended in an aerosol form and administered to the patient by a mechanical aerosol generator and a ventilation mask, mouthpiece, or hood.

Mechanism of action

The mechanism of action of this drug is not fully understood. Ribavirin appears to impair viral messenger RNA (mRNA) synthesis, probably by selectively inhibiting enzymes responsible for RNA replication. Inadequate viral mRNA production leads to impaired viral protein synthesis, which ultimately curtails viral replication.

Adverse effects

Ribavirin produces relatively few adverse effects when administered by inhalation. Most of the drug's action is confined to local pulmonary tissues, and severe systemic effects are rare. One adverse effect that may occur is local irritation of the eyes (conjunctivitis), due to the direct contact of aerosol with the eyes. This occurrence may be a problem if the drug is administered via some sort of hood or tent that encloses the patient's entire head.

Vidarabine

Antiviral efficacy and clinical use

Vidarabine (Vira-A) was the first systemic agent used to treat herpesvirus infections, including CMV, herpes simplex virus, and varicella-zoster virus. In the past, this drug was administered by continuous intravenous infusion to treat severe systemic infections caused by these viruses, but systemic use of vidarabine has been replaced by safer and less toxic agents. Vidarabine is currently used primarily to treat local viral infections of the eye (e.g., herpes simplex keratoconjunctivitis); it is applied topically by ophthalmic ointment to treat these infections.

Mechanism of action

Vidarabine appears to exert its antiviral effects in a manner similar to acyclovir. Both drugs selectively inhibit viral enzymes that are responsible for viral DNA replication.

Adverse effects

The primary problems associated with systemic administration of vidarabine include gastrointestinal distress (nausea, vomiting, diarrhea) and CNS disturbances (dizziness, hallucinations, mood changes). Ophthalmic application may produce local irritation (itching, redness, swelling) in some individuals.

Viral Resistance

As discussed in the last chapter, certain bacteria can develop strategies that render them resistant to drug therapy. This fact is true for other microorganisms, including most types of virus. Viruses can mutate and alter their structural or functional characteristics so that previously effective drugs will be unable to control specific viral infections adequately. It is beyond the scope of this chapter to address all the resistant viral strains, and how these strains acquired resistance against antiviral drugs. Viral resistance, like bacterial resistance, is a growing concern. Efforts should be made to limit the indiscriminate or inappropriate use of antiviral drugs, and to contain the spread of resistant viruses. Developing methods to overcome viral resistance using new drugs or different drug combinations is also a critical area of laboratory and clinical research.

Interferons

Interferons are a group of proteins that produce a number of beneficial pharmacologic and physiologic effects. These agents were first recognized as endogenous substances that exert nonspecific antiviral activity; that is, interferons enable healthy cells to resist infection from many viruses. Interferons produce other beneficial effects, including the control of cell differentiation, the limiting of excessive cell proliferation, and the modification of certain immune processes.

There are three primary classes of human interferons: alpha, beta, and gamma. Certain cells and tissues produce each primary interferon class. Of these three types, alpha and beta interferons are often grouped together as type I interferons; these type I interferons seem more important in terms of antiviral activity. Type II (gamma) interferons appear to be more important in regulating other aspects of the immune response and are responsible for promoting the growth of T lymphocytes and other responses promoting local inflammation.

The possibility that interferons can be used as pharmacologic agents has aroused a great deal of interest. Recombinant DNA techniques and cell tissue cultures have been used to produce sufficient quantities of interferons for clinical drug trials. The rationale is that exogenously administered interferons will produce antiviral and other beneficial effects in healthy cells in a manner similar to their endogenously produced counterparts. Some of the pertinent aspects of interferon action and clinical applications are presented below.

Synthesis and Cellular Effects of Interferons

Virtually all of the body's cells are capable of producing interferons, and these substances serve as an early step in preventing the virus from infecting healthy cells. Cells that have been infected by a virus produce interferons that are subsequently released from the infected cell. These interferons then travel to noninfected cells, where they bind to specific receptors located on the surface of the healthy cells. Binding of the interferon induces the healthy cell to synthesize its own antiviral proteins. Interferons apparently direct the healthy cell to synthesize the enzymes that inhibit viral messenger RNA and protein synthesis. Thus, even if the virus does penetrate into the healthy cell, the virus cannot replicate because of an inability to synthesize viral proteins.

The manner in which interferons control cell growth and proliferation is not fully understood. Interferons may limit excessive cell division by activating lymphocytes and other cytotoxic cells that combat the cancer, and by controlling specific gene segments in normal and cancerous cells. In particular, interferons may inhibit specific gene-regulatory segments of tumor cells known as *oncogenes*. The inhibition of oncogenes would attenuate the excessive proliferation and lack of cell differentiation typifying neoplastic disease. Interferons may also limit cancer growth by activating certain aspects of the immune system, including increased activity of natural killer cells and other cytotoxic cells that attack cancerous tissues.

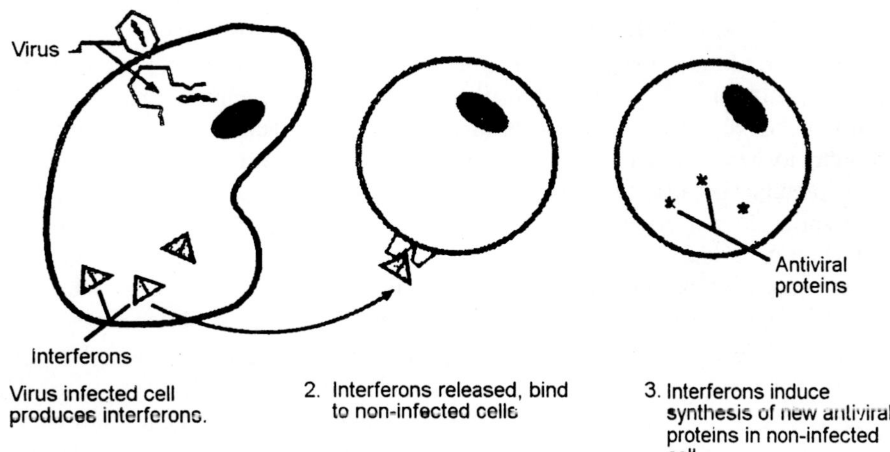

Fig. 12.3. Antiviral effects of interferons.

Pharmacologic Applications of Interferons

When interferons were first discovered, there was a great deal of optimism about their use as antiviral agents. Although early clinical trials with interferons were somewhat disappointing, their use as antiviral agents gained acceptance as more was learned about the three primary classes and subclasses of the interferons. We now realize that interferons cannot be used interchangeably as antiviral drugs, but that certain types of interferons can be administered to treat specific viruses. Currently, type I interferons (interferons alpha and beta) seem especially beneficial in treating hepatitis B and C infections. These interferons can also be injected locally to treat certain forms of viral-induced warts such as condylomata acuminate infections. The clinical use of interferons as antiviral drugs should continue to increase as more is learned about various interferon subclasses and other factors influencing their effectiveness. As mentioned, interferons also help control abnormal cell proliferation, and these drugs have been approved for use in certain cancers. Interferons are often used as part of the treatment for certain leukemias, lymphomas, and several other forms of cancer. Finally, certain interferons may decrease exacerbations of multiple sclerosis (MS). Specifically, interferon beta-1a (Avonex) and interferon beta-1b (Betaseron) may help reduce the incidence and severity of relapses in exacerbating-remitting MS. This effect seems to occur because these beta interferons modulate several aspects of the autoimmune response that initiates the pathological changes associated with MS. Although the details are unclear, it appears that type I interferons can reduce the activity of macrophages, lymphocytes, and other immune system components that are responsible for the autoimmune destruction of glial cells and neuronal structures in patients with MS.

Adverse Effects of Interferons

Interferons may cause flu-like symptoms including fever, sweating, chills, muscle aches, and general malaise. Other side effects such as loss of appetite, nausea, vomiting, diarrhea, and unusual tiredness can also occur, depending on the type of interferon and the dosage. Interferons may also cause behavioral side effects such as depression, presumably because these drugs inhibit serotonin activity in the brain. When interferons are administered by intramuscular or subcutaneous injection, some irritation may develop around the injection site. Finally, anti-interferon antibodies may be produced by the immune system, especially when interferons are administered for prolonged periods. These antibodies can neutralize the interferons, thus decreasing their effectiveness in controlling viral infections and other conditions such as cancer and MS.

Control of Viral Infection with Vaccines

Vaccines prevent viral infection by stimulating the endogenous production of immune factors that will selectively destroy the invading virus. Hence, the vaccine can be administered to healthy individuals to provide them with immunity from certain viral infections. A vaccine acts as an antigen that induces the immune system to generate virus-specific antibodies. The vaccine, however, does not cause any appreciable viral infection because the vaccine contains a virus that has been modified in some way so that it retains its antigenic properties but lacks the ability to produce infection. Vaccines, for example, typically consist of a whole virus or part of the virus (viral particle or fragment) that has been completely inactivated (killed vaccines) or partially inactivated (live attenuated vaccines). Thus, most antiviral vaccinations are accomplished by administering small amounts of the modified virus.

In general, it is somewhat easier to develop vaccines that prevent viral infection than to develop drugs that destroy the virus once it has infected human cells. This notion is reasonable when one considers that the virus is essentially coexisting with the host cell. As indicated previously, there are currently only a limited number of drugs that are able to selectively inhibit the virus without harming the host cell. A more practical strategy is to use vaccines to enable the body to destroy the virus before an infection is established.

At present, vaccines are available for several serious viral infections, including polio, smallpox, rabies, measles, mumps, rubella, hepatitis A and B, and influenza. In some situations, vaccination against certain viral infections is routine. For instance, schoolchildren must periodically show evidence of polio, measles, and other vaccinations according to state and local laws. In other cases, vaccines are administered prior to potential exposure to the virus or in high-risk groups. Influenza vaccinations, for example, are often administered to elderly and debilitated patients during seasonal influenza outbreaks.

Although vaccines exist for many serious viral infections, some drawbacks still exist. Some vaccines are only partially effective, and viral infection still occurs in a significant percentage of vaccinated individuals. Other vaccines, especially killed vaccines, often require periodic readministration (boosters) to help maintain antiviral immunity. In addition, certain types of viruses still lack an effective vaccination. For example, no vaccine is currently approved for the HIV that causes AIDS. Hence, the improvement of existing vaccines and the development of new vaccines remain two of the more important aspects of antiviral chemotherapy.

HIV and the Treatment of AIDS

HIV is a member of the retrovirus family. HIV impairs the function of certain cells in the immune system such as CD4+ (T-helper) lymphocytes. Destruction of immune system components often leads to the severe immunocompromised state known as AIDS. This virus exists in at least two forms: HIV-1 and HIV-2. Both forms of the virus are capable of causing AIDS, but HIV-1 is more prevalent. Hence, HIV-1 is also referred to informally as the "AIDS virus." Because there is currently no effective way to kill the AIDS virus in humans, there is no cure for AIDS.

AIDS is a life-threatening disorder because of the susceptibility of the immunocompromised patient to severe infections and certain forms of cancer. In particular, patients with AIDS often suffer from severe viral infections (CMV, various herpesvirus infections), bacterial infections (*Mycobacterium tuberculosis*), fungal infections (*Pneumocystis jiroveci*), and infections caused by various other microbes and parasites. Patients with AIDS also develop relatively unusual neoplastic diseases, such as Kaposi sarcoma.

Considerable neuromuscular involvement also occurs in patients with AIDS. Peripheral neuropathies, myopathies, and various CNS manifestations (dementia, other psychological manifestations) can occur directly from HIV infection or secondarily, due to some other opportunistic infection. Likewise, peripheral neuropathies are a common side effect of certain anti-HIV drugs (didanosine, stavudine, zalcitabine), and myopathies are a side effect of zidovudine therapy. Patients with HIV disease often have painful symptoms such as joint pain, back pain, and pain related to neuropathies and myopathies. Hence, HIV disease can often be regarded as a degenerative neuromuscular disorder from the standpoint of a rehabilitation professional. Therapists can therefore help improve function and decrease pain in patients with HIV infection and AIDS.

Individuals who are infected with HIV may remain very asymptomatic for several years before developing the full-blown clinical picture of AIDS. Even people exposed to HIV who do not initially develop AIDS carry the virus for the rest of their lives and are thus capable of transmitting the virus to others. Transmission of HIV from one individual to another occurs primarily through intimate sexual contact and through sharing intravenous needles. Transfusions of blood from HIV-infected donors are also a potential source of HIV transmission. Hence, practices such as safe sex, not sharing needles, and improved blood-screening techniques are crucial in preventing the transmission of HIV and the subsequent risk of developing AIDS.

The treatment of patients with AIDS and individuals infected by HIV is continually being modified as new drugs become available and more information is gained about the nature of the AIDS virus. Currently, the pharmacologic management of HIV-infected patients consists of two principal strategies: (1) controlling the proliferation and effects of HIV in individuals infected with this virus and (2) treatment and prevention of various opportunistic infections that attempt to take advantage of the compromised immune system in patients with AIDS. The pharmacologic methods used to accomplish these principal strategies are presented here.

Inhibition of HIV Proliferation in Infected Individuals

No drugs are currently available that selectively kill HIV in humans, hence the lack of a cure for this viral infection. Nonetheless, several antiviral drugs are given to inhibit the replication of this virus, thus decreasing the morbidity and mortality of HIV infection. These drugs are usually specific for the HIV-1 form of the virus, because HIV- 1 is more prevalent in people infected by HIV. Several pharmacologic strategies for treating HIV infection are currently available, and these strategies are discussed briefly here.

Zidovudine (Retrovir, AZT) was the first drug approved as an anti-HIV agent. Other agents that act like zidovudine were subsequently approved to prevent HIV replication. These drugs include abacavir (Ziagen), didanosine (Videx), lamivudine (Epivir), stavudine (Zerit), tenofovir (Viread), and zalcitabine (HIVID). As discussed in "Specific Antiviral Drugs," zidovudine and similar drugs are classified as NRTIs because they share a common mechanism of action; that is, these drugs inhibit the reverse transcriptase enzyme that HIV uses to synthesize viral DNA from viral RNA. This action impairs one of the early steps in viral replication, thus slowing the progression of HIV infection and the development of AIDS.

Protease inhibitors were the second major break-through in the pharmacologic treatment of HIV infection. Protease inhibitors are typically identified by generic names containing an "-avir" suffix. Protease inhibitors currently available include amprenavir (Agenerase), atazanavir (Reyataz), fosamprenavir (Lexiva), indinavir (Crixivan), lopinavir (Kaltetra; combination with Ritonavir), nelfinavir (Viracept), ritonavir (Norvir), and saquinavir (Fortovase, Invirase). As indicated earlier, these drugs impair the HIV protease enzyme that is responsible for several steps in HIV replication. Like the NRTIs, these drugs do not kill the virus but can slow its replication and prevent the spread of HIV to non-infected cells.

The third strategy developed to inhibit HIV replication is the NNRTIs. These drugs include delavirdine (Rescriptor), efavirenz (Sustiva), and nevirapine (Viramune). Like their nucleoside counterparts, NNRTIs also inhibit the reverse transcriptase enzyme's ability to perform one of the initial steps in HIV replication. The NNRTIs, however, directly inhibit the active (catalytic) site on this enzyme, whereas zidovudine and other NRTIs serve as false substrates that take the place of the substance (thymidine) normally acted on by this enzyme. Hence, NNRTIs provide another way to impair one of the key steps in HIV replication, and these drugs can be used along with other agents (NRTIs, protease inhibitors) to provide optimal benefits in preventing HIV replication and proliferation.

Finally, a group of agents known as HIV entry inhibitors is beginning to reach the market. These drugs impair the ability of the virus to attach to the host cell's surface, thereby inhibiting HIV entry into susceptible lymphocytes. If the virus cannot enter the cell, it cannot infect that cell or begin the process of viral replication. Enfuviritide (Fuzeon) is the first HIV entry inhibitor to be approved, and other drugs of this type will hopefully be available in the near future.

The arsenal of anti-HIV agents has therefore grown steadily since the development of the first anti- HIV drug (zidovudine). In addition, other drugs and strategies that inhibit HIV infection continue to be explored. As more is learned about the structure and function of this virus, drugs can be developed that impair specific steps in the absorption and replication of HIV in human cells. If clinical trials using these other drugs are favorable, they may also be approved for future use in individuals infected with HIV.

Anti-HIV Drug Combinations: Use of Highly Active Antiretroviral Therapy

Several anti-HIV drugs are often administered simultaneously to provide optimal inhibition of HIV replication and proliferation. The idea of combining several agents is referred to as highly active antiretroviral therapy, or HAART. HAART often involves the simultaneous use of at least three anti-HIV agents. A typical HAART strategy, for example, involves the use of two RTIs and one protease inhibitor. There are, however, many variations of the specific drug combinations used during HAART. Moreover, HAART regimens are continually being revised as new drugs reach the market or problems arise with existing strategies. Hence, the exact number and types of drugs used during HAART are selected based on the specific needs of each patient.

Regardless of the exact drugs used, there is ample evidence that HAART can successfully delay the progression of HIV disease in people infected with the virus. In many cases, strict adherence to HAART regimens can reduce the viral load (that is, the amount of viral RNA present in the bloodstream) to levels that are undetectable with current testing procedures. This fact does not mean that HAART has successfully eliminated the virus from the infected host or that the person infected with HIV has been cured. Even if HAART successfully reduces evidence of the virus in the plasma, the virus can be sequestered into T cells and other tissue "*reservoirs*" so that viral components cannot be detected in the bloodstream. Still, HAART regimens can prevent the progression of HIV infection and help sustain immune function by allowing increases in the number of functioning CD4 lymphocytes. The use of HAART is therefore associated with a substantial reduction in the incidence of AIDS and with improved clinical outcomes (fewer infections, decreased cancers, prolonged survival) in people who are infected with HIV.

HAART regimens are, however, associated with several problems and limitations. A certain percentage of people with HIV do not respond adequately to HAART; that is, HAART may not be very successful in producing a sustained and complete reduction in viral load in anywhere from 30 to 50 percent of patients receiving these regimens. The lack of effectiveness may be a consequence of poor adherence to the HAART regimen. Adherence to HAART is often difficult because of the potential for side effects with these drugs and because of difficulties in remembering the complicated dosage regimens associated with taking three or more agents. Resistance to anti-HIV drugs can also develop, especially if there is poor adherence to HAART regimens. As mentioned earlier, HAART does not completely eliminate the virus from the infected host, because some of the viral components remain sequestered within tissues, where they remain hidden from HAART drugs. Finally, the simultaneous use of several drugs during HAART increases the risk for drug-drug interactions, and likewise increases the chance for toxicity to the liver and other organs.

Nonetheless, HAART can suppress HIV disease in many people who are infected with this virus. Drug combinations can be used successfully for the long-term management of HIV disease, and they offer hope that people with HIV do not have to progress inexorably toward AIDS and death. Research continues to find the best way to combine existing agents and to incorporate new agents into a comprehensive and successful regimen for people infected with HIV.

HIV Vaccines

An HIV vaccine has not yet been successfully developed and approved for use in the United States. As indicated earlier, vaccines are typically an altered form of the original virus that is administered to stimulate the immune system, so that the immune system can recognize and destroy the virus if a person is exposed to it. Creation of an HIV vaccine is understandably a complicated endeavor, given the complexity of this virus and its tendency to evolve and mutate into different types of HIV. Nonetheless, the development of a safe, effective vaccine remains the best pharmacologic method for dealing with the spread of the virus, especially in underdeveloped nations that continue to experience a rise in the incidence of HIV and AIDS.

Hence, efforts continue to develop an HIV vaccine that will produce adequate immunity from HIV infection without severe untoward side effects. There is concern, however, that a successful vaccine may be very difficult to produce. For example, development of an HIV vaccine that is not 100 percent effective might give recipients a false sense of security; that is, a vaccine that confers only partial immunity (e.g., a 50 to 75 percent reduction in the risk of contracting HIV) might encourage the recipient to forgo other precautions, such as safe sex, not sharing intravenous needles, and so forth. Likewise, the question arises about whether a single vaccine will be successful in providing immunity from all the various HIV strains and subtypes. An HIV vaccine is urgently needed and would undoubtedly be received as one of the most important pharmacologic advancements of our time. The development of such a vaccine may be delayed, however, until we have a better understanding of HIV and how to best modify this virus into a successful vaccine.

We must therefore remember that zidovudine and other drugs currently available for treating HIV are not curative and may be helpful only in delaying or reducing AIDS-related deaths. A cure for AIDS, if possible, will take several years or even several decades before becoming a reality. As with many viruses, developing a vaccine against the AIDS virus is somewhat easier than making a drug that selectively destroys HIV. The development of an HIV vaccine, however, is probably still years away. Until a vaccine is developed, preventing transmission of HIV remains the best method of controlling the spread of AIDS.

Management of Opportunistic Infections

If HIV infection is not treated successfully, the body is open to infection from various other microorganisms. These infections are known commonly as opportunistic infections because microorganisms take advantage of the chance to infect people who lack normal immune defenses. Fortunately, newer anti-HIV drugs and the use of HAART regimens have reduced the risk of opportunistic infections. Hence, the best prevention against opportunistic infections is aggressive anti-HIV treatment that promotes T lymphocyte survival and helps maintain a functioning immune system. Still, some patients are prone to opportunistic infections, including patients who are newly diagnosed with HIV infection, or patients that cannot tolerate, respond to, or adhere to HAART regimens. Likewise, opportunistic infections are still a major cause of illness and death in areas of the world where HAART regimens are unavailable or unaffordable (i.e., developing countries). When immune function deteriorates beyond a certain point (typically less than 200 CD4 lymphocytes per microliter), these patients are said to have AIDS.

Because of a virtual lack of immunologic defenses, patients with AIDS often succumb to a variety of opportunistic infections. Essentially, these patients simply do not have the ability to fight off various viral, bacterial, and other microbial invaders. Consequently, much of the pharmacologic approach to the treatment of AIDS is associated with trying to curtail various infections by using the respective antimicrobial drugs that are currently available.

It is beyond the scope of this chapter to give a detailed description of the pharmacologic treatment of all the possible opportunistic infections that occur in patients with AIDS. Early recognition of infectious symptoms is crucial in helping initiate drug therapy before the infection becomes uncontrollable. Because patients with AIDS essentially lack endogenous defense systems, drug therapy must often be continued indefinitely, or the infection will recur. On the other hand, successful implementation or reinstitution of HAART strategies can restore immune function in certain patients, and drugs for opportunistic infections can sometimes be discontinued. Nonetheless, strategies for dealing with various infections are constantly changing, and drug therapy for HIV and opportunistic infections will surely be modified as new antimicrobial agents are developed and new evidence is provided about how these agents can be used in various infections.

Viruses present a unique problem in terms of the pharmacologic treatment of infectious disease. These microorganisms rely totally on the metabolic function of host (human) cells to function and replicate more viruses. Hence, there are currently only a limited number of effective antiviral agents that selectively kill or attenuate the virus without seriously harming the human cells. Developing and administering antiviral vaccines that stimulate the immunity of the host to specific viral infections is often more practical. In the future, the development of new antiviral agents and vaccines may help treat and eliminate viral infections that currently pose a serious health threat.

13

Drug Delivery Systems

In the in vitro–in vivo correlation (IVIVC) breakout session at the AAPS/FDA workshop on modified release (MR) parenterals in 2001, FDA reviewers stated that, in their personal opinion, the IVIVC of parenterals may be harder to develop but the process of developing the IVIVC and the process of demonstrating their validity had to be the same as MR oral products. The rationale was based on the fact that the IVIVC was going to be used for regulatory purposes such as a biowaiver and the development of release specifications. Over the last four to five years, the general belief remains the same—the development of an IVIVC for MR parenterals should follow the same process as a MR oral product. Although the design of IVIVC studies and the IVIVC modeling process have evolved, the fundamental principles of developing and validating an IVIVC has not significantly changed regardless of the type of delivery system. The purpose of this chapter is not to review the general principles of IVIVC, but instead, this chapter will address some of the special considerations that are required when developing an IVIVC for a controlled release parenteral product. Although the FDA guidance on IVIVC emphasizes the usefulness of Level A and multiple Level C IVIVC, this chapter will mainly address the development of a Level A IVIVC.

Special Considerations

Study Design

The study design for MR parenteral drug delivery systems should be similar to the design for oral formulations, if logistically possible. Typically, two or more formulations with different in vitro and in vivo release rates and formulation characteristics are administered to normal human volunteers. Patients may be used in the study if administration of the drug to normal volunteers is unsafe, which is more of a concern when administering a parenteral product, or the patient population significantly handles the drug and/or delivery system differently. The active drug in solution (defined here as the reference formulation) is also administered intravenously or through the same route of administration as the MR formulation in order to perform a Level A IVIVC. Although a complete crossover study is preferred, the logistical problems associated with running such a study may make the study impractical, given the time-course of in vivo delivery (e.g., implant delivery over a number of months). If the complete crossover study design is not possible, incomplete block and parallel designs have also been used. Regardless of the design, every subject should receive the reference formulation as the first arm of the study in order to define the unit impulse response and to ensure that a deconvolution or estimation of in vivo release can be performed, even if a subject drops out after receiving only one of three MR formulations.

In Vitro Release System

Although in vitro release (IVR) systems are well established for all types of oral formulations, standard IVR systems for MR parenterals do not exist. The literature reports a range of systems from the destructive test tube to the USP 4 or USP 7 apparatus. Although the IVR system is critical to the IVIVC modeling, this chapter will concentrate only on the modeling aspects.

In Vivo Release

With oral or any other systemic drug delivery system the in vivo release is typically estimated using the measurement of drug within the systemic circulation (i.e., studying the pharmacokinetics). However, with some parenteral products the delivery system is designed to administer drug locally. In this situation, the systemic measurement of drug does not represent what is occurring locally, or it may be difficult to obtain systemic measurements of drug because the concentration in the blood is below the limit of quantitation. For these local drug delivery systems, determining the amount of drug released over time requires invasive, destructive measurements of the delivery system to determine how much drug remains in the delivery system over time. This often cannot be determined in humans so the in vivo release must be determined in animals for the IVIVC (e.g., drug eluting stents). The FDA has been amenable to this approach, given the impossible task of measuring in vivo release in humans.

In Vitro–In Vivo Correlation Using More Complicated Modeling Approaches

For all parenteral IVIVC models, the author strongly recommends that at least three different formulations be studied in order to perform both internal and external predictability. In addition, with some MR parenteral dosage forms, in vitro release occurs over hours or days while complete in vivo release may take days, weeks, or months. The linear IVIVC models developed in the 1970s and 1980s could not deal with this time difference between the two releases. Over the last decade, time variant models have been introduced and used to deal with the differences in the time course of release. A model that has provided an enormous amount of flexibility in its ability to fit time variant and linear time invariant IVIVC data has been the model described by Gillespie and others. Both time shifting and time scaling can be described by the model, which allows the model to fit a wide variety of in vitro-in vivo profiles. The model used to describe both time shifting and scaling is presented in Equation 1:

$$x_{vivo}(t) = \begin{cases} 0 & t < 0 \\ & u = t \text{ for } t \leq T \\ a_1 + a_2 \cdot x_{vitro}(-b_1 + b_2 \cdot u) & u = T \text{ for } t > T \end{cases} \quad \ldots(1)$$

where x_{vivo} (t) = cumulative amount absorbed or released in vivo, x_{vitro} = cumulative amount released in vitro, a_1 = intercept for a linear IVIVC, a_2 = slope for a linear IVIVC, b_1 = coefficient representing a time shift between in vivo and in vitro, and b_2 = coefficient representing a time scaling between in vitro and in vivo. If b_1 = −1 and b_2 = 0, the IVIVC is the linear "point-to-point" model that has been reported in the literature over the years.

Predictable models have been developed using this approach for oral and parenteral delivery systems. The in vivo versus in vitro release of four formulations. Two of the formulations (K1, K2) have faster in vivo release than in vitro, while two of the formulations have faster in vitro release (K3, K4). Since an IVIVC now requires that one model be developed for two or more formulations, it would be impossible to develop one model to describe all four formulations using a conventional linear time invariant model. However, using Equation 1 to describe the shift and scaling, b_1 and b_2 can be estimated to obtain a single time variant model for all four formulations. The %PE of C_{max} and AUC for each formulation met the FDA criteria for internal predictability.

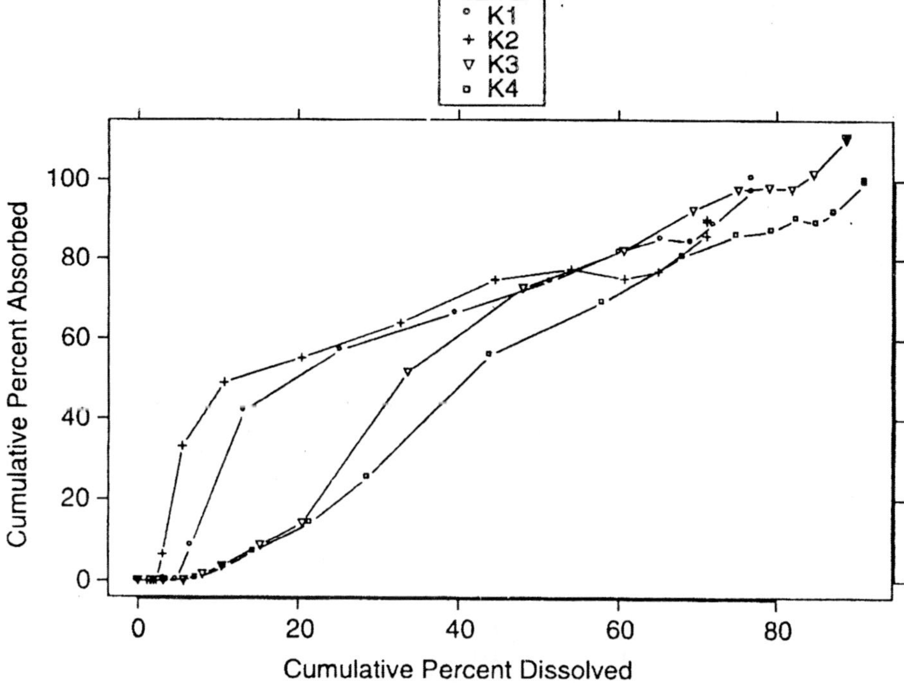

Fig. 13.1. Cumulative percent absorbed versus cumulative percent dissolved with time shifting.

EXAMPLES

Microspheres

Typically, there are two types of profiles that have been seen with MR microsphere delivery systems: Type 1 with one peak and continuous delivery and Type 2 with an initial burst peak and a second peak at a later time. The ideal approach to IVIVC modeling is to develop one IVIVC model for the total plasma profile. There are a number of reports on the in vitro–in vivo relationship for a single Type 1 formulation, but an IVIVC requires two ore more formulations. IVIVC models with two or more formulations have been developed for these Type 1 formulations but have not been reported in the literature. One of the few examples of investigating multiple formulations was reported by Van Dijkhuzien-Radersma et al. These investigators reported the in vitro and in vivo relationship for two formulations but did not develop a mathematical model for both formulations.

Investigators have attempted to develop a single IVIVC model for Type 2 plasma profiles using the two-stage deconvolution and the compartmental modeling approaches. In order to develop a single model, the IVR system must be able to correlate to the very fast absorption rate of the first plasma peak and the slower absorption rate of the second plasma peak. Although a significant amount of time has been spent in trying to develop an IVIVC and IVR system for formulations with a Type 2 profile, at the present time an example of this type of in vitro system or a validated IVIVC model describing both plasma peaks has not been reported in the literature.

For Type 2 plasma profiles, investigators have also attempted to develop an IVIVC for different parts of the plasma profile. This approach has been difficult because the first peak and second peak represent different release mechanisms from the dosage form and the magnitude of the second peak appears to be related to the magnitude of the first peak. Although acceptable IVIVC models have been developed for formulation development work, IVIVC models that meet the strict predictability criteria of the FDA IVIVC guidance have not been reported for the Type 2 plasma profile. The major problem appears to be in developing the relationship between the first peak and an in vitro release profile. The in vitro profile often represents more than the release of drug associated with only the surface of the microsphere, usually the major source of drug for the first plasma peak.

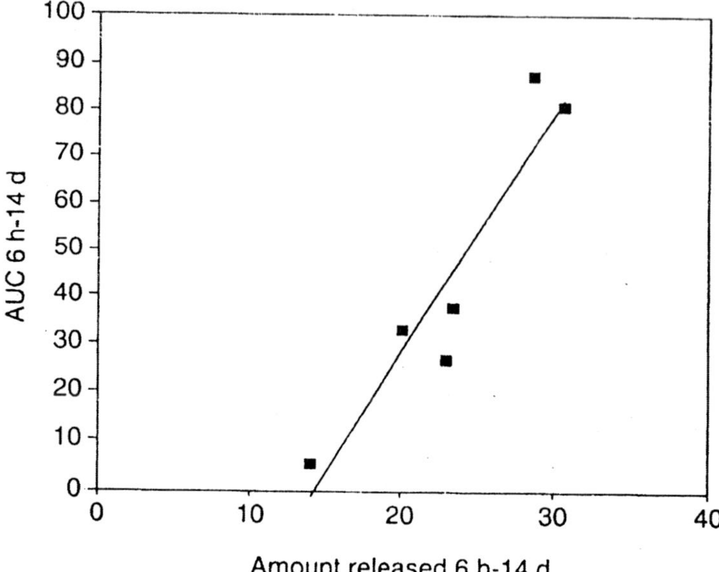

Fig. 13.2. Relationship between the amount of peptide released after the initial burst until day 14 and the AUC of plasma calculated for the same period of time (r=0.932).

IVIVC models describing the second peak (i.e., after the initial burst) have been successfully developed. Using a Level C correlation for in vitro and in vivo data after the initial burst, Blanco-Prieto et al. were able to develop a correlation for more than two formulations. The validity of the model, however, was not investigated for internal or external predictability. Time invariant, predictable Level A IVIVC models have also been successfully developed for the second peak. The IVIVC model met the strict predictability criteria of the FDA IVIVC guidance for both the C_{max} and AUC of the second peak.

Liposomes

Since liposomes have played a minor role as a parenteral MR delivery system over the years, there are no examples of a Level A IVIVC within the literature. Although the correlation between in vivo absorbed and in vitro release was for a single formulation, this example illustrates that the IVIVC methods reported within this book can be used for liposomes and that an IVIVC with more than two formulations may be possible for MR liposome drug delivery systems.

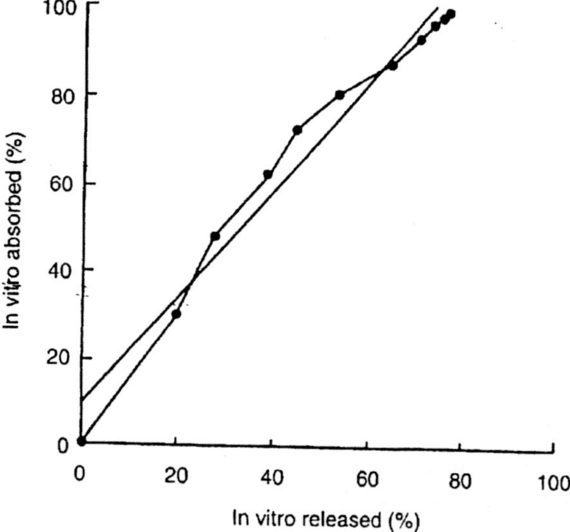

Fig. 13.3. Correlation of percentage of drug absorbed in vivo and percent drug released in vitro for bre-MVL (triolein/tricaprylin, 10/0).

Implants

The development of IVIVC models for implants has received the most attention within the literature. Chilukuri and Shah (10) were able to develop a relationship between in vivo and in vitro release for a single vancomycin implant product and Baro et al. were able to show a relationship for a single gentamicin formulation.

One of the few literature reports demonstrating a relationship between in vitro and in vivo release for more than one formulation has been reported by Negrin et al. The investigator manufactured implants and with slight differences in their in vitro release profiles evaluated the in vivo performance in animals. Negrin et al.'s investigation showed that all three implants followed a common in vitro to in vivo relationship. Unfortunately, the authors did not provide any information about an IVIVC mathematical model nor the predictability of the in vitro–in vivo relationship.

Fig. 13.4. Correlation of in vitro-in vivo release of vancomycin from GMS implants.

The FDA IVIVC MR guidance for oral products has been used to develop IVIVC models for parenteral products. This chapter has provided some of the specific aspects of IVIVC modeling that are relevant to MR parenteral drug delivery systems as well as selected examples to illustrate the possibility of developing an IVIVC for a parenteral product. Given the number of different parenteral delivery systems, it is not possible to discuss or present examples for each system but the basic principles presented here apply to all parenteral delivery systems. Within the literature there are a number of examples demonstrating that a relationship exists between the in vitro release of a single formulation and the in vivo release. There are few examples, however, of the in vitro to in vivo relationship being demonstrated for more than one formulation. In addition, the development of mathematical models that describe the relationships have not been provided for most of the single or multiple formulation examples within the literature. Although the actual IVIVC mathematical models have not been reported in the literature, the examples within this chapter demonstrate that it is possible to develop an IVIVC model for parenteral products that can be used throughout the development and regulatory cycle.

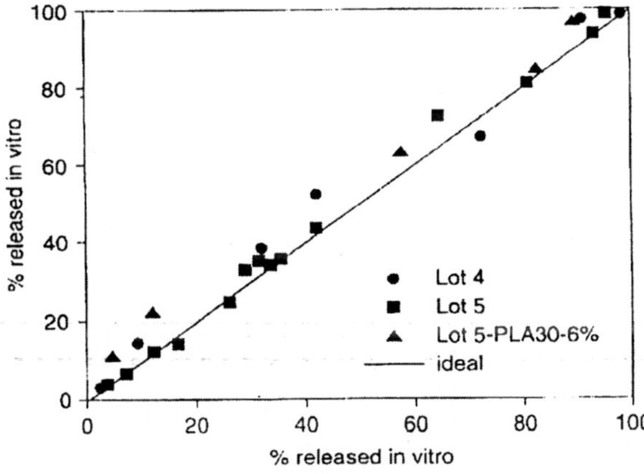

Fig. 13.5. In vitro-in vivo correlation obtained from different 1-week methadone base implants.

Transdermal Drug Delivery Systems

Transdermal delivery provides a potential noninvasive route of drug delivery, but only a small number of products are on the market. Skin, being a protective organ of the body, does not allow permeation of significant quantities of foreign substances into the body and the main barrier is the stratum corneum (SC). Only small and more lipophilic molecules could be delivered through skin until recently. However, the invention of novel transdermal delivery technologies such as iontophoresis, sonophoresis, electroporation, and microporation can now allow the delivery of hydrophilic small and macromolecules. Still, the commercial application of these technologies is difficult because of difficulties such as miniaturizing the devices. Iontophoresis has gained considerable importance in commercial development for systemic delivery of drugs due to the advantages of controlled and programmable delivery, and as a result some iontophoretic devices are in late stages of clinical development. An iontophoretic device has been approved by Food and Drug Administration for systemic delivery of fentanyl and another for local iontophoretic delivery of lidocaine. In vitro–in vivo correlation (IVIVC) in the case of transdermal drug delivery (TDD) is somewhat different compared to the oral route of administration. In most instances, steady state flux has been extrapolated to determine the in vivo plasma concentrations using pharmacokinetic (PK) modeling. IVIVC can help to achieve a mechanistic understanding of the drug delivery system. Unfortunately, until recently, the transdermal route has not been given enough attention as a potential delivery system by the industry even though a lot of academic research is being done. There are very few reports on IVIVC of transdermal delivery. The objective of this review is to make the reader aware of the theoretical aspects of skin permeation in passive and iontophoretic drug delivery systems, novel in vitro models for skin permeation studies, PK models that describe the transdermal delivery, and literature reports of IVIVC of TDD. This information will help further development of IVIVC of TDD systems.

Structure of Skin

Skin is the largest organ in the body and accounts for more than 10% of body mass. It consists of epidermis, dermis, and subcutaneous tissue. The SC is composed of the outermost nonviable cell layers of epidermis and is approximately 10 to 20 μm thick. It is composed of 15 to 25 flattened, stacked, hexagonal, and cornified cells embedded in intercellular lipid. Each cell in SC is approximately 40 μm in diameter and 0.5 μm in thickness. Dermis is about 0.1 to 0.5 cm thick and composed of collagenous fibers and elastic connective tissue matrix of mucopolysaccharides. Dermis contains an extensive vascular network with a blood flow rate of 0.05 mL/min/cc and is the layer responsible for systemic absorption of drugs delivered through the skin. Appendages such as hair follicles lie deep in the dermis.

Principles of Diffusion

Passive Transdermal Delivery

For drugs to be absorbed through the skin, they should be dissolved in the vehicle from which they will partition out, then permeate through the SC, and reach the systemic circulation via absorption by the blood capillaries under the epidermis. Permeation through the SC is usually the slowest process and, therefore, the rate-limiting step. However, there are some transdermal patches available with rate-controlling membranes in which diffusion through the membrane or matrix is slower than skin permeation and thus will be the rate-limiting step. Passage of the drug molecules through the skin can be described by Fick's laws of diffusion. The flux of a drug through the skin is dependent on the saturation solubility of the drug in the formulation vehicle. Flux can be described by the following equation:

$$J = \frac{DK}{h}(C_v - C_b) \qquad \ldots(2)$$

where D is the diffusion coefficient of the drug through the skin, K the partition coefficient, h the thickness of the skin, C_v the solubility of drug in the vehicle, and C_b the plasma concentration.

Iontophoretic Drug Delivery

Iontophoresis involves the delivery of ionic drug molecules under electric fields. The drug molecules will take the least resistance pathways, such as through hair follicles. There are two components to the iontophoretic delivery: electrorepulsion and electro-osmosis.

$$J_{\text{iontophoresis}} = J_{\text{electrorepulsion}} \pm J_{\text{electro-osmosis}} \qquad \ldots(3)$$

where J refers the flux of the drug molecule in each component, electrorepulsion is the simple repulsive force between similar charges, and electro-osmosis is the convective solvent flow in the direction of anode to cathode because of the current passage.

Skin is negatively charged at physiological pH and acts as a cation- selective membrane for the permeation. The direction of electro-osmosis can be changed by altering the membrane's electrical properties by preferential binding of cations to the fixed negative charges in the membrane. Electro-osmosis facilitates the passage of cationic species, but inhibits that of anionic species. It can be used to deliver polar and neutral solutes. The relative importance of electrorepulsion and electro-osmosis depends on the physicochemical and electrical characteristics of the membrane.

Theories of electrotransport

Iontophoretic transport of monovalent cations and anions can be approximately predicted by the modified Nernst–Planck model, which is modified to account for the influence of convective solvent flow.

The steady state flux ($J_{\Delta\psi}$) during iontophoresis in a porous membrane can be written as follows:

$$J_{\Delta\psi} = \varepsilon\left\{-\left(D\frac{dC}{dX} + \frac{C_Z F}{R_{gas}T}\frac{d\psi}{dx}\right) \pm vC\right\} \qquad \ldots(4)$$

where ψ is the electric potential in the membrane; F, Faraday's constant; R_{gas}, the gas constant; T, the temperature; v, the average velocity of the convective flow; ε, the combined porosity and tortuosity factor of the membrane; C, the concentration; x, the position in the membrane; and z, the charge number.

The predictions of the fluxes from this equation are consistent with the induction of pores in iontophoresis. A better appreciation of the meaning of the equation may be achieved by considering the case of a nonelectrolyte in which the charge $z = 0$, and Equation 4 is reduced to:

$$J_{\Delta\psi} = \varepsilon\left\{-\left(D\frac{dC}{dX}\right) \pm vC\right\} \qquad \ldots(5)$$

This is similar to Fick's first law of diffusion with the porosity and tortuosity of the membrane and the effectie convective flow added in the equation.

In the case where the permeant molecular radius is of the order of magnitude of the membrane pore radius, hindrance considerations must be included and Equation 4 can be rewritten as follows:

$$J_{\Delta\psi} = \varepsilon\left\{-\left(HD\frac{dC}{dX} + \frac{CzF}{R_{gas}T}\frac{d\psi}{dx}\right) \pm WvC\right\} \qquad \ldots(6)$$

where H is the hindrance factor for simultaneous Brownian diffusion and migration driven by electric field and W is the hindrance factor for permeant transport via convective solvent flow. Equation 6 is called modified Nearnst - Plank equation (8).

The steady state flux for passive transport ($J_{passive}$) across a porous membrane can be expressed as:

$$J_{passive} = \frac{DC_D\varepsilon H}{\Delta x} \qquad \ldots(7)$$

where H is the hindrance factor for passive diffusion; C_D, the concentration of the solute on the donor side; and Δ_x, the effective thickness of the membrane. After integration of Equation 4, the steady state flux can be expressed as: For anions

$$J_{\Delta\psi} = \frac{C_D\varepsilon HD\{[Wv/(HD)] + [K/\Delta x]\}}{\exp\{[Wv(\Delta x)/(HD)] + K\} - 1} \qquad \ldots(8)$$

For cations

$$J_{\Delta\psi} = \frac{C_D\varepsilon HD\{[Wv/(HD)] - [K/\Delta x]\}}{1 - \exp\{[K - Wv(\Delta x)/(HD)]\}} \qquad \ldots(9)$$

where $K = (zF\Delta\psi)/(R_{gas}T)$ and $\Delta\psi$ is the applied voltage across the membrane.

Enhancement factor (E_{total}) due to iontophoresis can be determined by the following equation:

$$E_{total} = \frac{J_{\Delta\psi}}{J_{passive}} \qquad ...(10)$$

In another study by Li et al., the average effective pore sizes induced by the electrical field was measured around 12Å, which were of the same order of magnitude as those of pre-existing pores determined from the conventional passive diffusion experiments. Li et al. showed the correlation between the electromobilities predicted and observed by the model. They suggested that the modified Nernst–Planck models predictions are satisfactory only when the electromobilities and the effective molecular size of the molecules are known.

Kontturi and Murtomaki proposed a model with two penetration routes for iontophoresis: one aqueous and one lipoidal. The mathematical form of the model is as follows:

$$J_p = J^w + J^o \qquad ...(11)$$

$$J_{if} = E \times J_p + J^o \qquad ...(12)$$

where J^w and J^o are the fluxes across the aqueous and organic pathways, respectively; J_p and J_{if} are the total passive and iontophoretic fluxes, respectively; and E represents the iontophoretic transport. Hirvonen et al. confirmed the predictability of the model and confirmed the idea that hydrophilic drugs experience the greatest benefit from iontophoretic delivery, whereas the flux enhancement of lipophilic drugs remains low.

Manabe et al. proposed the hydrodynamic pore theory for iontophoretic drug transport. They assumed parallel permeation pathways, pore and lipid pathways. Pore pathways are the main routes for hydrophilic drugs, as explained by the pore theory, and the net flux of a drug at steady state (J) can be described as the sum of each pathway flux:

$$J = J_L + J_P \qquad ...(13)$$

where J_L and J_P represent the flux through lipid and pore pathways, respectively.

In vitro Models of Skin Permeation Studies

Franz Diffusion Cell Set Up and Novel Modifications

For in vitro transdermal and topical absorption studies, Franz diffusion cells are widely used compared to the other methods. They consist of a donor and receptor compartment with the membrane of interest clamped between the two compartments. They can be either static or flowthrough, based on how the receptor phase is replenished, and provide a cost-effective evaluation method. But the inherent problem with static Franz diffusion cells is the lack of microvasculature, which is present in the in-vivo situation and helps in rapid clearance of the drug. It is particularly a problem when poorly soluble drugs are tested by these methods. For poorly soluble drugs, the drug concentration may reach closer to saturation solubility and, thus, the assumption of sink conditions may no longer be valid. To avoid these problems, flowthrough cells were designed in such a way that the receptor buffer is continuously removed. Flux is calculated as the linear slope of the cumulative amount delivered versus the time profile in standard Franz diffusional cell experiments. Permeability coefficient (P), using the steady state flux (J), can be derived by the following equation:

$$J = A \cdot P \cdot \Delta C \qquad ...(14)$$

where A is the surface area and ΔC the difference in the donor and receptor concentration.

However, in the case of flowthrough diffusion cell experiments, the collector volume, receiver cell volume, flow rate, and sampling interval may modify the apparent flux data. Additionally, these parameters may influence the finite dose flux profiles and the infinite dose diffusional lag times. In general, the concentration in the receiver (C_r) of a flow-through diffusion cell versus time (t) in the case of infinite dose can be studied by the following equation:

$$V_{rec} \cdot \frac{dC_{rec}}{dt} = J \cdot A - F_{rec} \cdot C_{rec} \qquad \ldots(15)$$

where V_{rec} is the volume of receiver chamber; J, the flux of drug out of the skin; A, the diffusional area; and F_{rec}, the flow rate of the receptor fluid.

In the case of finite dose studies, the flux increases to steady state flux and then decreases. Thus, the apparent flux profiles can be fitted to a bi-exponential function by the following equation:

$$J = A \cdot (e^{-K_1 \cdot t} - e^{-K_2 \cdot t}) \qquad \ldots(16)$$

where K_1 and K_2 represent the apparent increasing and decreasing rate constants of J. The first derivative of Equation 15 gives the value of maximum J, corresponding to the flux at steady state.

Tanojo et al. proposed a modification to the flowthrough diffusional cells. In the modified cells, the contact between the membrane and the receptor chamber was optimized by a spiral channel, which formed when the membrane was clamped between the donor and receptor compartments. Thus, the concentration of donor can be ensured throughout the experimental period by a separate flowthrough system. These cells have the unique advantage of using both finite and infinite doses in the donor. This design eliminates any stagnant domains in the compartment and sink conditions, and proper mixing in the receptor compartment is assured. The cumulative amounts reached plateau for p-amino benzoic acid through human SC in the case of a finite dose, due to the depletion of the drug in three hours, whereas it increased throughout the 16 hours that the constant donor concentrations were maintained. Bosman et al. developed Kedler cells, which can be used in combination with the automatic sample preparation with extraction columns system. These are the automated alternative to the static Franz cells. These cells consist of inlet, donor, and receptor compartments. This design has advantages of automated sampling, reduction of air bubble entrapment, mimicking the in vivo situation by the continuous flow of receptor buffer, and smaller areas of skin can be used for experiments. They showed the comparative results of Kedler cells with Franz cells for the permeation of dexetimide.

Isolated Perfused Porcine Skin Flap

Riviere et al. developed an isolated perfused porcine skin flap (IPPSF) model, which consists of porcine skin isolated with the microcirculation. This method can be used to determine in vitro absorption and metabolism within the skin. Pigskin has the potential disadvantage of excessive fat, and this allows the drug to distribute into the fat rather than into the actual sampling compartment. The possible necrosis of the excised skin during the long experimental conditions may affect the in vitro flux of drugs. To avoid this problem, Venter et al. developed an in situ adapted diffusional cell model in nude mice, which they compared with the static Franz cell data. In this method, a modified diffusion cell was implanted under the dissected dorsal skin of the animal. The skin was dissected with the least bleeding possible and which represents minimal disturbance of blood supply to the specific skin area. The skin was clamped between the donor and receptor chambers and consisted of intact cutaneous micro-vasculature. Histological observations showed that necrosis occurred in both epidermal and dermal regions in the excised skin pieces. They observed a higher flux in vitro compared to the in situ situation and could be due to the structural changes in the excised skin.

IN VIVO MODELS OF SKIN PERMEATION STUDIES

A variety of animal models were used both for in vitro and in vivo skin absorption studies. Commonly used excised skin membranes for diffusion studies are from hairless rats, hairless mice, fuzzy rats, guinea pigs, rabbits, and human. Of all of the aforementioned cases, human skin is ideal, but because of availability and ethical constraints there is a need for a good animal model that can mimic human skin. All the animal species differ in hair follicle density per unit area and SC thickness. Generally, thickness of the SC increases with the size of the animal. There are several conflicting reports comparing different animal species for in vitro permeation, but the results show that the permeation is more subjective to the drug and no generalized conclusions can be made. Wester and Noonan suggested that pig and monkey were the most predictive models for percutaneous absorption inhuman. Niazy observed that a species difference in penetration-enhancing effect of a zone and the enhancement factor was in the order rabbit skin > human skin > rat skin> guinea pig skin > hairless mouse skin. Panchagnula et al. investigated the permeation characteristics of a lipophilic and hydrophilic molecule across various animal models in vitro. By comparing the lag times and permeability values of both compounds, they suggested that the guinea pig, hairless guinea pig, and Brattleboro rat were good models for transdermal absorption studies. They did not find any qualitative or quantitative relationship between number of hair follicles and permeability of either of the compounds. Artificial composite membranes composed of silicone and poly 2-hydroxy ethyl methacrylate were also investigated as an alternative to skin membranes.

Composite membrane permeabilities for a wide range of drugs with diverse physicochemical properties were compared and reasonable correlation was found between the calculated and observed permeability coefficients. Shed snakeskin was considered to have a close correlation with the permeation rates of drugs through human SC and they are devoid of hair follicles, and thus can be used for mechanistic studies. But the thickness and permeability characteristics differ in different species of snakes and thus they showed that the snakeskin is not a good model for human skin. Rittirod et al. demonstrated metabolic differences in the in vitro skin experiments. They showed that the differences in permeation profiles of ethyl nicotinate among the species tested was primarily due to the differences in the esterase activity, and thus when extrapolating the skin permeation data to human skin, skin metabolism should be considered. Hikima et al. demonstrated the differences in hydrolase activity in different animal species in vitro and they suggested that the skin of the hairless rat and the hairless mouse might be good models to simulate clinical situation of hydrolytic activity. Recently, cultured skin was used as alternative to the excised animal skin.

Excised animal skin has the disadvantages of high variability and a lack of viability. Suhonen et al. investigated an epidermal cell culture derived from rat keratinocytes for permeability characteristics. They showed that the organitryptic ketinocyte culture may give a very close estimate on human epidermal membrane permeabilities over a large range of lipopholicities and molecular weights. These cultures are devoid of appendages and, thus, may not be useful to investigate iontophoretic drug delivery. Monteiro-Riviere et al. used the human epidermal keratinocytes to demonstrate an irritant induced cytokine release. This method has a good potential to investigate the drug-skin interactions. Grafe et al. demonstrated a pH dependent carrier mediated transport of clonidine in human keratinocytes cultures. They proposed that after the passage through the SC, the transporter might contribute to the passage of clonidine.

Pharmacokinetic Models for Transdermal Drug Delivery

Drug delivery through skin is a complex phenomenon due to the complexity involved in the skin structure. The ultimate aim of the PK modeling is to predict the future state of a system, which plays a major role in optimizing the dosing regimens and toxicological consequences.

Diffusion Model

Berner derived a PK model for passive diffusion of drug from the device with finite and infinite doses. The transdermal device consists of a stirred-drug reservoir and a rate controlling membrane in contact with the SC. It was assumed that the membrane is in equilibrium with the drug reservoir.

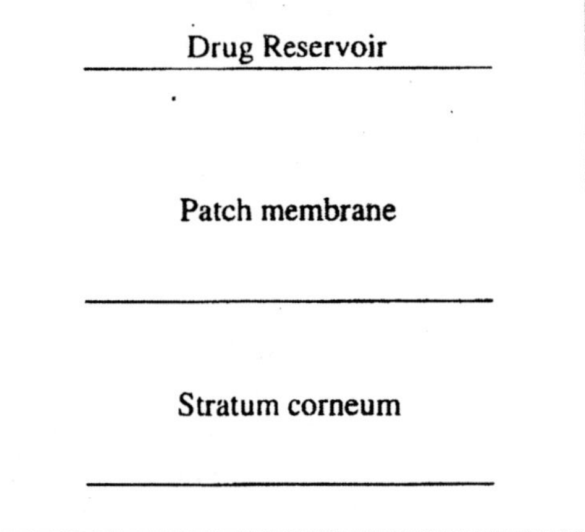

Fig. 13.6. Transdermal devices with infinite dose.

Collection of urine sample after transdermal patch application is the easiest and noninvasive way to monitor the fate of the drug in the body.

Total amount excreted in urine (M_u) can be related to the steady state flux (J_{ss}) as

$$M_u^a(t) = \frac{k_u A J_{ss}}{K}(t - t_L^D - 1/K) \quad \ldots(17)$$

where M_u^a is the asymptotic limit of M_u; k_u, the urinary excretion rate; A, the surface area of the patch; K, the elimination rate constant; t, the time; and t_L^D, the lag time to reach steady state diffusion.

Steady state blood concentrations can be obtained as

$$C_b = \frac{AJ_{ss}}{KV_d} \quad \ldots(18)$$

where C_b is the blood concentration and V_d the volume of distribution.

PK lag time (t_L) can be calculated as

$$t_L = \frac{1}{K} + \frac{l_s^2}{6D_s} \quad \ldots(19)$$

where l_s is the thickness of SC, and D_s the diffusion coefficient of the drug through SC

PK lag time is composed of PK contribution, which is the lag time for diffusion across the SC. This is precisely the result for the PK lag time for the skin permeation alone.

Parallel Infusion Model

This model assumes that transdermal patch provides two simultaneous drug infusions resulting from the burst effect and parallel controlled maintenance infusion. The transdermal patch has a temporary compartment due to the burst effect other than drug reservoir. The burst infusion (F_{fst}) and the maintenance infusion (F_{inf}) will contribute to the total drug input into the body.

Plasma concentration (C) can be represented as:

$$V \cdot \frac{dC}{dt} = F_{inf} + F_{fst} - Cl \cdot C \quad \ldots(20)$$

Cl and V represent total body clearance and volume of distribution, respectively.

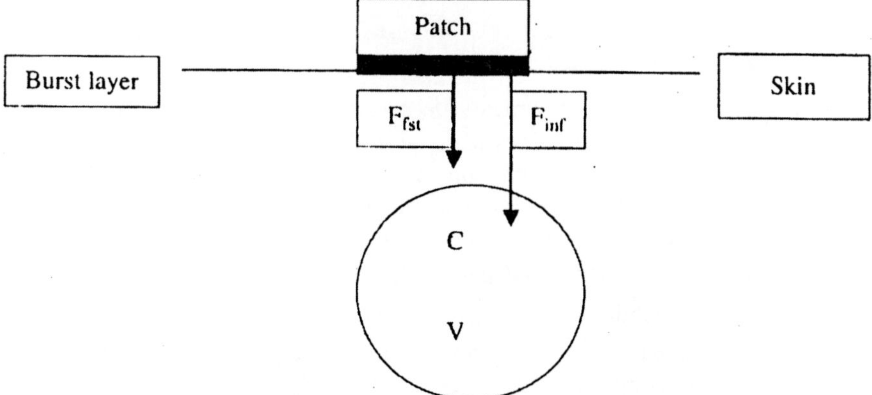

Fig. 13.7. Pharmacokinetic model with parallel infusions.

F_{fst} and F_{inf} are defined as:

$$F_{fst} = \frac{\text{Dose}_{fst}}{\text{Time}_{fst}} = \frac{\text{Released dose} - \text{Dose}_{inf}}{\text{Time}_{fst}} \quad \text{...(21)}$$

$$F_{inf} = \frac{\text{Dose}_{inf}}{\text{Time}_{inf}} \quad \text{...(22)}$$

where Time_{fst} and Time_{inf} are the times of burst and maintenance infusions; Dose_{inf} and Dose_{fst} are the doses delivered in maintenance and burst infusion periods.

Multicompartment Model Describing Intradermal Kinetics

Nakayama et al. developed a six compartmental model considering skin and muscle layers as different compartments. They showed that the skin and muscle layer below the patch act as a different compartment compared to the contralateral skin and muscle layers. In Figure 13.8, V and C represent volume of distribution and drug concentration in each compartment, respectively. Cl indicates the clearance between the tissues and tissue or plasma. The subscripts d, vs, m, and p reveal the donor cell, viable skin, muscle, and plasma compartments, respectively.

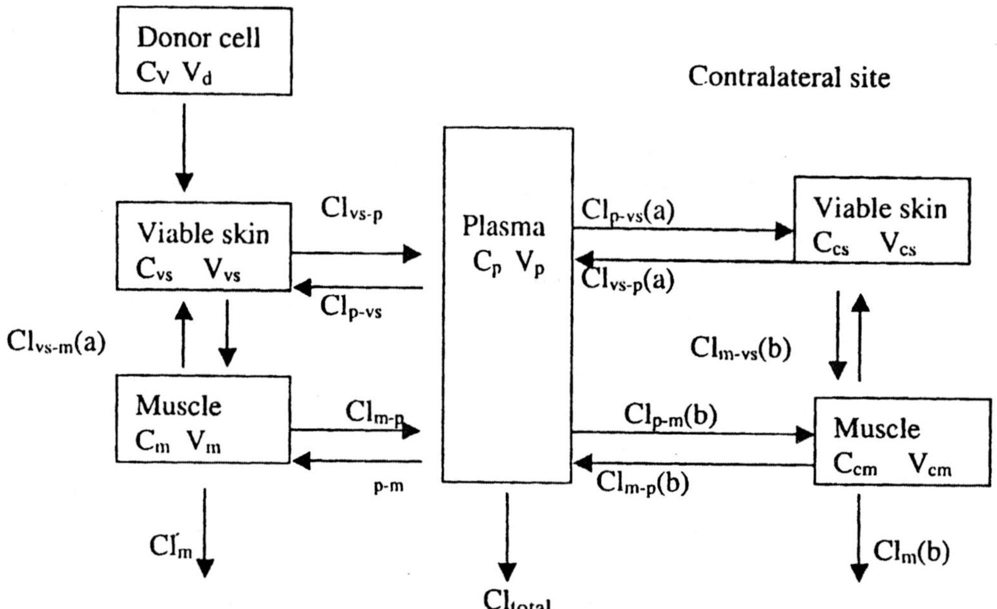

Fig. 13.8. Six compartmental model for intradermal disposition kinetics.

Differential equations for the compartments described earlier give the drug distribution in each tissue compartments. In this model, the values of $Cl_{vs\text{-}m}$ and $Cl_{vs\text{-}p}$ could be the indices for the efficiency of the systemic delivery or the local delivery and they showed that 20% antipyrine in the viable skin after topical application can directly penetrate into the muscle layer below the application site. This model could be used to evaluate the fractional contribution of the direct penetration and the blood supply to the deeper muscle layer below the patch application site.

Population Pharmacokinetic Model

Auclair et al. proposed a PK model to calculate population PK parameters of nitroglycerin and its metabolites after transdermal administration. They used a one-compartment model with a first-pass, mixed-order release. This model showed a very good fit to the observed data following transdermal

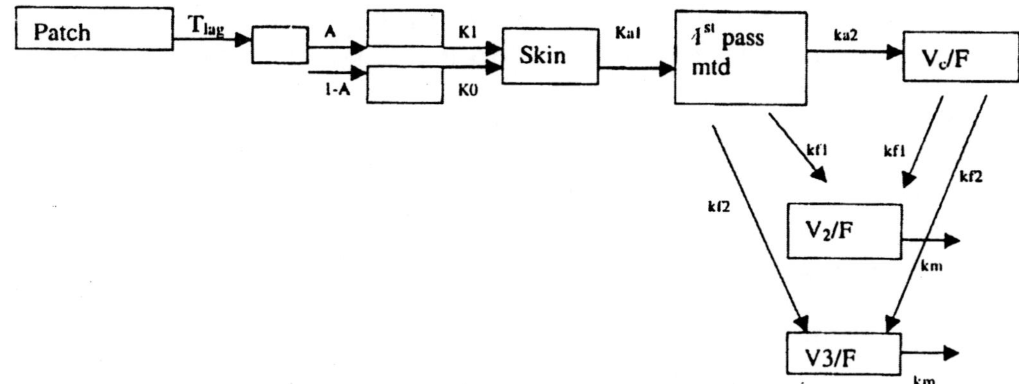

Fig. 13.9. Population pharmacokinetic model.

nitroglycerin in human volunteers. Due to the reservoir and membrane in the transdermal device, a mixed-order release gave a better fit than the assuming first-order or zero-order release alone. A lag time is needed in this model because time is needed for equilibrium to be made between the patch and the skin, and for the skin reservoir to be filled before the appearance of the drug in the systemic circulation. This model has an advantage in a head-to-head comparison between different formulations of nitroglycerin by minimizing the errors resulting from the fluctuations in the plasma concentrations and differentiating the formulations in terms of onset of action and drug elimination.

Physiologically Based Pharmacokinetic Model

Tashiro et al. developed a modified physiologically based PK (PBPK) model to show the effect of iontophoresis on drug transfer from skin to cutaneous blood. It has been shown that cathodal iontophoresis of ketoprofen resulted in a higher cutaneous plasma concentration than the systemic concentration, demonstrating the transfer of ketoprofen from skin to cutaneous blood. Transfer rate of the drug from skin to cutaneous blood (R_{sc}) can be defined as:

$$R_{sc} = Q_b(C_{vein} - C_{artery}) \quad \ldots(23)$$

where Q_b is the flow rate of cutaneous blood; C_{artery}, the drug concentration in the arterial blood entering cutaneous circulation; and C_{vein}, the drug concentration in the venous blood leaving cutaneous circulation.

In Equation 23, C_{artery} and C_{vein} can be substituted by blood and plasma concentration in systemic vein and cutaneous vein ($C_{b,systemic}$, $C_{p,systemic}$ and $C_{b,cutaneous}$, $C_{p,cutaneous}$, respectively) and Equation 23 can be rewritten as:

$$R_{sc} = Q_b \frac{C_b}{C_p}(C_{p,cutaneous} - C_{p,systemic}) \quad \ldots(24)$$

This model can be used for kinetic analysis of local disposition in TDD. They showed that iontophoresis induced the change of drug transfer to cutaneous blood flow and the change may depend on the application period and magnitude of electrical current.

Convolution/Deconvolution Methods

Deconvolution can be used to determine the input function into the systemic circulation. Bioavailability can be estimated by the integral of this input function. If the disposition of the drug after intravenous bolus administration is $w(t)$ and input rate is $I(t)$, the response function $r(t)$ can be considered as a cumulation of various intravenous doses, assuming that the presence of drug does not affect its kinetics. Thus, the relation between the input rate, intravenous bolus or unit impulse response, and response function can be written as the convolution function (Eq. 25):

$$C = r(t) = I(t) * w(t) \quad ...(25)$$

where C is the plasma concentration and equal to $r(t)$ (the response to the input function) and * the convolution operator.

Deconvolution is the opposite mathematical operation of convolution and can be described by Equation 26.

$$I(t) = r(t)//w(t) \quad ...(26)$$

where // is the deconvolution operator.

Phase Plane Methodology

Dokoumetzidis and Macheras investigated the phase plane method to characterize absorption kinetics of drug delivery systems. In this method, phase plane plots consist of dC/dt versus concentration (C) using concentration (C) and time (t) data. The shape of the phase plane plot is indicative of output and input kinetics. Input rate can be related to concentrations:

$$\text{Input} = \frac{dC}{dt} + K_e C \quad ...(27)$$

where K_e is the first-order elimination rate constant.

They calculated the ratio of the slopes of absorption and elimination phases and compared to the value 2, a theoretical minimum for the ratio of the slopes. Zero-order absorption kinetics will have a patent discontinuity between absorption and elimination phases, and similar slopes for the data above and below the x-axis. By modeling errant data, they showed that the ratio of slopes (r) indicates the absorption kinetics. A $r < 2$ represents the presence of zero order kinetics and $r > 2$ represents the presence of first order of Michaelis–Menten kinetics. Additionally, this method allows for the construction of fictitious "*cumulative concentration-time*" profiles by calculating the area under the curve of the input rate for each time interval. When each of these quantities is divided by the total area, this provides the "*normalized fictitious concentration-time*" profile, which has all the qualitative features of the classical percent absorbed versus time plots.

In Vitro-In Vivo Correlation of Transdermal Drug Delivery

Some focused published examples to predict in vivo blood levels using the models described earlier will provide more practical insight into the utility of the models. Examples for passive and iontophoretic drug delivery will be discussed as separate categories.

Passive Transdermal Delivery

Physiologically based pharmacokinetic model

Macpherson et al. developed a PBPK model consisting of four compartments: (i) rapidly perfused tissues, (ii) slowly perfused tissues, (iii) liver (major route of elimination), and (iv) plasma to predict the in vivo blood levels of benzoic acid (BA) after transdermal delivery. Schematic representation of the model is given subsequently. In vitro percutaneous absorption studies were performed using flowthrough diffusion cells and the skin was perfused with oxygenated HEPES-buffered Hank's balanced salt solution, pH 7.4 at a flow rate of 1.6 mL/hr to keep the tissue viable. The transdermal input rate $I(t)$ was calculated from the following first-order, one-compartment absorption model:

$$I(t) = \frac{\left[K * K_a * \alpha\left(e^{-K*t} - e^{-K_a*t}\right)\right]}{K_a - K} \quad ...(28)$$

where K is the elimination rate constant from skin; K_a, the absorption rate into the skin; and α, the scaling parameter. The parameters in the model were calculated by fitting the in vitro data to the above model using SAS computer program. Differential equations for the PBPK model in different tissues were written and the blood levels in the plasma compartment can be written as:

$$V_b * \left(\frac{dC_b}{dt}\right) = \left[\frac{(Q_r * C_r)}{P_{(r/b)}}\right] + \left[\frac{(Q_s * C_s)}{P_{(s/b)}}\right] + \left[\frac{(Q_l * C_l)}{P_{(l/b)}}\right] + I(t) - (Q_b * C_b) \qquad \ldots(29)$$

where C_b, C_r, C_s, and C_l, and Q_b, Q_r, Q_s, and Q_l represent the concentration of BA in blood, rapidly perfused tissues, slowly perfused tissues, liver, and blood flow to the respective compartments. Partition coefficient between the different tissue compartments were described by $P_{r/b}$, $P_{s/b}$, and $P_{l/b}$. Volume of tissue compartments were either calculated experimentally or obtained from the literature. Partition coefficients were calculated by experimental methodology. The input rate $I(t)$ calculated from the in vitro experiment was utilized in Equation 28. The developed model was capable of predicting plasma BA levels that would result from topical exposure to finite doses of BA.

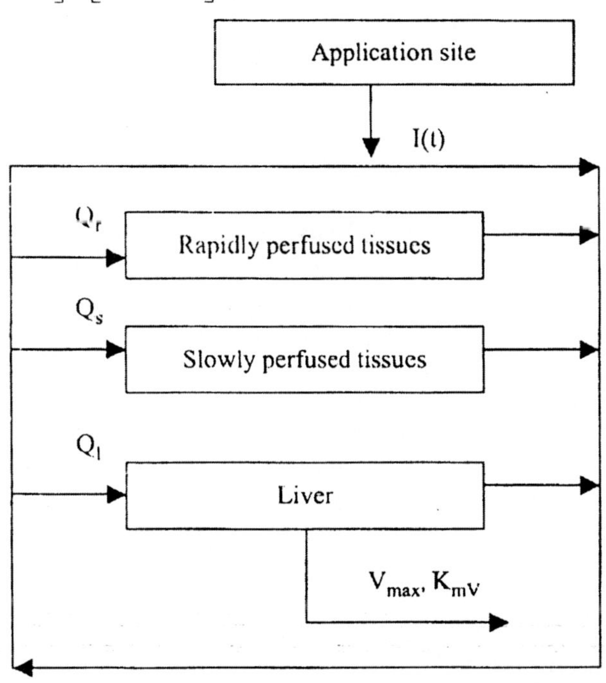

Fig. 13.10. Physiologically based pharmacokinetic model developed to predict plasma levels of benzoic acid (BA) in hairless guinea pigs after topical exposure to a finite dose.

Two-compartment model

A two-compartment model with zero-order absorption was used to predict in vivo concentrations of a synthetic cannabinoid after transdermal delivery in guinea pigs. The patches were applied until the steady state plasma concentrations were achieved. Basic PK parameters were calculated from the plasma concentration-profile after intravenous administration of the cannabinoid. Steady-state plasma concentrations were calculated from the following equation:

$$C = \frac{J_{ss}S}{V_c K_{el}}\left[1 + \frac{\beta - K_{el}}{\alpha - \beta}\exp(-\alpha t) + \frac{K_{el} - \alpha}{\alpha - \beta}\exp(-\beta t)\right] \qquad \ldots(30)$$

where α and β are the distribution constants; V_c, the volume of distribution of the central compartment; and K_{el}, the elimination rate constant obtained from intravenous administration. J_{ss} is the steady state flux observed in the in vitro permeation studies using hairless guinea pig skin.

Convolution method

Qi et al. predicted in vivo plasma concentrations of 2,3,5,6-tetramethylpyrazine (TMP), following transdermal application by the convolution methodology. The unit impulse parameters A, B, a, b were calculated by intravenous administration of the compound and model fitting. A weighting function was estimated from the in vitro permeation data. TMP release showed a biphasic pattern with a burst release phase during the first four hours followed by a slow release phase from four to six hours, and further slower release phase from 6 to 24 hours. In order to include the effect of diffusion changes, a multiple-constant input in convolution procedure was followed. Convolution was performed by the following equations for all the phases:

If $0 \le t \le t$

$$C(t) = \frac{J_1 A}{a}(1 - e^{-at}) + \frac{J_1 B}{b}(1 - e^{-bt}) \qquad \ldots(31)$$

If $t_1 \le t \le t_2$

$$C(t) = \frac{J_2 A}{a}\left[1 - e^{-a(t-t_1)}\right] + \frac{J_2 B}{b}\left[1 - e^{-b(t-t_1)}\right] + \frac{C(t_1)}{A+B}\left[Ae^{-a(t-t_1)} + Be^{-b(t-t_1)}\right] \qquad \ldots(32)$$

If $t_2 \le t \le t_3$

$$C(t) = \frac{J_3 A}{a}\left[1 - e^{-a(t-t_2)}\right] + \frac{J_3 B}{b}\left[1 - e^{-b(t-t_2)}\right] + \frac{C(t_2)}{A+B}\left[Ae^{-a(t-t_2)} + Be^{-b(t-t_2)}\right] \qquad \ldots(33)$$

Iontophoretic Drug Delivery

IVIVC of iontophoretic delivery is more controversial due to the conflicting reports. Generally, a higher in vivo flux has been reported than in vitro flux in various reports. Most of these differences were ascribed to the intrinsic ion concentration of the skin This could be due to the faster in vivo clearance of drug from the skin due to the cutaneous microcirculation and the presence of an ion reservoir in the skin that may compete for charge transport with the drug and the depletion of this reservoir in turn may contribute to the lag-time before a steady iontophoretic flux is achieved. Conventionally used Franz-diffusion cells have relatively smaller area than the actual patch studies in vivo. The amount of drug adsorbed per unit area could have a negative impact on the drug flux. Geest et al. studied the iontophoretic delivery of arbutamine and found that the IVIVC is highly dependent on the experimental conditions. Several mechanisms that contribute to the overall transport may effect in vitro and in vivo transport rates to a different degree.

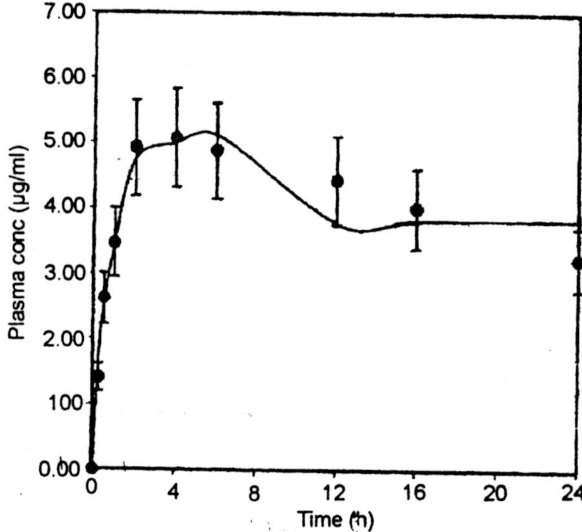

Fig. 13.11. Transdermal delivery of 2,3,5,6-tetramethylpyrazine (TMP) after a single 24-hour application of TMP-TTS (300 mg/30 cm²).

Isolated perfused porcine skin flap model to predict in vivo concentrations

Riviere et al. utilized IPPSF model to predict iontophoretic delivery of arbutamine in humans. The in vivo PK parameters were calculated using an intravenous infusion of arbutamine in human. The observed concentrations of drug in the venous efflux from IPPSF versus time were normalized by the concentration of applied drug concentration, electronic dose, and electrode area. These input profiles were then renormalized by the in vivo conditions by multiplying with the concentration of drug in vivo, electron dose, and electrode area. The resultant input function was fed in the systemic model and thus these input profiles served as a continuous function and produced a simulated plasma concentration-time window with the following equation that was computed iteratively (two minute intervals):

$$M_t = \frac{U(t)}{K_{el}}(1 - e^{-K_{el}t}) + M_0(t)e^{-K_{el}t} \qquad \ldots(34)$$

where M_t is the mass of drug in the body at time t; $U(t)$, the drug input (IPPSF output) rate; and $M_0(t)$, the initial drug mass determined from the previous iteration. Dividing $M(t)$ by steady-state volume of distribution yields the predicted concentration of drug in plasma. This model predicted the in vivo plasma concentrations well. But the authors warn that the model must be validated for other drugs as the effect of drugs on the cutaneous blood circulation will in turn effect the over all results.

Cutaneous microdialysis

The microdialysis technique to measure skin concentrations of drugs has been widely reported in the literature. It was portrayed as a minimally invasive method and more suitable than the current methods of drug assessment in the skin. Ault et al. investigated the effect of probe implantation in skin in vitro–in vivo histological examination and microdialysis delivery in fuzzy rats. There was no inflammation or edema formation immediately after the probe insertion. However, increased infiltration of lymphocytes was observed after six hours of implantation and during the entire experiment (72 hours). Noticeable changes in the cells surrounding the probe were observed 32 hours of probe implantation. Groth and Serup investigated the probe insertion trauma on skin perfusion and erythema skin thickness in human. They reported that insertion with a 21 G needle increased blood flow and skin erythema, and baseline blood flow was recovered after 90 to 120 minutes. Ultrasound imaging studies showed a 38% relative skin thickening due to the probe. Similar experiments in hairless rats resulted in the probe placement around 1 mm in the skin and significant skin thickening (30%) was observed. The edema developed after 15 to 30 minutes after insertion and it was preferred to start microdialysis procedure after 30 minutes of probe insertion. Mathy et al. investigated the in vivo tolerance of skin after subcutaneous and dermal microdialysis probes in rat using bioengineering methods such as transepidermal water loss (TEWL), Laser Doppler velocimeter, and Chromameter. Dermal insertion of a probe using 26 G needle did not show any physical damage to the skin. Subcutaneous probe insertion did not show any significant changes in the skin characteristics. Elongation of the cells surrounding the probe was observed after 24 hours of probe insertion. Recently, we utilized subcutaneous microdialysis to show IVIVC of granisetron after iontophoretic delivery. We compared the area under the curve from time 0 to t (AUC_{0-t}) values of microdialysate data to the in vitro cumulative amounts delivered. A good correlation was observed. This method could be potentially evaluated clinically for transdermal and topical bioequivalence of commercial drug products.

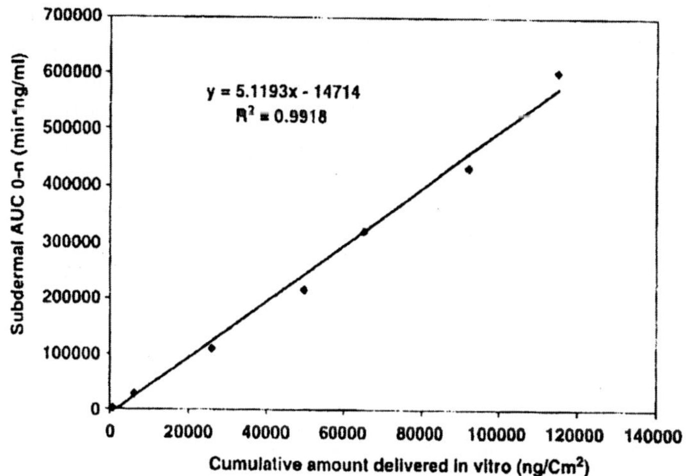

Fig. 13.12. In vitro-in vivo correlation of iontophoretic delivery of granisetron using cutaneous microdialysis.

IVIVC of transdermal delivery is more dependent on the experimental conditions and the nature of the molecule of interest, in case of Iontophoretic delivery, but is better established in passive transdermal delivery. However, the variability of human skin thickness and resulting differences in the permeation of drugs is a major problem that still needs to be addressed. It is sometimes hard to optimize the formulations due to inherent variability in the in vitro techniques. More comprehensive research should be done in this area to come up with better techniques to accurately predict the permeation characteristics of drugs from different formulation. Current in vitro methods are not sufficient for product development purposes but are good for candidate selection purposes. One major aspect of transdermal delivery is the irritation caused by the drugs. There is no reported method available, currently, for the in vitro method to evaluate the skin irritation potential of drug molecules, and researchers should be looking into this issue so that many more drug candidates could be screened for their irritancy potential in the drug discovery stages. More drug candidates could be marketable if TDD is also considered as a major route of drug delivery, as many drugs fail clinical development due to high first-pass metabolism.

Oral Drug Delivery

The correlation between the in vitro dissolution performance of an oral dosage form, particularly those employing proprietary delivery technologies, to the corresponding in vivo performance has long been an important goal for the pharmaceutical scientist. However, in more recent times, interest in the field of in vitro–in vivo correlations (IVIVC) has grown, reflecting the potential of this methodology as a tool for optimizing formulation development as well as a tool for supporting applications to regulatory authorities. This chapter will focus primarily on the development, validation, and application of IVIVC models for oral dosage forms for both regulatory applications and for formulation development.

Almost a decade has passed since the publication of the 1997 FDA Guidance on IVIVC for oral modified release (MR) products. In this time, both companies and the regulatory agencies have gained valuable experience in the development, validation, and application of IVIVC models. As with other disciplines, "*best practise*" has evolved since the IVIVC guidance was first published, although many of these practises are not formally documented. This chapter will also endeavor to highlight the current state of play regarding IVIVC and oral drug delivery.

IVIVC and Extended Release Dosage Dosage Forms

The concept of IVIVC for extended release (ER) dosage forms that allows scientists to predict the expected bioavailability for an ER product based on its in vitro dissolution profile has long been discussed by the pharmaceutical community. Over the years, a number of seminal workshops and publications have tracked the progress made in this area. A 1987 ASCPT/DIA/APS/FDA-sponsored workshop concluded that the available science and technology at that time did not permit consistently meaningful IVIVC for ER dosage forms and encouraged IVIVC as a future objective. The workshop also concluded that in vitro dissolution testing could only be considered useful for stability, process control, minor changes to formulations, and changes in manufacturing site. The following year, 1988, saw the publication of a USP PF stimuli article in which the classification of IVIVC models into Levels A, B, and C was established — a classification that is still in use today. A report from an ASCPT/DIA/APS/FDA-sponsored workshop in 1990 concluded that, although the science and technology available did not always allow for meaningful IVIVC, the development of such models was considered an important objective on a product-by-product basis, and procedures for the development, evaluation, and application of an IVIVC were described.

The report also included the suggestion that proposed in vitro dissolution specifications should be validated by conducting a bioequivalence study involving two batches with in vitro dissolution profiles representative of the upper and lower specifications. Another ASCPT/DIA/APS/FDA-sponsored workshop in 1993 resulted in a report that provided further information related to IVIVC. The objectives of an IVIVC were identified as being the use of in vitro dissolution testing as a surrogate for bioequivalence (BE) testing, as well as being an aid in the setting of dissolution specifications. This report concluded that in vitro dissolution might be used as a sensitive, reliable, and reproducible surrogate for bioequivalence testing. The report also supported the concepts contained in USP chapter 1088, which described appropriate techniques for Level A, B, and C correlations and methods for establishing dissolution specifications. The report from the 1993 workshop also found that IVIVC could be useful for changes other than minor changes in formulation, equipment, process, manufacturing site, and batch size.

Quite clearly, the 1993 workshop report reflected the increased confidence within the pharmaceutical industry at that time in the use of IVIVC to estimate the in vivo bioavailability characteristics of an ER drug product and the willingness to rely on in vitro dissolution testing and IVIVC to serve as a surrogate for bioequivalence studies. All this is in marked contrast to the conclusions only six years earlier of the 1987 workshop.

The heightened awareness of IVIVC and its potential application to both the formulation development process and the support of regulatory submissions for ER dosage forms culminated with the publication in 1997 of the FDA Guidance for Industry—ER oral dosage forms: development, evaluation, and application of IVIVCs. This guidance describes the levels of correlations that can be established, but more critically also established the varying degrees of usefulness of the different levels of IVIVC. The guidance also provides information on issues related to study design and conduct, how IVIVC models are to be evaluated, and the practical applications of IVIVC.

The 1997 FDA guidance on IVIVC and oral ER dosage forms still serves today as the only specific guidance on IVIVC. However, the principles and applications laid down in this document should serve those interested in developing IVIVC for alternate dosage forms, particularly those that utilise controlled release technology.

IVIVC and Immediate Release Dosage Forms

Historically, attempts to successfully develop IVIVC models for oral immediate release (IR) dosage forms have been less successful than for controlled release or sustained release dosage forms, particularly for Level A IVIVC models. A number of factors contributed to the lack of success: in vitro dissolution evaluation of IR dosage forms frequently only included one to three time-points, making the development of Level A models almost impossible; many of the IR dosage forms did not exhibit dissolution-rate limited absorption; the relationship between in vitro dissolution and in vivo absorption frequently appeared to be nonlinear as in vivo absorption could not "keep up" with in vitro dissolution. This last factor did not preclude the development of Level A models but at the time, Level A models were defined as "point-to-point" relationships and were anticipated to be linear. As a consequence, IVIVC was not attempted for many IR dosage forms because of the low expectation for success.

However, our understanding of this apparent lack of success with IVIVC for IR dosage forms has increased with the advent of the biopharmaceutical classification system (BCS). As discussed elsewhere in this compilation, the BCS, as defined by Amidon et al. provides a framework for classifying drug substances based on their aqueous solubility and intestinal permeability. The BCS takes into account the three major factors that govern rate and extent of absorption from IR solid oral dosage forms: dissolution, solubility, and intestinal permeability. On this basis, drug substances are classified into four classes: (i) class I for substances with both high solubility and permeability, (ii) class II for substances with low solubility and high permeability, (iii) class III for substances with high solubility and low permeability, and (iv) class IV for substances with both low solubility and permeability.

For drug substances in class I, an IVIVC is anticipated if dissolution is slower (i.e., rate controlling) compared to gastric emptying. Otherwise, a limited or no correlation is expected for rapidly dissolving formulations of a class I drug substance. For class II drug substances, an IVIVC is expected if in vitro dissolution is similar to in vivo dissolution rate. For drug substances in class III, absorption (permeability) is the rate-controlling factor, not dissolution. Therefore, only a limited or no correlation between in vivo absorption and in vitro dissolution rate is anticipated. Finally, no correlation is expected for class IV drug substances unless in vivo dissolution is rate controlling.

The BCS has helped us understand some of the historical lack of successful IVIVC attempts for IR dosage forms and also helps us to anticipate the likelihood of success for future drug substances, based on their classification.

Regulatory Framework for IVIVC and Oral Dosage Forms

Although the 1997 FDA guidance is the only specific IVIVC guidance to be published to date, for any pharmaceutical scientist with an interest in the area of IVIVC, there are a number of additional guidances that are associated with this area that provide the framework for the regulatory application of IVIVC. These include the guidances on scale-up and post approval changes (SUPAC) for both modified release and IR solid oral dosage forms. There is also guidance on the waiver of in vivo studies for IR solid oral dosage forms based on the biopharmaceutics classification of the drug. The recent guidance on bioavailability and bioequivalence studies for oral products also provides information on the application of IVIVC models.

The Committee for Proprietary Medicinal Products (CPMP) within the European Agency for the Evaluation of Medicinal Products (EMEA) has also issued a note for guidance on the pharmacokinetic and clinical evaluation of modified release oral products that provides some information on the development and evaluation of an IVIVC.

A review of these guidances should quickly inform the scientist that the area of IVIVC requires the collaboration of formulators, analytical chemists, pharmacokinetists and regulatory personnel to provide an integrated approach to the development and application of IVIVC models in both the formulation development and regulatory submission process.

At present, no specific guidance has been issued dealing with IVIVC and oral IR dosage forms. However, the applications of IVIVC for oral IR dosage forms are discussed in both the FDA Guidance for Industry on dissolution testing of IR dosage forms and in the SUPAC-IR guidance.

Development and Validation of Level a IVIVC Models for Oral Dosage Forms

Before discussing the application of IVIVC models to the development of oral dosage forms, it is worth spending a few moments briefly reviewing the development and validation of such models.

The 1997 FDA IVIVC guidance for extended-release oral products defines an IVIVC as "a *predictive mathematical model*" that describes the relationship between an in vitro property of an ER dosage form (usually the rate or extent of drug dissolution or release) and a relevant in vivo response (e.g., plasma drug concentrations or the amount of drug absorbed). Originating from the USP stimuli article, IVIVC models have been classified into different main categories: Levels A, B, and C. The category of IVIVC model depends entirely on the analysis performed—in all cases, the same in vitro (dissolution-time data) and in vivo data (plasma concentration-time data) are collected. Critically, the usefulness of an IVIVC model, in terms of both internal decision making during drug development programs and for regulatory submissions, is determined by the category of model.

Level C models are simple single-point relationships between the amount dissolved in vitro at a particular time or the time required for in vitro dissolution of a fixed percentage of the dose, for example, $t_{50\%}$ and a summary parameter that characterizes the in vivo time course, for example, C_{max} or AUC. By its very definition, Level C IVIVC models need at least three formulations and it is important to note that a Level C correlation does not reflect the complete shape of the plasma concentration time curve.

Multiple Level C models relate one or several pharmacokinetic parameters of interest to the amount of drug dissolved at several time points along the dissolution profile, such as the amount released at certain time points or the time to release a certain percentage, that is, $t_{50\%}$. Multiple Level C models can be useful in identifying critical dissolution time points to assist in setting dissolution specifications.

According to FDA Guidance, multiple Level C models can be as useful as Level A models and both the the FDA and CPMP suggest that if multiple Level C models can be developed, a Level A IVIVC is also likely. However, our experiences suggest that multiple Level C correlations may not be acceptable to all regulatory authorities.

Level B IVIVC models use the principle of statistical moment analysis. For example, the mean in vitro dissolution time could be compared to the mean residence time or mean in vivo dissolution time. Such models are considered to be the least useful for regulatory purposes and will not be discussed further.

Finally, Level A IVIVC models describe the relationship between the entire in vitro dissolution time course and the entire in vivo response time course for example, the time course of plasma-drug concentration or amount of drug absorbed. From a regulatory viewpoint, these models are considered to be the most informative and are recommended. Therefore, the focus of this section will be on the development and evaluation of Level A IVIVC models for oral dosage forms. The development and evaluation of a Level A IVIVC model can be broken down into a series of steps:

1. Selection of appropriate formulations
2. Obtaining in vitro dissolution data for these formulations
3. Design and conduct of the in vivo study itself
4. Data analysis

The likelihood of obtaining a successful outcome to the development of an IVIVC model can be increased by considering the first three topics listed above. The reader is directed to a comprehensive review by Shepard et al. of the issues related to study design considerations for IVIVC studies. Therefore, the present chapter will confine itself to a brief overview of the development and validation of Level A IVIVC models to facilitate the later discussions regarding the applications of such models.

Level A IVIVC models have historically been developed using a two-stage approach. The first stage involves deriving the in vivo release profile from the observed plasma concentration data using a suitable deconvolution method and the second stage involves the modelling of the relationship between the derived in vivo release and the in vitro release data.

Since the release of the 1997 IVIVC guidance, experience gained from both regulatory submissions and subsequent discussions at scientific meetings, a number of key issues regarding the two-stage approach have emerged: firstly, it is expected that the deconvolution procedure takes place on an individual subject basis. That is, the in vivo release profile should be obtained for each individual, rather than averaging the concentration-time data before performing the deconvolution procedure. Following the individual deconvolution, the average in vivo input function is obtained and it is this entity that is subsequently correlated with the average in vitro dissolution data to obtain an IVIVC model. The output of the IVIVC model itself is a single predicted in vivo input function for each formulation.

In order to validate the model, the output from the IVIVC model needs to be translated into concentration-time profiles for each treatment and this is done by performing the reverse operation of deconvolution, namely convolution. The result of the convolution procedure is a single predicted concentration-time profile for each formulation from which summary parameters AUC and Cmax are obtained and compared to the corresponding parameters derived from the average observed data.

For internal predictability, the IVIVC model is used to predict the AUC and C_{max} for each of the formulations or batches used in the development of the model. To satisfy the FDA criteria, the AUC and C_{max} absolute percent prediction error (%PE) should be no greater than 15% for any single formulation and the mean absolute percent prediction error (MAPPE) should be less than 10% for each parameter. Where the MAPPE falls within 10% to 20%, the IVIVC model is considered to be inconclusive and external predictability should be conducted.

To demonstrate external predictability, the IVIVC model is used to predict the AUC and C_{max} of a formulation or batch that was not included in the original model development. This could be a formulation that was evaluated in the same study as those formulations used in the model development or it could be a formulation evaluated in a separate study to that used to develop the IVIVC. The criteria for external predictability are that the %PE should be less than 10%. Therefore, these criteria may be perceived as being more stringent that those for internal predictability, in that a formulation can have a %PE of up to 15% for internal predictability but must be less than 10% for external predictability.

Although the criteria for IVIVC model validation discusses AUC and C_{max} only, our recent experiences indicate that regulatory agencies also place emphasis on how well an IVIVC model predicts the entire plasma concentration time course, for example, how well does the model predict the time at which the maximum concentration is observed and how well the IVIVC model describes the terminal phase of the data.

Application of IVIVC

The various applications of IVIVC for oral dosage forms are all based on the same principle—that is, a validated IVIVC model allows us to predict the impact of changes to a formulation on the in vivo performance without having to conduct a BE study.

In the absence of a validated IVIVC model, the management of change to a dosage form is typically done according to the following procedure. For example, the new manufacturing process or revised formulation is used to produce the new dosage form, which is subjected to in vitro dissolution testing. Based on the results, a decision is then taken whether to proceed with a standard two-way, crossover BE study between batches produced with the new and the existing process/formulation. If the two products are demonstrated to be bioequivalent, then the new process/formulation is substituted for the existing one in the development program. However, if BE cannot be demonstrated, the cycle starts all over again. More costly though are the implications of the bioinequivalence on the drug development program, being more severe the further down the development program the change is made.

Having a validated IVIVC, the process is similar, but now the decision regarding BE is taken on the basis of the results of the in vitro dissolution test and the IVIVC model, by predicting concentration-time profiles for the batches produced with the new and the existing process/formulation and determining the differences.

Thus, although the most obvious saving between the two approaches may be financial in terms of the money saved in not performing BE studies, the bigger saving is in time. An IVIVC model allows the impact of a change on the in vivo performance to be determined in a matter of minutes or hours, rather than in months. In the current drug development climate, this is critically important as it avoids decisions being taken at risk, pending the results of a BE study. Thus, the value of having an IVIVC in the oral dosage form development program is that it allows more timely and reliable decisions to be taken regarding the potential impact of changes on the in vivo performance of the dosage form.

One critical point regarding the application of IVIVC models is that the predicted concentration-time profile and corresponding parameters for the new process/formulation should not be compared to historical observed data for the existing process/formulation. The rationale for this is quite simple: any IVIVC model has an associated error in terms of its ability to predict data. For validated IVIVC models, the error has been quantified and demonstrated to satisfy the criteria outlined in the guidance and discussed earlier in this chapter. For example, a validated IVIVC model predicts AUC for the target formulation with an associated prediction error of 10%. A second site manufactures a batch of the same target formulation and in vitro dissolution testing shows it has an identical profile to the formulation manufactured at the current site. However, comparison of the IVIVC model-predicted AUC for the batch from the new site and the observed AUC for the batch from the current site reveals an apparent 10% difference. So, for identical in vitro dissolution profiles, a 10% difference in AUC is apparently predicted. Clearly, this represents the already quantified prediction error associated with the IVIVC model. Using the IVIVC model to predict the in vivo performance for both batches would show no difference in AUC, as anticipated from identical in vitro release profiles. This approach is also consistent with the notion that an IVIVC model acts as a surrogate for a BE study. Were such a study to be performed, a batch from each of the current and new manufacturing sites would be evaluated in the same study.

Regulatory Application of IVIVC for Immeduate Release Dosage Forms

As previously discussed, successful development of IVIVC models for IR dosage forms may be limited to those drug substances in either class II or III, according to the BCS. Despite this apparent limitation, IVIVC, where developed, can be applied for IR dosage forms for regulatory purposes.

In the 1995 SUPAC-IR Guidance, the use of an "*acceptable IVIVC*" is discussed to support the waiving of a full BE study where a change requires in the in vivo BE documentation. Such documentation is only required for a Level 3 change in components and composition or a Level 3 change in the manufacturing process (i.e., change to a different campus). IVIVC models can also be applied to the development of in vitro dissolution specifications for IR dosage forms.

Regulatory Application of IVIVC for Extended Release Dosage Forms

The IVIVC guidance for ER oral dosage forms discusses in some detail the applications of an IVIVC. The guidance does stress, however for these applications, that predictability of the IVIVC model must have been established if it is to serve as a surrogate for in vivo testing. The IVIVC guidance refers the reader to the SUPAC-MR guidance for industry, where the requirement for BE documentation for various levels of scale-up and post-approval changes. Where such documentation is required, the need to conduct a formal study may be waived in the presence of an established IVIVC. Presently, under SUPAC-MR, an IVIVC may be used to support a waiver for the following changes: (i) a Level 3 change in a nonrelease controlling excipient, (ii) a Level 2 change in release controlling excipient for a drug with a narrow therapeutic index, (iii) a Level 3 change in release controlling excipient, (iv) a Level 3 change in manufacturing site, and (v) a Level 3 change in manufacturing process.

The FDA IVIVC guidance also discusses how an IVIVC can be used to justify a biowaiver request for the approval of lower strengths or new strengths. In these cases, the IVIVC should have been developed using the highest strength and the new strengths should be compositionally proportional or qualitatively the same, have the same release mechanism, and have similar in vitro dissolution profiles.

Importantly, the IVIVC guidance from the FDA also qualifies the application of IVIVC models as a surrogate for an in vivo study, based on the number of formulations/release rates used in the development of the IVIVC and whether the drug has a narrow therapeutic index. For example, an IVIVC developed with only two formulations/release rates is more limited in its applications than an IVIVC developed with three or more formulations/release rates. Similarly, the demonstration of external predictability strengthens the case of applying IVIVC as a surrogate for a BE study, particularly where the model has been developed with just two formulations/release rates or where the drug has a narrow therapeutic index. Clearly, the greater the confidence in an IVIVC, the wider it can be applied in a regulatory setting.

As well as the possibility of using an established IVIVC to waive the requirement to conduct a BE study, the SUPAC-MR Guidance for Industry also discusses how an IVIVC can reduce the amount of in vitro dissolution documentation required to support Level 2 changes to a formulation or process. For all MR oral dosage forms, in the presence of an established IVIVC, only application or compendial dissolution testing should be performed (i.e., only in vitro release data by the correlating method needs to be submitted).

The FDA IVIVC Guidance for Industry outlines how a Level A IVIVC can be applied for the setting of dissolution specifications. Using the IVIVC model, predicted C_{max} and AUC are obtained for the fastest and slowest release rates that are allowed by the dissolution specifications such that a maximal difference of 20% exists. Ensuring a maximal difference of 20% in the predicted C_{max} and AUC for the upper and lower specifications is considered the optimal situation. The guidance suggests that an established IVIVC may permit the setting of wider specifications, dependent on the predictions of the IVIVC (i.e., as long as the differences in the predicted C_{max} and AUC for the lower and upper limits do not exceed 20%). This was re-affirmed in a presentation at a recent advisory committee for pharmaceutical science meeting.

The 1997 guidance did suggest a less optimal, but still acceptable, situation where the specifications ensure lots exhibiting dissolution profiles at the upper and lower limits are bioequivalent to the clinical/ bioavailability lots or to an appropriate reference standard. The implication was that the difference in the predicted C_{max} and AUC between the lower and upper specifications could be greater than 20% as long as both were bioequivalent to the target. However, our recent experience suggests that proposed dissolution specifications that fail to ensure a maximal difference of 20% in the predicted pharmacokinetics for the upper and lower specification limits are not currently acceptable to the FDA. The advisory committee for pharmaceutical science meeting in May 2005 also suggested that external validation is not required for the application of an IVIVC model in setting dissolution specifications. However, our recent discussions with the Agency suggest this only applies to models that are considered to be straightforward. More complex IVIVC models, especially those developed to account for dissolution rate-dependent changes in the in vivo performance of an ER product, may require evidence of external validation before the model can be applied to dissolution specifications.

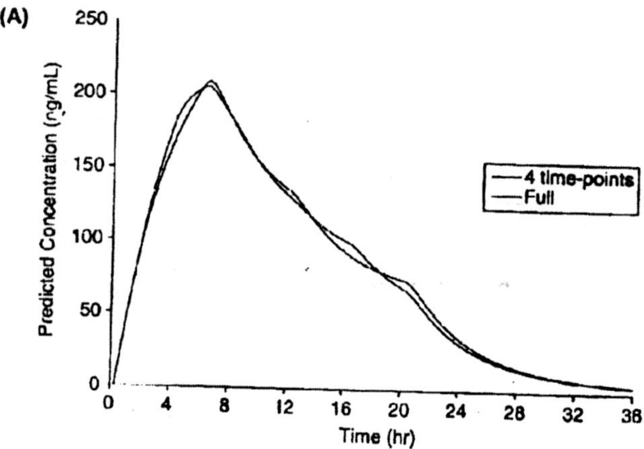

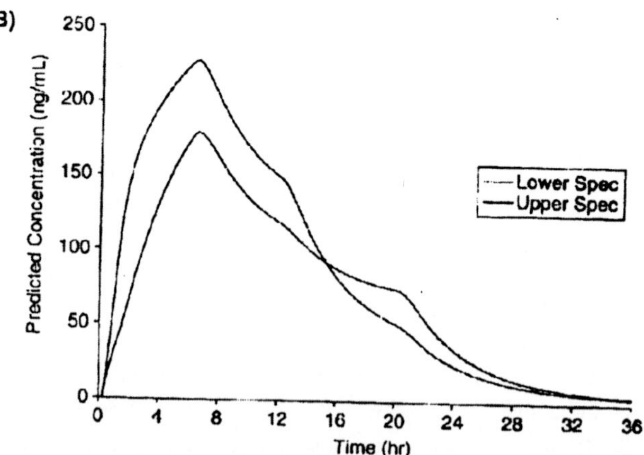

Fig. 13.13. A–Predicted concentration-time profile for the target formulation using either the full dissolution profile; B–Predicted concentration-time profiles for the lower and upper dissolution specifications.

Application of IVIVC for Development of In vitro Dissolution Specifications

This case study briefly illustrates how a validated Level A IVIVC model for an ER dosage form was applied for the development of in vitro dissolution specifications. The IVIVC model was developed using in vitro dissolution data sampled at eight time points over 20 hours. The established model was firstly used to identify which time point(s) was critical for an accurate prediction of C_{max} for the target formulation around which the specifications were to be established. By omitting each time point in turn, predicting C_{max} and comparing the predicted value to the value obtained using the full dissolution profile, the IVIVC model quickly indicated that only the six-hour time point was critical for the prediction of C_{max}. The IVIVC model was used to demonstrate that the concentration-time profile for the target formulations could be described using only four time points. The predicted profiles and corresponding PK parameters were then obtained for the lower and upper specifications by convolution through the established IVIVC model.

Application of IVIVC for the Justification of a Level 3 Site Change

The following case study briefly described how an established IVIVC model was used to justify a Level 3 site change in manufacturing site, a change that would require documentation of BE according to SUPAC-MR, in the absence of an IVIVC model. The target formulation was manufactured at the proposed commercial manufacturing site and the in vitro dissolution profile compared to a batch of the identical formulation manufactured by the clinical trial supply site. The concentration-time profile and corresponding PK parameters for each batch were predicted using the established IVIVC model and shown to be bioequivalent, that is, both AUC and C_{max} within 20%.

Both case studies clearly illustrate the application of an established IVIVC model, allowing in vitro dissolution testing to serve as a surrogate for BE studies so that the impact of changes in a formulation or changes in site of manufacture can be assessed quickly and allow the development program to continue.

In the same way that postapproval changes can be supported using an IVIVC, changes made during the preapproval process may also be justified using in vitro dissolution data and an established IVIVC. However, companies need to consider the potential risk of utilizing an IVIVC that has yet to receive approval from a regulatory agency to support such pre-approval changes. Clearly, the more robust the IVIVC model, the greater confidence the company can have in its application in the pre-approval environment. For example, was the model developed using three or more different formulations/release rates? Has external predictability, in addition to internal predictability, been

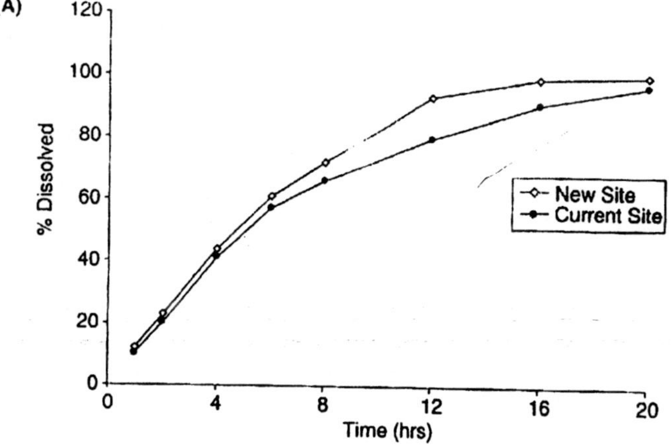

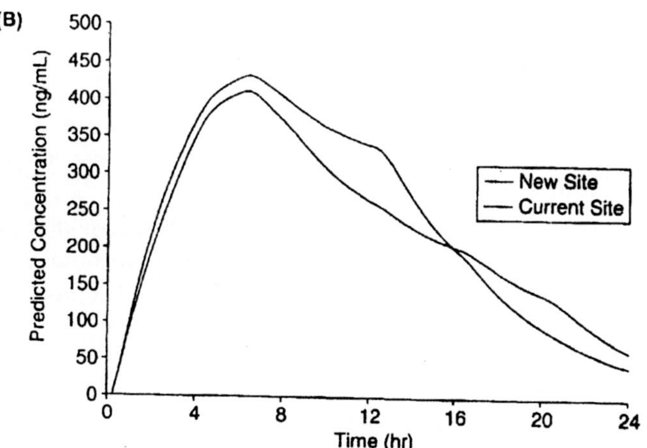

Fig. 13.14. A-In vitro dissolution profiles for a 50 mg formulation manufactured at the current and proposed new sites. B-Concentration-time profiles predicted from the in vitro dissolution profiles using an in vitro-in vivo correlaions models.

demonstrated for the model? Frequently, companies now present IVIVC models at end of phase II-type meetings with regulatory agencies, and outline how they intend to incorporate such models into their BE strategy, for example, bridging the clinical trial material and the final to-be-marketed formulation. While these meetings do not provide a definitive or binding opinion from the agencies, sponsors do obtain valuable feedback as to the likely acceptance of basing a BE strategy on a particular IVIVC, and for this reason, introducing IVIVC and the intended applications at such meetings is highly recommended.

Timing of an IVIVC within a Formulation Development Program

Not surprisingly, the application of an IVIVC to any oral dosage form development is dependent on when, during the program, the IVIVC study or studies are conducted to allow a model to be developed. The timing of such studies frequently reflects the prevailing view of IVIVC within a company. For those companies that view IVIVC as being a powerful tool to assist the formulation development, a study designed to permit the development of an IVIVC model may be conducted very early in the formulation development program. A range of formulations considered sufficiently wide to allow a meaningful IVIVC model to be developed are evaluated in vivo. Typically, one of the formulations will represent what is believed to meet the product specification and formulations having either faster or slower release rates are also included in the study. If one of the formulations does meet the product specifications, the IVIVC can be used to assist the further optimization and scale-up of that formulation. If none of the formulations meets the specifications, the IVIVC can be used to guide the formulation developments and help identify formulations that more closely match the product specification. Incorporating the IVIVC model development early into the formulation program allows the model to be refined and expanded as further data become available.

Other companies are less aggressive in the application of IVIVC and tend to view IVIVC as a tool for supporting changes to an already identified target formulation. Developing an IVIVC late in the formulation development program usually requires the manufacture of formulations designed to be sufficiently faster or slower than the target to be evaluated in a prospectively designed study to allow for a meaningful IVIVC to be developed.

However, a review of the formulation development program may help identify a suitably wide range of formulations that have been evaluated over a series of early develop studies that could then be combined into a single IVIVC. For example, early studies evaluating ER dosage forms would need to include an IR reference in each study in order to develop an IVIVC using the traditional deconvolution-based approach. Therefore, although IVIVC may not be a primary or even secondary objective of early formulation development studies, attention should be paid to the design of such studies that may permit the use of data obtained from these studies to be used for IVIVC analyses later in the development program.

Rohrs et al. approach the timing of IVIVC within an ER formulation development program from the viewpoint of the in vitro dissolution methodology. They suggest obtaining in vivo data on ER formulations as early as possible in the development program as any changes in the dissolution methodology are easier to implement early on the drug development before a large historical and stability database has been generated. They also recommend that samples from early formulations should be retained for any future in vitro methodology development.

14

TABLETING

Introducing high-speed tableting in 24-hr shifts has tremendously increased productivity, which in turn places heavy demands not only on the tablet presses and the compressibility of the tableting materials but also on precision with respect to dimensions and the wear resistance of the toolings (punch and die sets). Furthermore, in many cases of high tableting-speeds, adhesiveness of tablets to the toolings becomes a problem in the course of long-term production. Tableting materials need to be optimized in line with new demands. At the same time, tooling requirements with respect to adhesion-reducing finish have become more important than ever.

Special attention must be paid to handling and maintaining the tool sets during their entire lifetime. Not only does timely mechanical work-over prolong their total lifetime, but also trace patterns of wear on the tooling itself can be indicative of numerous different events during production, inter alia pressures that are generally too high, inadequate lubrication resulting in excessive friction, blockage of pressure rollers, tilted punches, or dies. Furthermore, worn-out punches not only affect the quality of the tablets (increased variation of mass, reduced surface shininess etc.), but can also cause serious problems in the process (powder loss with dust sticking to lubrication oil as well as excessive wear of the tablet press itself). Scratched surfaces can lead to grave problems with tablets sticking to the punches at the discharge point, making tablet production impossible. A deviation in the length of a lower punch translates directly into mass variability in the tablet batch; variation in the length of the entire set also leads to varying compression forces and consequently affects the dissolution properties of the tablets.

On the other hand, tablet tooling design opens up for many possibilities for overcoming common tableting problems that cannot be solved by modifying the materials or the compression process, such as lubrication problems which in general are also a function of tooling size and shape.

In the following text, only examples and principles will be discussed. Mentioning or omitting a specific make or model does not constitute any value judgment. Comprehensive recommended publications are "The Tablet Specification Manual'' with respect to technical and practical problems of tooling, and for all aspects of tableting including development of tableting materials, optimization of compression cycles, and handling of tooling "Die Tablette."

GENERAL TERMINOLOGY OF TOOLING

A set of tooling consists of upper punch, lower punch, and die. The upper punch has a shorter stem; the lower punch stem is longer because it travels longer distances up and down in the die for filling, compression, and ejection, thereby sealing the die hole from below during the entire process of compression.

In single-punch tablet presses (reciprocating tablet presses), the punches are fixed to the punch holders which travel up and down, and in many cases fixation screws are used. Each make has its own holder design for punches and dies, and consequently for the tooling sets as well. Therefore little can be said in general terms, but it would appear that on the whole the remarks on the rotary press tooling apply correspondingly.

In rotary tablet presses, only the dies are fixed in the die table, whereas the punches are vertically mobile and are not fixed to a holder. They slide up and down in the turret bores, driven by cam tracks guiding the punch heads. The dwell time, i.e., the period during which the tablet is under full compression, is determined by the diameter of the flat part of the punch head.

The amount of clearance (space) between interacting parts like punch/die and barrel/turret guide, depends on the tolerance range (deviation from theoretical dimensions due to practical manufacturing reasons) of tooling dimensions. The clearance between the die wall and the punch tip affects the tableting process as well as the mechanical properties of the finished product: while the powder is compressed, air needs to be released, and when the compressed tablet is moved upwards within the die bore, friction on the die walls is affected by the clearance.

A deviation in the overall length or the working length of a lower punch in a set of punches for a rotary press translates directly into mass variability in the tablet batch; a deviation of not more than ±0.1 mm can lead to a mass variability of 2% in the case of small tablets. Moreover, variability of the lengths of both lower and upper punches affects the variability of compression forces with consequences for tablet dimensions, their tensile strength, and dissolution behavior. In the case of a short lower and upper punch, overfilling would not necessarily lead to an increased force signal.

Tooling for Single-punch Presses and Compaction Simulators

Nowadays, single-punch presses are, in general, only used in R&D, but hardly in pharmaceutical production. Useful research tools are instrumented special hydraulic presses, "*compaction simulators*," which allow for online measurements of forces and displacements during the tableting process. Compaction simulators are in many cases designed to accommodate standard single-punch tooling, which is specific for each machine type, e.g., Korsch EK0, Kilian SP300. Dimensions of the tooling and tolerances thereof are up to the press and tooling manufacturer.

Two-piece configuration—i.e., a punch with interchangeable punch tips—is common for single-punch presses as, in general, single-punch tooling is less exposed to abrasion and—compared to tooling for rotary presses—can relatively be aligned easily. In the case of two-piece tools, the lower punch tips are not rigidly fixed but allow for some tilting in order to avoid excess friction in the die bore. Multiple tools comprise several punch tips on a single holder in order to increase productivity. They have been common for single-punch presses used in small-scale production, particularly in the form of multipiece tools, where any cracked tip can be exchanged separately.

Tooling for Rotary Tablet Presses

The punch consists of head, neck, barrel, and stem. The barrel diameter and the overall length are determined by the machine turret dimensions. The working length (i.e., overall length minus any cup depth at the punch tip) determines thickness and mass of the tablets and needs to be controlled regularly. The variation in working length should be within ±10 μm to ensure low variability of tablet properties. The die depth should also be accurately cut in order to guarantee a flush fitting with the die table.

International Standards

Standardization of tooling dimensions has been agreed to facilitate interchangeability between presses and to reduce the number of spare parts. In many cases, a certain press is available with different turrets in order to standardize tooling within a tablet manufacturing company irrespective of the make of tablet presses used in R&D and production, respectively. A special turret for R&D on which all standard tooling can be used on one and the same turret is available from Pharmachine India. It allows to interchange punches and dies of any sizes for trial compression.

There are two main standards: (1) B-tools with subcategories EU19/TSM 19/Japan Norm; (2) D-Tooling, also called EU1, TSM 1, which are classified according to the dimensions of the barrel diameter, overall length, and the overall diameter of the punch head. D-tooling is thicker than B-tooling; European toolings (both B- and D-types) are longer compared to TSM types. The head angle or head radius (in the case of "*domed heads*"), respectively, determines the lead under the compression roller. The head flat determines the dwell time of the compression event (i.e., the period during which the tablet is under maximum pressure), which should preferably be long so as to yield mechanically resistant tablets. The head flat must in all cases be smaller in diameter than the neck in order to guarantee pressure transmission onto the whole punch. Neck shape and neck diameter are determined by the dimensions of the cam track. The head thickness needs to be precisely cut in order to ensure a smooth gliding of the punches through the cam track and, in the case of lower punches, to guarantee a reproducible dosing of granule in the die as well. There is another head shape to the D-tooling called Fette EU1 441, which is characterized by the absence of a neck and a larger head diameter (38.00 mm) allowing for increased dwell times.

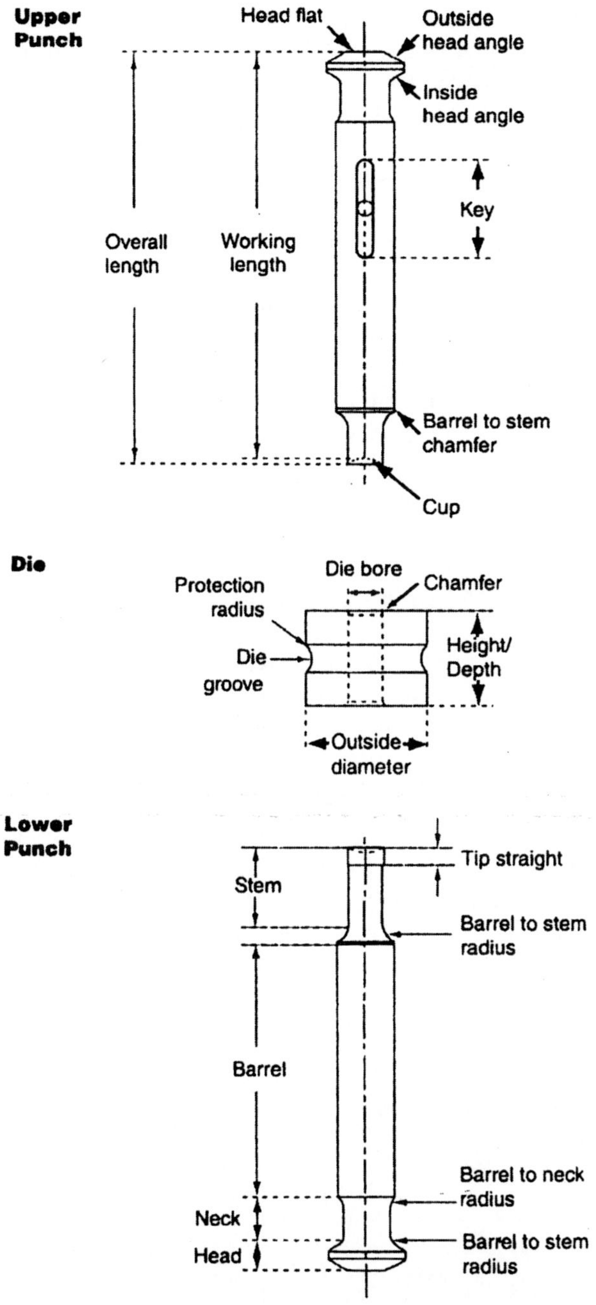

Fig. 14.1. General terminology of tooling for rotary tablet presses.

A further subcategory of B-tooling, which is referred to as B2-type, has the same barrel diameter as the standard B-type, but the overall length of the lower punch is smaller. B2 is used on some older presses, but not manufactured any more. There is yet another variation on standard B-type tooling, where the overall diameter of the die is smaller. The die diameter determines the maximum tablet diameter as well as the maximum number of die bores in the case of multiple tools. A larger die is more resistant although pressure is not directly applied to it but only by lateral extension. The height (depth) of the die ensures a flush fitting with the die table. The overall die diameter—nominal size and manufacturing tolerances—enables a tight fit in the turret avoiding lateral movement, which is also supported by the die groove accommodating the locking screws. A protection radius or protection shoulder prevents damage to the die locking screw or scoring of the die pockets in the turret caused by burrs or sharp edges on the die. The die bore should be made as close to its nominal size as possible because it is this, which determines the tablet size, not the punches. A bore chamfer provides a lead for the upper punch to enter the die. Any clearance between the die wall and the punch affects the tableting behavior, as entrapped air will escape through the gap when pressure is applied.

Die bore tapers with a conical opening have the same effect as the clearance. Tapered dies are more expensive than standard dies. Tapers can be applied to both ends of the bore to allow for an inversion of the dies. Tapered dies not only let air escape, but also assist ejection as the stress is gradually released by ejecting to an increasing diameter thereby preventing capping and generally increasing the tensile strength of the tablets. Furthermore, their use also allows higher machine speeds.

Shaped punches—all other shapes than round ones—and multitip punches need to have keys on their barrel in order to prevent any rotation. Keys are available in two configurations: the Woodroff key and the flat key can be distinguished by the shape of the slot milled into the barrel where the key is in many cases screwed into position. The vertical position of the key on the punch barrel and the length of the key itself are determined by the turret dimensions in such a way as to allow for clearance in the punch-guide keyways. The optimum angle of the key with respect to tablet shape is determined by the

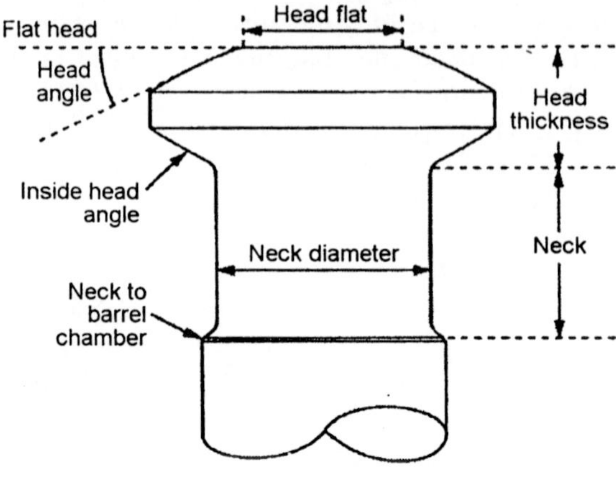

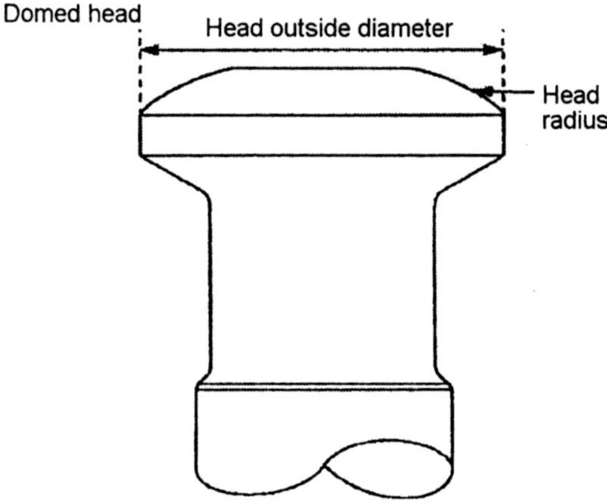

Fig. 14.2. Punch head terminology.

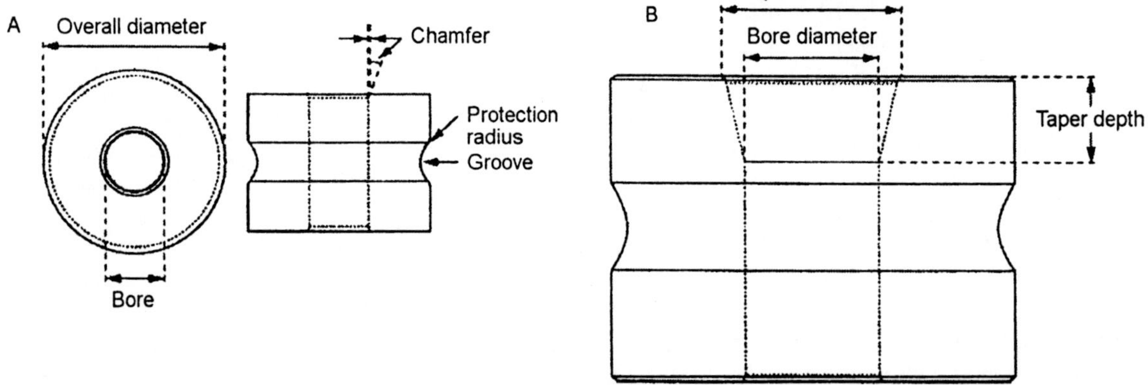

Fig. 14.3. Die terminology: A–Standard die, B–Tapered die.

rotation direction of the tableting machine and the design of the take-offence at the discharge point with respect to the punch tip, and therefore not standardized. Tablets hitting the fence with a corner should be avoided; they should rather hit it with a flat face in order to ensure proper discharge without fragmentation. Common configurations for punch keys and their lengths can be found in Tablet Specification Manual.

Barrel flutes, usually on round upper and lower punches, are vertical sharp-edged grooves along the length of the punch barrel. During production, they would rotate and thereby scrape off possible depositions of material in the punch guideways.

Fig. 14.4. Terminology of tolerances and clearances between punches and dies.

Several types of dust caps and sealings fitted to the barrel-to-stem chamfer are available to prevent contamination of the tablets by machine oil dripping from the upper punch. Alternatively, punch bellows in silicone rubber fitted into special seal grooves for Euro-standard are available.

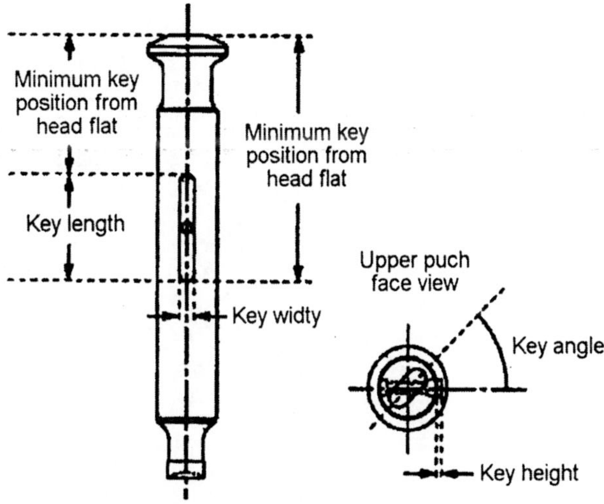

Fig. 14.5. Keys on punches: terminology.

Special Tooling

Some makes of tablet presses have their own tooling specifications allowing for longer dwell times and higher compression forces, such as the Fette EU1 441 mentioned earlier, and Kilian 25/32, with subtypes in die shape, i.e., grooved and slotted, which are depicted together with standard types in a tooling identification chart. Most tablet presses from the manufacturers cited are alternatively available with turrets for standard size tooling. Two-piece configurations with interchangeable punch tips can also be used in punches for rotary presses. Special care and experience are necessary as these punches can be difficult to assemble and align; they are mostly used with multiple tools in order to increase productivity, thus offsetting additional costs. Korsch has a special machine for solving sticking problems, where the entire punches are rotated before and after the compression phase in order to prevent adhesion. These punches have a cogwheel around their neck. From Manesty a special rotating-head tooling is available which enables the punch head of shaped tooling to rotate in order to increase the lifetime of punches and cams. By IMA, a special high-speed machine design has been developed. Feeding happens at the center, taking advantage of increasing centrifugal forces. This design requires special tooling, which is made in two pieces. This means that only the punch tips need to be changed, which saves time in this special machine. Instrumented punches and dies, which enable online measurement of forces on the punch and relative displacement or acceleration, electrical resistance, and acoustic release as well as measurement of die wall forces, are special tools used exclusively in research.

Punch Tips

First of all, one has to make a general distinction between round and shaped tablets. It is impossible to maintain an infinite sharp edge as this would wear off immediately; the figure also shows how a land is introduced by polishing the punch tip in order to increase its pressure tolerance. The land/cup connection can be designed as a sharp corner, a standard curvature (radius), or a blend radius.

In order to avoid sticking, it is recommended to avoid corners. Compared to the profile of the land/cup connection, an alteration of the common connection between the bevel and the flat by rounding the beveled edge of flat-faced punches, thus reducing the possibility of sticking of material to the sharp edge, has been proposed to reduce sticking problems.

Break lines are most often bisects or quadrisects, whereas engravings often comprise characters and graphic objects facilitating identification of the tablets. Engravings on tablets can be embossed or debossed, the punch has to be the respective opposite, and the characters and figures are mirrored. In many cases, break lines and engravings trigger sticking problems. In order to quantify the pull-off force of a tablet sticking to a punch surface, a special instrumentation was developed and used for the optimization of the angle between the engravings and the surface. As sticking in most cases starts at the lateral faces of the engravings due to shear forces occurring there during compression, the authors quoted above generally recommend a small angle of the stroke to the surface. This is in contrast to findings of Sabir, Evans, and Jain, who recommend an angle of 90°, but their study lacks conclusiveness as the steep angle tooling, unlike the reference tools, was chromium-plated. Waimer et al. used a cone for their measurements, and it can be assumed that engravings comprising a greater number of lateral faces per area would need even more attention. Empirically, it is recommended to avoid sharp corners as in characters like "A" and to use radii instead; tooling manufacturers have their special rounded character type sets. For film coating, the profile of the engravings must be particularly flat-angled in order to ensure wetting with the coating material. The maximum area on the surface of the tablet that can be used for engravings depends on the cup depth.

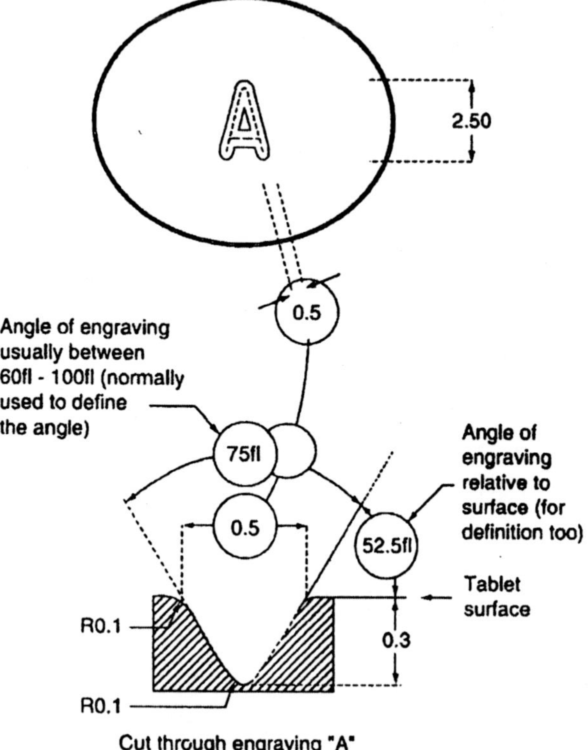

Fig. 14.6. Terminology of engravings, exemplified by the character "A".

Requirements for break lines have been increased during the past years. All break lines must ensure that the tablet breaks into equal parts and lines for decoration purposes are not legal any more. Guaranteeing a reproducible crack is not trivial as the powder located right under the break line is exposed to the highest compression stress and most compaction and is therefore in many cases mechanically strongest. Therefore, break lines should not be too deep, and notching of the outer tablet wall serves to ensure a defined crack line. Notching requires coves in the die wall and, consequently, punch rotation has to be prevented. The shape, angle, and depth of bisects with regard to the shaped tablet surface has been optimized in order to facilitate the breaking of tablets by pressing them against a hard pad with one finger.

In bigger tablets other than those commonly used pharmaceutically, the requirements for reproducibility are lower, which, e.g., makes it possible to press a trough into the tablet surface so that a second mixture of tensides for dish-washing can be applied after tableting. The punch can be designed as an interchangeable cone made from synthetic material. Multiple tools have several punch tips on one and the same barrel; the corresponding die has as many bores in order to increase productivity. One disadvantage results from the more delicate handling of the tools, but multiple tools are definitely useful for small tablets in order to increase productivity. Minitablets of 2 mm diameter are produced as a substitute for pellets and offer the advantage of better reproducibility of filling into capsules as well as better reproducibility of their specific surface area, which is important for the coating process and the subsequent reproducible release of the active drug. Multiple punch tips are frequently manufactured as multiple tools in a several-piece punch design. A 19-fold punch set is available and working in standard production of minitablets.

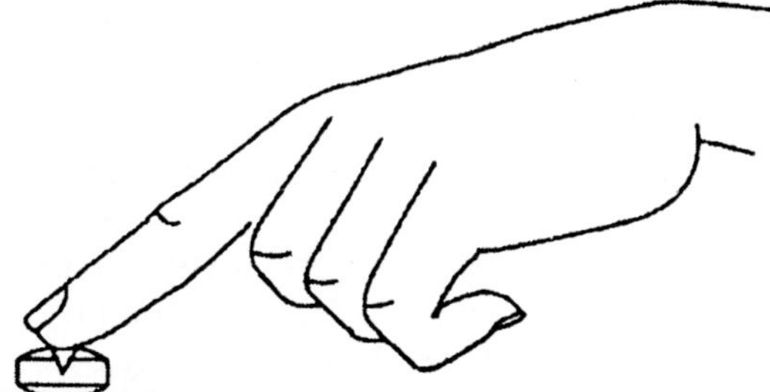

Fig. 14.7. Method for dividing pressure-sensitive tablets into equal parts.

Materials, Manufacture, Finish, and Pressure Tolerance

Materials and Manufacture

Steels are basically classified as carbon and alloy steels which are defined by national and international standards, e.g., ASTM and DIN. Carbon steels contain less than 1.65% manganese, 0.6% silicon, 0.6% copper, plus boron and deoxidizers as well as carbon as the principal additive increasing hardness. Manganese also increases hardness, particularly the ability to be hardened by tempering, and is present in all steels. Silicon acts as a deoxidizer. Alloy steels exceed these limits or contain additional elements, e.g., chromium, vanadium, tungsten, molybdenum, nickel, and cobalt. A high-nickel content increases resistance to corrosion caused by HCl released from drug salt. The composition of special steel types for tooling, their provenance, and their thermal treatment are part of the trade secret of tooling manufacturers.

A high abrasion resistance usually corresponds to high hardness of a steel type, whereas its ductility and toughness is low and vice versa: very hard tooling may fracture, ductile material may wear off quickly. Hardness and ductility do not only depend on the chemical composition of the steel but also on its heat-treatment (tempering). A second tempering procedure for punch tips, which is computer-controlled and carried out at high temperatures in a vacuum furnace, softens the material and prevents fracture.

Punches usually have a longer lifetime than dies if they are made from the same material; that is why manufacturers often choose different steel qualities. The surface of a die bore can become smoother or rougher during its use. The ejection force does not— apart from the composition of the tableting material and the compaction force—necessarily depend on roughness of the die wall, but to a high degree depends on the metal type of the die.

For specific tableting tasks, the tooling manufacturer will be able to provide optimum tool properties. It may be helpful in this respect to supply him with a sample of the tableting material in question.

440C has the highest chromium content (17%), which increases wear resistance. D2 and D3 have a high-chromium content (12%) and are additionally carbon-rich (over 1.5%). Chromium and carbon together form stable carbide, which increases hardness. S1 contains tungsten (2%), which makes heat-treatment easier.

Finish

Adhesion, sticking, picking, and filming on punches and dies can in many cases be avoided by a suitable surface finish of the tooling. In some cases, the surface is smoothened during continuous use of punches, whereas in other cases, depending on the material compressed, e.g., in the case of crystalline lactose, small scratches may occur on the punch tips after a few thousand compression events. On those small scratches and defects in the surface, corrosion will start. Tolerances for the surface finish of tooling are also specified by manufacturers and in international standards. Any roughness of the finishing is below 1 μm peak-to-valley height, and particularly punch-tip faces and die bore walls are polished to achieve lower tolerances.

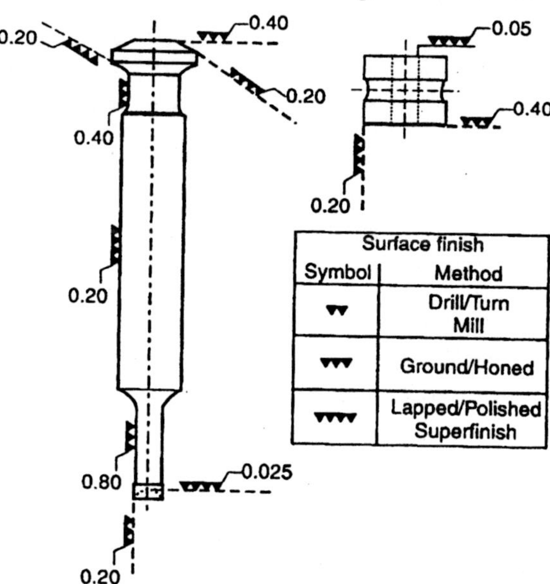

Fig. 14.8. Surface finish of punches; tolerances for top-to-valley differences (in μm).

Coatings and Platings on Punch Tips

Reduced ejection forces can help to avoid both lamination and capping and give tablets a shiny surface as well as high mechanical strength. Internal lubrication (lubricants added to the tableting material) is counter-productive not only because its admixture is another critical step in production, but also because the most effective lubricants are hydrophobous and make the tablets softer and increase disintegration time as well as dissolution rate. Attempts to coat the tooling with fluid or solid lubricants just before each compression event are relatively complicated with respect to machinery, reproducibility, dust formation, and GMP demands, e.g., batch definition. In many cases, an easier alternative may be to apply a finish to the punches that reduces friction by special coating or plating of the punch tips so that ejection forces are reduced. Another reason for coating the punches may be to decrease the adhesiveness of tablets to the punches as this does not necessarily decrease with reduced ejection forces. It may also be necessary to increase corrosion resistance in cases where aggressive chemicals are compressed. A critical demand on all coatings and platings is their wear resistance. The thickness of the coat must be taken into account as it affects clearances and tolerances. As this is also a part of the trade secret of manufacturers and specialized companies, little is published on this subject.

Hard chromium plating is applied galvanically with a thickness of approximately 30 μm. It should not be confused with blank chromium plating, which consists of several layers of other metals with a very thin chromium layer on top and is not suitable for tooling. Hard chromium platings, although appearing shiny and smooth, are more porous than the blank coatings, brittle, and in many cases not sufficiently wear-resistant. Moreover, any transition of traces of chromium into the product would be totally unacceptable for pharmaceutical use. Not in all cases do they have the desired effect with respect to sticking.

Nodular thin dense chromium is an FDA-approved coating which is applied to the entire punch and all its faces. Chromium can be implanted into the surface in the form of chromium nitride at a depth of up to 1 μm by nitrogen ion bombardment of the surface. This treatment proved to have a favorable effect on sticking problems and makes the surface relatively wear-resistant. Titanium can be applied in the same way in the form of TiN. This treatment leaves the tools in a "bronzed" appearance because the surface is relatively rough as seen in the electron microscope. Increased hardness and greater wear and corrosion resistance is achieved, but the effect on friction is smaller than in the case of CrN. Nickel–chromium–boron alloying coat applied on both punches and dies has been described and compared to untreated tools. Surprisingly, depending on the material under compression, the coating had the expected effect, or there was a total lack of effect, or they even increased ejection forces. The authors concluded that anyway, the tablets were superior in appearance.

Titanium carbide is by far the hardest material available for the treatment of surfaces. Teflon coating has not proven to be wear-resistant enough to tolerate tableting. Carbon in layer thickness of 0.1 μm–10 μm, doped with hydrogen in 5 at.%–30 at.% has proven to be extremely wear-resistant and to prevent sticking of tablets. The amorphous carbon layer is applied by CVP (chemical vapor deposition), which can also be used to apply coatings of metal, alloy, carbide, and nitride. It generally yields lower adhesion and superior wear resistance of the coatings, but the high temperatures necessary for the process (1000°C) would soften the steel and distort it. Ion plating is an alternative ensuring low adhesion and minimum distortion of the punches.

Alternative Materials

Inserted (lined) dies are fitted with an insert (liner) in the outer shell of the metal and consist of a much harder material such as tungsten carbide or a ceramic. Liners are used for compression of abrasive or corrosive materials. The outer shell of steel protects the harder, more brittle liner from possible failure, e.g., by the die locking screw.

Maximum Pressure Tolerance

The pressure tolerance depends on the smallest diameter of the punch, e.g., the backing-off lathe at the punch tip and the cup depth. It is calculated from the load capacity of the tool steel.

Lifetime

Fatigue failure is cumulative because any over-stress inflicts microscopic damage. It correlates with the maximum stress in each loading cycle: a 25% reduction in stress may prolong the lifetime tenfold. It is advisable not to exceed the stress level over the maximum allowable limit for infinite lifetime; it is much better to change the design of the punch-tip cup in order to eliminate fatigue failure. Average lifetime is most affected by granule composition and lubrication properties, lying between 200,000 and several millions of compression events.

Principal reasons for termination of punch life are damage to heads and tips, rolled-in or burred tip edges, pitted faces, distorted and/or flatted bisects or engravings, and undersized tip lands. For dies, it is the wear in the die bore that terminates lifetime, whereas for carbide lined dies it is often distortion leading to die screw groove. Increased clearances accelerate wear, e.g., by extrusion of powder between punch and die. During lifetime the deflection of the upper punch in the turret can double, which leads to rolled-in punch tips. Cam design and cam track tolerances determine wear on punch heads with smaller tolerances used on modern machines prolonging punch life.

Maintenance of Punch Sets

Sets of toolings, i.e., upper punch, lower punch, and die, should not be interchanged. Therefore, they are usually marked by engraved numbers, punches at the neck, dies on the outer wall. Special care must be taken when toolings are fitted to the tablet press. Fitting instructions usually follow with the manual for the respective press. In general, careful aligning is crucial. Special maintenance kits useful for changing punches and containing a set of aids are available from press manufacturers and tooling manufacturers. Immediately after the end of the production campaign, and in the case of long-lasting production cycles also during runs (e.g., daily), tooling should be carefully cleaned. Unless a special washing machine is used, warm soap water and a soft brush are suitable for thorough cleaning; if necessary, a few minutes in an ultra-sound bath can be helpful. Be careful not to scratch the surfaces! Upon rinsing with warm water, ethanol or isopropanol is used to remove any remaining oil. Removing punches and dies for washing takes a lot of time. Some tablet presses are constructed in a way that enables interchangeability of the whole turret including tooling, and the cleaning of the turret takes place in a fully automatic washing machine at the same time as the rest of the tablet press is cleaned in place, which very much reduces turn-over-time, especially if two separate turrets are available.

Tooling should not be touched with bare fingers after washing, and usually all the tooling is thoroughly coated with an acid-free oil in order to prevent corrosion. Instead of expensive commercial products, paraffin and vaseline in pharmacopoeial quality are also suitable. Some users want to avoid all oiling as oil may contribute to sticking problems; in this case punches are washed with alcohol, possibly dusted with magnesium stearate, and stored in a humidity-controlled atmosphere.

Surface roughness and alteration in tooling dimensions are results of use and wear. Tooling surfaces should be frequently checked (magnifying glass). Timely polishing will prolong the lifetime of the tooling. Polishing can be done conventionally by hand on a lathe using ultra-fine polishing paste, polishing wool, and felt or a polishing brass brush. Alternatively, one can use cost-effective "*drag finishing*" machines, which drag and rotate punches and dies through a granulate consisting of slightly abrasive particles coated with a special paraffin base. This process takes about 1 hr, depending on the abrasiveness of the granulate. The process does not round off the tooling but only decreases surface roughness and can be used whenever tooling appears dull or discolored. Furthermore, the punch barrels are polished too, which may help to prevent rough motion of the punches.

The wear pattern on punch heads, punch tips, and in die bores may indicate specific problems during tableting. Measuring dimensions of punches and dies is a task which has to be performed frequently and can be carried out computer-aided. Dimensions to be checked are overall length, cup depth, working length, diameters, tip diameter, and die bore dimensions. Use a micrometer. For estimating the clearance of the upper punch in the turret and wear of the turret guide, it is easiest to measure the deflection of the upper punch tip, which should be approximately 100 μm. If it is more than 0.3 mm, the punches and/or guides are worn out. Wear is unavoidable and it alters the dimensions of the tooling sets with time. It is, therefore, recommendable to use spare sets of tooling in regular turn-over in order to equalize wear of all tooling sets. Storage cabinets for tooling should be clearly laid out for individual punch sets and protect them from clashing, dust, and humidity. Cabinets where punches lie or hang are available in many models made from different materials and with different degree of airtightness. A special tooling utility case system, consisting of individual punch and die trays enabling the combination of as many trays as needed, has an open design for easy inspection and cleaning.

Demands from GMP and the necessity of connecting tool sets to tablet products led to the introduction of "tooling management" with the help of special software, where information on each individual encoded punch and die set is collected to provide a tooling life record. The software may be installed on a mobile trolley and the code on each individual tool will be checked while it is set onto the machine. Many common tableting problems (e.g., sticking, capping, and corrosion) which cannot be overcome by optimizing the properties of the tableting material and/or the compression cycle, can possibly be solved by changing the tooling design. Options are the form, the material and/or the finish of the respective toolings. Although there are software programs available for designing any possible punch tip shape and for theoretically calculating tablet volumes, surface areas, and other useful features, this is no guarantee for being able to compress the respective tablets in practice. Moreover, it may be difficult to imagine on the basis of a punch design how the tablet itself would look like. For this purpose, simulated prototypes made quickly and inexpensively from a special plastic material can be bought under the trade name Elizatab. As tooling manufacturers have been working with effective tablet designs for many years, it is generally recommendable to ask their advice whenever questions arise as to the design of tooling or tablets.

Tablet Formulation

The best new therapeutic entity in the world is of little value without an appropriate delivery system. Tableted drug delivery systems can range from relatively simple immediate-release formulations to complex extended- or modified-release dosage forms. The most important role of a drug delivery system is to get the drug "delivered" to the site of action in sufficient amount and at the appropriate rate; however, it must also meet a number of other essential criteria. These include physical and chemical stability, ability to be economically mass produced in a manner that assures the proper amount of drug in each and every dosage unit and in each batch produced, and, as far as possible, patient acceptability (for example, reasonable size and shape, taste, color, etc., to encourage patients to take the drug and thus comply with the prescribed dosing regimen). The discovery of new therapeutic entities always initiates excitement, but the contributions of the formulation specialist are either not well understood or are often taken for granted and thus remain "unsung." However, the drug and its delivery system cannot be separated. The general design criteria for tablets are given as follows:

1. Optimal drug dissolution and, hence, availability from the dosage form for absorption consistent with intended use (i.e., immediate or extended release)
2. Accuracy and uniformity of drug content.
3. Stability, including the stability of the drug substance, the overall tablet formulation, disintegration, and the rate and extent of drug dissolution from the tablet for an extended period.
4. Patient acceptability. As much as possible, the finished product should have an attractive appearance, including color, size, taste, etc., as applicable, in order to maximize patent acceptability and encourage compliance with the prescribed dosing regimen.
5. Manufacturability. The formulation design should allow for the efficient, cost-effective, practical production of the required batches.

That tablets can be formulated to uniquely meet these criteria accounts for their emergence as the most prevalent oral solid dosage form. Although several different types of tablets may be distinguished, they are mostly made by compression, intended to be swallowed whole and designed for immediate release. This paper presents a systematic approach to the design and formulation of immediate-release compressed tablets.

Modern Tablet Formulation Design and Manufacture

Tablet dosage forms have to satisfy a unique design compromise. The desired properties of rapid or controlled disintegration and dissolution of the primary constituent particles must be balanced with the manufacturability and esthetics of a solid compact resistant to mechanical attrition.

Excipients are critical to the design of the delivery system and play a major role in determining its quality and performance. They may be selected to enhance stability (antioxidants, UV absorbers), optimize or modify drug release (disintegrants, hydrophilic polymers, wetting agents, biodegradable polymers), provide essential manufacturing technology functions (binders, glidants, lubricants), enhance patient acceptance (flavors), or aid in product identification (colorants). Thus a tablet formulation is not a random combination of ingredients, but rather a carefully thought out, rational formulation designed to satisfy the above criteria. A long list of possible excipients is available to the formulation scientist, but certain external factors such as cost, functional reliability, availability, and international acceptance govern their selection. For example, although the official compendia provide standards for identity and purity of excipients, monographs may not provide tests to assure their functionality. For instance, the NF monograph for Compressible Sugar provides no test for compressibility. The monograph for Lactose USP does not address the many particle size and tableting grades meeting monograph standards. The NF monograph for Pregelatinized Starch refers to grades that are "compressible and flowable in character," but provides no specifications or tests for these properties. Nor do the monograph tests for disintegrants and lubricants necessarily relate to their functionality. The need to provide functionality tests or tests for properties clearly related to functionality may be as important as controlling identity and purity. This point has been made even more apparent in recent years with the emergence of multiple sources of such modern excipients as direct- compression filler-binders and the various classes of "super" disintegrants.

A major problem currently being faced by multinational firms and others who market in the international arena, is the lack of universal acceptability of excipients in different countries. The selection of excipients for international markets is often a compromise between functional efficacy, local restrictions, and cost and availability in the countries where the product is to be made. In recent years, the globalization of the pharmaceutical industry has brought about an intense interest in developing harmonized pharmacopeial excipient standards, Good Manufacturing Practices (GMP) for excipient manufacture, and safety evaluation guidelines for new excipients to eliminate or avoid trade barriers between different countries. The International Pharmaceuticals Excipients Council (IPEC), which consists of producers, users, and pharmaceutical scientists, was launched in 1991 to assist regulatory authorities in the United States, Japan, and Europe with harmonization. The separate organizations later formed in the United States, Europe, and Japan are now known as TriPEC and include, as of 1993, more than 100 excipient and pharmaceutical firms.

Preformulation

The objective of preformulation studies is to develop a portfolio of information about the drug substance to serve as a set of parameters against which detailed formulation design can be carried out. Preformulation investigations are designed to identify those physico-chemical properties of drug substances and excipients that may influence the formulation design, method of manufacture, and pharmacokinetic-biopharmaceutical properties of the resulting product. Following is a generalized preformulation protocol appropriate for tablet dosage forms. For certain tests, it is assumed that the drug substance is multisourced (a previously new chemical entity whose patent has expired and which is available to the generic market) for which a USP monograph exists.

Identity and Purity

The study of any drug substance must start with the determination of identity and purity. Such tests are necessary to identify degradents and contaminants and may include organoleptic tests for color, odor, and taste. Purity tests can be found in the USP for almost all marketed compounds. Alternative methods can be employed only if they are validated against the USP procedure. Tests other than potency, which can help to identify or determine the purity of compounds, are melting point, specific rotation, pH, heavy metals, residue on ignition, etc. Impurities can occasionally affect stability, and metal contamination can catalyze chemical reactions. Impurities can also alter the color of drug substances. Techniques can be utilized to give a quantitative estimate of impurities such as the impurity index (II) and the homogeneity index (HI). An ordinary impurity test can be found in the USP that estimates impurities by thin-layer chromatography (TLC).

Crystal Properties and Polymorphism

Many drug substances appear in more than one polymorphic form. The form is determined by certain conditions during the crystallization step. Occasionally drug substances are precipitated in such a way that molecules do not organize themselves in any set pattern, resulting in an amorphous powder. It is also possible for solids to entrap solvents stoichiometrically to form solvates.

Even though they are chemically identical, the different polymorphic forms of a compound are associated with different free energies, and, therefore, have different physical properties that can impact significantly on product performance. These include differences in solubility and dissolution rate (affecting bioavailability), solid-state stability (affecting potency), deformation characteristics (affecting compactibility), and particle size and shape (affecting powder density and flow properties). The form with the lowest energy is more stable than the others. Although the other polymorphs are thus energetically unfavored, if kept dry, they may persist indefinitely and are called "*metastable.*" A metastable form may be preferred, particularly for its ability to dissolve more rapidly.

Polymorphic transformation can take place during pharmaceutical processing, such as particle size reduction, wet granulation, drying, and even during the compaction process. Tests employed to determine crystal properties include differential thermal analysis (DTA), differential scanning calorimetry (DSC), and X-ray diffraction.

Particle Size, Shape, and Surface Area

Probably no characteristics of a drug substance are more important than particle characteristics in determining its performance in a formulation. This is particularly true in those cases where the drug is a poorly soluble non-electrolyte or a free acid form with poor solubility at low pH values. Such drugs are likely to exhibit dissolution-rate-limited absorption, and if dissolution does not take place rapidly enough, a therapeutic concentration in the body fluids may never be achieved, the peak plasma concentration may be significantly delayed, or much of the drug may bypass that region of the gastrointestinal (GI) tract where absorption is best. Particle size reduction (e.g., micronization) is often utilized to enhance dissolution rate. Small particles present a larger surface area per unit weight to the dissolution media and hence dissolve more rapidly than large particles. Particle size and surface area are two of the most important properties determining the solubility rate of a drug and thus potentially its bioavailability. There are numerous examples of bioavailability problems and bioinequivalence due to the inappropriate particle size of the drug substance.

Particle size and shape also play an extremely important role in the homogeneity of powder blends and the unblending of powders in a mixer. Segregation in handling or during the compaction process has a significant effect on the content uniformity of the finished products. Particle size can also affect the stability of a drug substance in that it governs the surface area available for oxidation and hydrolysis. Surface area is critical for interaction with excipients in tablet dosage forms and can greatly affect stability. Methods to determine particle size and shape include light microscopy, scanning electron microscopy, sieve analysis, and various electronic sensing-zone particle counters. Methods available for surface area measurement include air permeability and various gas adsorption techniques.

Bulk Powder Properties

Bulk powder properties are extremely important in pharmaceutical processing. Knowledge of the true and bulk densities of the drug substance as well as of the excipients is extremely useful in

1. Providing perspective as to the size of the final tablet and the size and type of processing equipment needed,
2. Anticipating problems in the physical mixing of powders and the homogeneity of intermediate and final products because significant differences in true densities can result in segregation,
3. Anticipating problems in flow properties, since that property is affected by density, and
4. Identifying differences in different lots and raw materials from different suppliers because different polymorphic forms can be expected to exhibit different true densities.

A comparison of true particle density, apparent particle density, and bulk density can provide information on total porosity, interparticle porosity, and intraparticle porosity. Methods include true particle density measurements via helium pycnometry, mercury intrusion porosimetry, and poured and tapped bulk density.

The influence of sorbed moisture on chemical stability and the flow and compaction of powders and granulations is well established. The moisture content and hygroscopicity of excipients is particularly important as total product processing as well as finished product stability can be affected. Hygroscopicity, moisture-sorption isotherms, and equilibrium moisture content can be determined by thermogravimetric analysis and Karl Fisher titration methods.

The compactibility of relatively large-dose drug substances and formulations is another important property. Compactibility is of less concern for smaller-dose drugs for which direct compression fillers may be able to compensate for a lack of ability to form mechanically strong compacts. An instrumented tablet press or compaction simulator may be used to assess the relationship between the mechanical strength of the compact and the force (or pressure) employed to form the tablet. This relationship is the easiest of all compaction measurements to establish and provides important information on the ability of the material to form practical compacts. Measures of compact mechanical strength include hardness (or crushing force), tensile strength, and friability. Other more complex studies, more easily and perhaps best done using a compaction simulator, include measurement of the work or energy of compaction, pressure–density analysis, strain-rate sensitivity, and elastic recovery. The Athy–Heckel analysis can provide information on deformation mechanism and give an estimate of the mean yield pressure of the material. A comparison of yield pressures determined at different punch speeds can give information on the strain-rate sensitivity of the material. If the major components of the formulation (including the drug) are strain-rate sensitive, the tablets produced on a high-speed production press may exhibit lamination or capping. Excessive elastic recovery may also indicate such tablet failure. The Hiestand indices (bonding and brittle fracture) may be used to assess the compactibility of materials under laboratory conditions.

For the evaluation of flow properties the following test methods may be used:

1. Angle of repose
2. Minimum orifice diameter
3. Carr index
4. Flow rate and
5. Direct observation of weight variation during tableting runs.

The ultimate goal of flow analysis is to identify the powder or powder blend that provides the least weight variation in the finished tablet. The more fluid the powder is, the more efficiently and reproducibly it should fill the die cavities of a tablet press. This more efficient and reproducible die fill should be reflected in increased tablet weights and reduced intertablet weight variation.

Solubility and Permeability

In many cases, the rate of dissolution in gastrointestinal fluids is the rate-limiting step in absorption. The bioequivalence requirements established by the FDA define low solubility as "...<5 mg/mL in water, and slow dissolution rate to be <50% in 30 minutes." However, the solubility of a drug should be considered together with its dose; that is, even a very poorly soluble drug having a sufficiently small therapeutic dose may completely dissolve under physiological conditions. Thus, Amidon et al. have defined a "high solubility" drug as one which at the highest human dose is soluble in 250 ml (or less) water throughout the physiological pH range (1–8) at 37°C. A "low solubility" drug is thus one which requires more than 250 ml of water to dissolve the largest human dose at any pH within the physiological range. The likelihood of having bioavailability problems requires both a consideration of the dose and a solubility volume of the drug and its permeability. Amidon et al. created a Biopharmaceutics Drug Classification System (BCS) based on estimates of these two parameters:

1. Class I: High solubility and high permeability
2. Class II: Low solubility and high permeability
3. Class III: High solubility and low permeability
4. Class IV: Low solubility and low permeability

A jejunal permeability of at least 2-4 $\times$ 10^{-4} cm/s, measured in humans by an intubation technique, is considered "*high permeability*." For many substances, this permeability corresponds to a fraction absorbed of 90% or better. The classification system provides a logical basis for estimating the risk of bioavailability problems. For example, Class I drugs (e.g., propranolol HCl, metoprolol tartrate) are expected to exhibit few bioavailability problems. On the other hand, Class II drugs (e.g., piroxicam) are more likely to exhibit dissolution-rate-limited absorption problems. Class III drugs (e.g., atenolol) are more likely to be prone to absorption (permeability) rate-limited absorption. Class IV drugs (low solubility–low permeability) present formidable obstacles to bioavailability. An in vitro–in vivo correlation (IVIVC) is expected only in the case of Class II drugs. An IVIVC could be expected for Class I drugs if the dissolution rate is slower than the gastric emptying the rate. With a sufficiently rapidly dissolving Class I drug, little or no IVIVC is expected because gastric emptying (not dissolution) would be the rate limiting step. Little or no IVIVC is expected for Class III or Class IV drugs.

The FDA has adopted the BCS in developing a guidance that provides relaxed policies on scale-up and postapproval changes of immediate-release oral solid dosage forms (SUPAC-IR). For certain changes, requirements depend on the drug class, with the most liberal policies for Class I drugs, less liberal policies for Classes II and III drugs, and the least liberal policies for Class IV drugs.

The intrinsic dissolution rate (IDR) of drugs is frequently measured in preformulation tests by the rotating disk method or Wood's apparatus. An automated IDR system, based on a modification of a standard dissolution apparatus, allows for attachment to the stirrer of a die in which the pure drug has been compressed with the tablet face flush with the bottom surface of the die. The IDR may be used to detect different polymorphs as well as to judge the risk of a drug exhibiting dissolution-rate-limited absorption. Kaplan suggested that an IDR of higher than 1 mg $cm^{-2}min^{-1}$ indicated that dissolution-related absorption problems were unlikely, whereas an IDR lower than 0.1 mg $cm^{-2}min^{-1}$ indicated dissolution-rate-limited absorption.

Drug-Excipient Compatibility Studies

A knowledge of the interaction of drugs and excipients is essential in the initial formulation of a product. It may also be necessary later on during processing scale-up, when problems arise, to determine if incompatibilities exist which affect manufacturing or stability. Drug-excipient interactions are often directly related to the moisture present in one or another of the components or to the humidity to which the formulation is exposed during processing or storage. These studies are always carried out at accelerated temperature and humidity conditions, even though it must be recognized that some interactions are physical (melting and volatilization) and not chemical and that accelerated aging may not be predictive. Tests for excipient drug interactions are usually conducted on blends of the pure drug and excipient in ratios similar to those in the final dosage form. For example, excipient-to-drug ratios are higher for filler-binders than for lubricants and disintegrating agents. These studies are often performed with the help of a factorial or fractional- factorial experimental design. Powders are physically mixed and may be granulated or compacted to accelerate any possible interaction. Samples can be exposed in open pans or sealed in bottles or vials to mimic product packaging. Evaluation of samples includes:

1. Visual inspection for changes in color or texture.
2. Both HPLC and TLC are commonly employed with unstressed samples being used as controls. In general, only qualitative results are important initially.
3. Differential thermal analysis is applied and the appearance or disappearance of one or more peaks is noted. Isothermal microcalorimetry can also be employed as well as a thermal activity monitor (TAM) technique.

Compatibility studies are essential in characterizing both raw materials and finished formulations. It has been argued that binary drug-excipient screening studies are inefficient, unrealistic, and ignore processing variables. A better approach may be to carefully select potential excipients based on known chemistry and published compatibility data, and perform miniformulation stability studies.

Formulation Design

Based on the preformulation information, decisions can be made regarding formulation design and process strategy. Initial guidance may be provided by the proposed dose. Relatively low-dose drugs can often be tableted by direct compression, a term that is applied to the process by which tablets are compressed directly from blends of the active ingredient and suitable excipients. No wet or dry granulation is required, although the drug may occasionally be sprayed out of solution onto one of the excipients to ensure uniform dispersion of drug in very low dosage. Larger doses of poorly compactible drugs may be granulated prior to tableting. The process steps required and the choice of excipients are often governed by other properties of the drug.

Analysis of Critical Variables and Formulation Development

Based on the analysis of the preformulation data, likely excipients are selected and small batches may be produced. The number and size of the batches depend on the availability of the drug substance. The batches are intended to assess the feasibility of the formulation, including the types and levels of excipients, as well as the process and its operational variables, such as order of addition, mixing times, compression force, granulation time, etc. The goal is to develop a formulation and process that meets the criteria set forth earlier under Objectives.

MANUFACTURE

Traditionally, tablets have been made by granulation, a process that imparts two primary requisites to formulations: compactibility and fluidity. Both wet granulation and dry granulation (slugging or roll compaction) are used. Regardless of whether tablets are made by direct compression or granulation, the first steps, milling and mixing, are the same; the subsequent steps differ.

The wet massing of powders is typically carried out in high-shear mixers prior to wet screening. The wet granules are often dried in fluidized-bed equipment, enhancing the efficiency of the process. Alternatively, wet granulation may be carried out in fluid-bed drier-granulators in which the liquid phase is sprayed onto fluidized powders while the hot air flow dries the granules. This process reduces the number of handling steps and the time and space needed for granulation; it can be automated.

Regardless of the granulation method, the comparative simplicity of the direct compression process offers obvious advantages, such as

1. Economy
2. Elimination of heat and moisture
3. Optimization of tablet disintegration
4. Stability

The most obvious advantage of direct compression is its greater economy, owing to reduced processing time, less equipment and space required, less process validation, and lower energy utilization.

Generally, only blending and compression are required, although prior micronization of the drug may be needed. Unlike wet granulation, processing does not require heat or moisture, which can be detrimental to drug stability. Moreover, direct compression avoids the high pressures associated with slugging or roll compaction. In addition, disintegration is optimized because directly compressed tablets produce primary particles upon disintegration, rather than granules, which must deaggregate to liberate primary particles. Finally, direct compression tablets often exhibit fewer long-term problems of chemical stability or changes in dissolution.

Although there are many significant advantages of direct compression over granulation, there also are important limitations:

1. Uniform blending and prevention of unblending of low-dose drugs.
2. Fillers often are costlier than fillers used in granulation.
3. Physical properties and functional specifications are more critical; properties of raw materials must be defined and carefully controlled.
4. Limitations in producing colored tablets.
5. Dust problems.
6. Limitations in the dilution capacity of fillet- binders.
7. More sensitive to lubricant softening and over-mixing than granulations.

Limitations in the dilution capacity of excipients can make the direct compression of large-dose, poorly compactible drugs impractical. Lubrication is often a compromise between the amount and type needed for adequate lubrication and their adverse effect on compactibility. Content uniformity is of greater concern in direct compression tableting, particularly with low- dose drugs. Since the drug is not "locked" into granules, direct compression blends are subject to unmixing in subsequent processing steps. In addition, drugs are often micronized prior to blending to enhance their dissolution rate, and the resulting high surface-to-mass ratios may lead to difficulty in flowing and mixing due to surface interactions. Another important limitation is that unlike granulation, which tends to compensate for variability in excipients, direct compression is heavily dependent upon reproducible properties of the excipients (and the drug). Raw material standards must be carefully defined and address functionality. Lot-to-lot variations in both the drug and the excipients must be avoided. The cost of raw materials and their testing is higher in direct compression.

Thus, direct-compression tableting requires careful attention to the choice of excipients, appropriate flow properties, and blend homogeneity, and to the interplay of formulation and process variables that can affect both compactibility and drug dissolution.

Excipients

The design of the formulation and selection of excipients is especially critical in tablet dosage forms. Products can vary from a relatively simple aspirin tablet containing aspirin and starch to more complex systems that might contain fillers, binders, disintegrating agents, glidants, lubricants, and coating agents. Modified release introduces even more complexity. The appropriate selection of excipients and their concentration are clearly critical to both the ability to manufacture tablets as well as to their performance as a drug delivery system.

Manufacturability

Excipients function to provide compactibility, lubrication, flow properties, disintegration efficiency, wetting, etc. Poor choice of excipients may give rise to poor characteristics (hardness, appearance), which can be important in packaging, storage, and patient acceptance. Problems with excipients may arise from variations in source or lot, particularly in formulations made by direct compression. Examples of excipient problems include variation in performance between Hoc cellulose and microcrystalline cellulose relative to particle size, flow, and compactibility, or different polymorphic forms of sorbitol (α, β and γ) resulting in tablet hardening. Differences in lactose particle size and modification (spray-dried or anhydrous) can provide differences in surface areas over which a lubricant is distributed. Anhydrous lactose hydrates at high humidities with increase in size.

Biopharmaceutics

The formulation of a tablet can affect its bioavailability. Particular care should be given to low-dose poorly soluble drugs, especially those that are micronized. Drugs with low water solubility should never be formulated solely with insoluble fillers, including calcium salts (calcium sulfate, calcium phosphate) which are only soluble at very low pH. Differences in solution rate between hydrated and non-hydrated forms of calcium salts as well as between dibasic and tribasic forms may also be important. In some cases, excipients complex with drug substances such as calcium salts with tetracycline. Varying the ratio of soluble to insoluble fillers in tablets can significantly alter the dissolution pattern of poorly soluble drugs (weak acids and non-electrolytes), but has little effect on weak bases, which are soluble in gastric fluids.

The type and amount of disintegrating agent can also be important. Differences in source (corn, potato, rice) as well as variations in amylopectin–amylose ratios result in variable disintegration times. The fact that starch included within granules is not as effective as starch added between granules has led to tablets with good disintegration but poor dissolution. Incorporation of super-disintegrants (crospovidone, croscarmellose, sodium starch glycolate) has improved dissolution from both direct-compression and wet-granulation formulations. Both croscarmellose and sodium starch glycolate can complex with small amounts of cationic drugs in water, but not in physiologic fluids. The type and amount of binder used in granulations affects dissolution rates. Many binders are hydrophilic polymers whose solubility and solubility rate depend upon molecular weight. Quality control tests such as viscosity may be necessary as part of raw material testing of polymeric substances. However, an advantage of the granulation process is that it results in a wetting of drug surfaces, which enhances drug dissolution once the granules have disintegrated. Wetting agents such as sodium lauryl sulfate can significantly improve the dissolution of drugs of poor water solubility formulated into direct compression tablets.

Perhaps the greatest source of concern in excipients is with lubricants, particularly magnesium stearate, which is not only hydrophobic but also has a laminar crystal structure. When blended with other ingredients, it tends to make them hydrophobic by delaminating to coat their surfaces. The problems with magnesium stearate are thus highly process dependent. For example, blending time differences of as little as 2 min can significantly alter the dissolution pattern of finished tablets. Because direct-compression formulations have a higher specific surface area, the same amount of magnesium stearate blended for the same length of time makes direct-compression tablet matrices more hydrophobic than matrices made from granulations. The degree of shear imparted by different mixers during processing significantly affects the distribution of magnesium stearate. The characteristics of magnesium stearate vary from supplier to supplier and sometime within the same supplier. It is essential to draft raw material specifications and strictly adhere to Standard Operating Procedures (SOPs) during the manufacture of products containing this lubricant. Establishing purchasing specifications beyond those listed in the National Formulary, such as bulk and tap density, powder fluidity, particle size, surface area, degree of hydration, and morphology is desirable.

Effects of Manufacturing Processes on Formulations

Numerous unit processes are involved in making tablets, including particle size reduction and sizing, blending, granulating, drying, compaction, and (frequently) coating. Various factors associated with these processes can seriously affect content uniformity, bioavailability, or stability. Some of these are given in the following list:

1. Particle Size Reduction
   - Non-uniform particle size can lead to segregation problems
   - Development of electrostatic forces inhibits complete blending
   - Changing the crystalline state can affect solubility
2. Blending
   - Non-homogeneous distribution of drug substance is the result of poor blending or unblending
   - Overblending of lubricant lowers dissolution rates and affects compactibility
3. Granulation
   - Non-homogeneous distribution of binder and drug substance gives drug-rich or drug-poor fines
   - Decomposition of drug substance due to residual moisture
   - Uneven granule size (too many or to few fines) leads to compaction or uniformity problems
4. Tableting
   - Uneven compaction pressures affect dissolution
   - Loss of mix quality in hopper and feed frame gives poor content uniformity
   - Additional shearing of lubricant in feed frame lowers dissolution rates
5. Coating
   - Non-uniform or incomplete coverage of tablets and beads results in different dissolution patterns

When validating new equipment or procedures, the sampling techniques must reflect the quality of the material being tested, the blend of powders, moisture in granulation, or coating integrity. Another potential source of problems in manufacturing is reprocessing or reworking. Reworking may be required when finished products fail to meet hardness, content uniformity, disintegration, dissolution, or appearance specifications. Reworking procedures must be in writing and are often part of New Drug Applications (NDAs) and Abbreviated New Drug Applications (ANDAs). Although practiced less today than in past years, given the high cost of some drug substances, reworking continues to be justified, but may involve the following problems: overdistribution of lubricant leading to poor compactibility and dissolution; distribution of particles of coating in the reprocessed tablet may lower the dissolution rate; and loss in compactibility due to work hardening of direct-compression fillers, particularly at higher initial compaction pressures. Reworking is less likely to cause dissolution problems with water-soluble drugs.

Systematic Formulation Development

Previously, pharmaceutical experimenters were rarely afforded the luxury of using expanded experimental designs. Time and manpower constraints, imposed by an ever-quickening pace to market, have prevented the thorough examination and full understanding of most commercial formulations. Although the pace of formulating pharmaceutical systems has not lessened recently, a rapid turnaround means formulators must quickly gather information and base final decisions on that information. The window for error is narrower, and the formulator can no longer afford to use empirically gathered data to obtain the critical dosage form information needed for a marketable formulation. Systematic development approaches are also desirable to provide data in anticipation of the use of SUPAC (scale up and post-approval changes) regulatory policies by providing for the establishment of a research database that can help justify such changes to regulatory agencies. Enormous progress has been made in the direction of systematic formulation development through the use of such statistical tools as multivariate analysis and response surface methodology, and artificial intelligence.

Experimental Design

In the long term, an efficient experimental design saves time and avoids costly mistakes, and some pharmaceutical firms have departments devoted to the preparation of experimental designs and their analysis. If a statistician is not available, a myriad of commercial experimental-design software packages are on the market (SAS, JMP, STATGRAPHICS, DESIGN EXPERT) with which a formulator can design experiments on a personal computer. These same packages can also aid in data analysis and presentation. The early phase of such a statistical experimental design approach may include screening designs such as two-level full or fractional factorial designs or Plackett-Burman designs. The number of experimental runs is reduced by intentionally confounding some experimental effects. Ultimately, the screening design narrows the number of potential variables for further study.

The latter phase of such as a central experimental design approach might include response surface methodologies to optimize a formulation such as a central composite or Box-Behnken design. Such methods allow experimenters to assess the effects of several variables at one time without having to study every possible unique combination of variables. This way, a systematic identification of critical variables and an optimization of the formulation and process can be obtained. Response surfaces are generated, which give formulators a graphic demonstration of the effect of variables on various responses, such as drug dissolution. The designs and models available to experimenters are numerous and the proper choice depends on the number of variables and the possible responses. General references for experimental design can be consulted as well as design software manuals, if a statistician is not available for advice.

Artificial Intelligence Approaches

Among the artificial intelligence approaches that have been used to provide support for the formulation process are expert systems and artificial neural networks. An expert system (ES) is an intelligent computer program that attempts to capture the expertise of specialists who have knowledge and experience in a well-defined domain. They are designed to simulate an expert's problem solving process. Developed more than 20 years ago for other applications, expert systems are a relatively new idea in pharmaceutical technology. In rule-based systems, the knowledge is highly structured and often represented as a set of rules that express the relationship between several pieces of information in the form of conditional statements. These statements specify actions to be taken or advice to be followed. Such systems can shorten development time, simplify formulations, provide the rationale for decisions taken in arriving at a formulation, serve as excellent teaching tools for novices, and accumulate and preserve the knowledge and experience of experts. ESs suffer from the limitation that they are not creative. They can only deal with situations that have been anticipated. They must be designed to handle every contingency. Examples include expert systems developed for formulating tablets, for process troubleshooting, and for the selection of a mixer.

Used in other disciplines for about 40 years, artificial neural networks (ANNs), like ESs, have only recently been applied to pharmaceutical development. ANNs are computer-based programs that attempt to simulate certain functions of the biological brain, such as learning, generalizing, or abstracting from experience. They have the ability to discern relationships or patterns in response to exposure to facts ("learning."). ANN models may be viewed simply as multiple nonlinear regression models. Through ANNs, the data and information generated during experimental work may be transformed relatively easily into knowledge that would enable the formulator to at least construct a few domain specific rules, even though confined, for future cases. However, ANN effectiveness is limited by the training data selected. One limitation is that, in most cases, ANNs lack explanation capability and there is difficulty in obtaining justification for results. Examples of applications to product development include predicting model granulation and tablet characteristics from knowledge of material and process variables, and predicting drug release from immediate release formulations. The development of a hybrid system, i.e., an Expert Network, that integrates ANNs and ESs has the potential of taking advantage of the strengths of both ANNs and ESs and avoiding the weaknesses of either.

Formulation Development

Whether working in a large established laboratory or a small research organization, formulators are well advised to take an overall look at the development process to assess the most rational approach to their particular needs and resources. Among many approaches to rational tablet formulation, the strategy used by researchers at the University of Maryland in collaboration with FDA scientists examines the drug product development process in light of the SUPAC guidance. This generalized plan focuses on the assessment the possible influence of formulation and processing variables on bioavailability and manufacture. The model begins with the preformulation stage wherein information is obtained on the physicochemical and biopharmaceutic properties of the drug. One outcome of the preformulation study should be the identification of the biopharmaceutic class (BCS) in which the drug falls since this will provide important guidance in making formulation decisions. For multisourced drugs, the different sources are considered. The preformulation study results in a portfolio of information, which provides guidance in formulation design and in the development of appropriate hypotheses to be tested and the critical variables studies that follow.

In the critical variables analysis phase, a statistical experimental design is created intended to assess critical formulation and process variables in relatively small-scale manufacture. In these studies, the ranges of composition variables are chosen to at least encompass those noted in the recommendations of the AAPS–FDA Workshop on Scale-up of Immediate Release Oral Solid Dosage Forms or SUPAC. This phase is usually preceded by a development phase during which variables and levels to be studied are determined and the exact method of manufacture is established. Experimental formulations are assessed at least in terms of dissolution performance, content uniformity, and weight variation. On the basis of these studies, the specific formulations to be manufactured for biostudy are selected.

In the small-scale clinical manufacturing phase, formulations are manufactured under GMP conditions for possible clinical testing. These will be manufactured on a larger scale than those in the previous phases. An experimental design is chosen; however, if some of the variables can be eliminated based on the earlier experiments, the number of formulations produced may be reduced. The intent of the biostudy phase is to establish an in vitro–in vivo relationship. If an appropriate correlation can be established, dissolution may serve as a surrogate for biostudies in the interpretation of what is significant and what is not among the variables studied. In the scale-up phase, larger runs of formulations are manufactured. The formulations are selected to determine if the larger scale will enhance the significance of certain variables. The statistical analysis of the data provides the opportunity to predict changes in dissolution performance resulting from incremental changes in one or more formulation or process variable at a time (e.g., the level of an excipient or the time of mixing). The development model presented here may differ from some formulation research programs in that biostudies may not be performed on small-scale batches. The major advantage of early biostudies is the potential for early IVIVC and subsequent surrogate use of dissolution testing in further work.

15

Dry Powder

Drug delivery to the lung has been historically aimed at controlling local respiratory disease where the central airways may be as suitable a target for drug deposition as the deeper lung. With little exception, currently marketed inhalation products provide therapy for asthma, chronic obstructive pulmonary disease (COPD), and bronchitis. More recently, however, there has been significant interest in using the lung, and in particular the deep lung alveolar surface, as a portal to the systemic circulation for drugs not readily administered orally. Therapeutic targets have therefore broadened substantially because pulmonary delivery is recognized for its potential to provide a non-invasive alternative to injection. New delivery systems capable of delivering drug in particles or droplets small enough to reach the peripheral or deep lung are under intense development to meet these new therapeutic targets.

Historical Overview

Delivery of drugs to the lung depends on administration by any one of three methods: nebulizer, metered- dose inhaler (MDI), or dry powder inhaler (DPI). The nature of the drug substance and its therapeutic target may dictate which lung-delivery dosage form is more appropriate for the drug. Nebulization, for example, requires that the drug dissolve well in an aqueous medium at a concentration suitable for convenient dosing. Drugs developed as MDIs must dissolve or suspend well in a non-aqueous propellant medium at a concentration appropriate for doses metered in volumes generally less than 100 μl. For DPIs, the physical properties of the drug substance determine the ease with which processing will yield a stable powder that can be effectively aerosolized in milligram quantities by the inhaler device to deliver the proper drug dosage.

Nebulizers

Nebulizers have a long history in pulmonary delivery. Although generally effective, traditional nebulizer systems require lengthy (10–20 min) administration periods during which drug solution is delivered with relative inefficiency using an external power source. More convenient hand-held systems are currently in development and offer the convenience of portability and metered-dose administration. Depending on drug solubility and dose, these systems may require multiple actuations to deliver an effective dose.

MDIs

Since the 1970s, MDIs have dominated inhalation delivery, especially in the United States. MDIs are more convenient to use than nebulizers, generally offering 100–300 metered doses per pocket-sized canister. Limitations to the reliability of their therapeutic effectiveness, however, typically arise from the need for the patient to coordinate MDI actuation with breath inhalation and from the deposition of a sometimes significant amount of drug, driven by the propellant blast, to the back of the throat instead of the lung. Then, in the late 1980s, the chlorofluorocarbon (CFC) propellants used in MDIs were identified as agents contributing to the depletion of the ozone layer. This led to industry-wide reformulation efforts still underway to replace CFCs with environmentally more friendly propellants.

DPIs

The technical challenges of MDI reformulation have contributed to a growing interest in the potential of DPI technology for the development of new products that satisfy similar therapeutic, market, and environmental needs.

The DPI device presents medication to the patient as a dry powder in a form that can be inhaled orally for delivery to the target lung tissues. The delivery system should assist in the generation of very fine particulates of medication in a way that enables them to avoid the impaction barriers that normally operate in the lung to prevent the ingress of potentially harmful particles. These barriers include the oropharynx and, for deep lung delivery, the air-conducting bronchi and bronchioles.

Studies have shown that to clear the oropharyngeal impaction barrier (comprising the mouth, throat, and pharynx), particles with aerodynamic diameters smaller than 5 μm are required. Only particles with aerodynamic diameters less than 3 μm will reach the terminal bronchi and the alveoli in significant numbers. Therefore, the particle diameter required to be produced by the delivery system will depend to a great extent on the intended target lung tissue. Lung deposition is also affected substantially by the specific inhalation dynamics of the patient, which, in turn, are influenced by the delivery device. This article addresses various attributes of the dry powder inhalation product, from intrinsic material properties to final product performance.

More simple in concept than implementation, DPI technology is rapidly expanding to address a broadening therapeutic need as well as market opportunity. Characteristics of the ideal DPI system will include most or all of the following attributes:

1. Simple and comfortable to use;
2. Compact and economical to produce;
3. Highly reproducible fine-particle dosing;
4. Reproducible emitted dose;
5. Physically and chemically stable powder;
6. Minimal extrapulmonary loss of drug, with low oropharyngeal deposition, low device retention, and low exhaled loss;
7. Multidose system;
8. Powder protected from external environment and can be used in all climates and protected from moist exhaled air;
9. Overdose protection; and
10. Indicate number of doses delivered and/or remaining.

Outline

Fine particle powders can be produced by various methods such as micronization or spray drying. The physicochemical nature of these fine particles generally defines the stability of the bulk powder, which in turn is critical to the long-term effective performance of the dry powder product. The section Fine Particles and the Solid State is an introduction to better understanding the fundamental properties that underlie the behavior of bulk powders.

Drug containment in DPIs falls into two categories: unit dose, in which the dose is premetered during manufacture, and reservoir, in which the drug dose is metered during dose administration.

Some devices store multiple unit doses for convenience. The next section, Devices: Forming the Dry Powder Aerosol, considers the various means of aerosolizing powder in the context of device design history and functionality. Advantages and disadvantages of different design types are considered.

Performance and Regulatory Requirements describes various ways of characterizing the dry powder aerosols and provides information on product quality performance requirements and how these attributes must be reflected in registration applications.

The Role of DPIs in Therapy briefly addresses factors affecting the therapeutic profiles of drugs delivered by DPI profiles. The article concludes with DPIs: *A Burgeoning Industry*, which surveys the DPI products on the market in 1999 and a selection of those known to be under development. Thoughts on the potential of the DPI dosage form in future therapeutic applications conclude the article.

Fine Particles and the Solid State

Crystalline and Amorphous (Glassy) States

Pharmaceutical solids can generally be described as either crystalline or amorphous (or glassy). In fact, the actual solid phase composition of a pharmaceutical formulation is usually characterized by an intermediate composition composed of both crystalline and amorphous character. In a multicomponent system such as a solid formulation comprising drug and excipient(s), certain components or even a single component may be amorphous. Because the amorphous form of a material is always a less stable, higher-energy form than its crystalline counterpart, the distinction between these forms relates to thermodynamic stability of the solid.

Crystalline materials are characterized by a three- dimensional, long-range order that translates into a distinct and unique molecular pattern that can be characterized by X-ray diffraction (XRD). The molecular arrangement of the glassy state resembles that of the liquid state and lacks three-dimensional order. Thus, the classically glassy state has been designated as amorphous, that is, without structure. Pharmaceutical operations commonly used in the manufacture of DPI formulations, such as milling, spray drying, and lyophilization (freeze drying), produce materials possessing amorphous character.

Milling of crystalline materials introduces or increases amorphous character as the result of the significant mechanical activation that takes place during the process, including friction, deformation, attrition, and agglomeration. The extent of disorder, or amorphous character, introduced by the milling process depends on the behavior of the material and its inherent resistance to the milling-imposed stresses, the amount of energy imposed by the process, and the time scale of energy release. Solid particles formed from the liquid phase, as in spray drying or freeze drying product from solution, are predominantly amorphous materials.

Crystalline materials exhibit a characteristic melting point at which they convert into a liquid form, whereas amorphous materials show no such defined transition. Rather, amorphous materials change on heating from a brittle glassy state to a rubbery state over a narrow temperature range known as the glass transition temperature, or T_g. Orders of magnitude of change in properties such as viscosity and molecular mobility take place near the T_g for amorphous materials; the temperature dependence of these properties near the T_g is typically non-Arrhenius. Glassy to rubbery transition is also associated with a stepwise change in the heat capacity. Thus, the T_g of an amorphous material may be determined using a differential scanning calorimeter where a stepwise change in heat flow (corresponding to a change in heat capacity) is observed during sample heating. For many hydrophilic drugs and excipients, water acts as a plasticizer, increases molecular mobility, and reduces the glass transition temperature. It is not uncommon for as little as 2–3 wt% water to depress the T_g by 30–40°C. The physical and chemical stability of a glassy material decreases as it approaches the T_g because of that mobility. Thus, the presence of water promotes instability. The rate at which a compound crystallizes from an amorphous state will likewise increase as the temperature of storage approaches T_g and as moisture content is increased.

Effect of Physical State on Stability of Dry Powder Formulations

The impact of even subtle changes in physical properties of a DPI formulation can lead to substantial changes in aerosol behavior. Moisture uptake by the hydrophilic components of the formulation can lead to surface dissolution and liquid bridging between particles. This in turn leads to crystal growth, particle fusion, and an increase in particle size, which can result in strongly diminished aerosol performance. Powder densification under vibration during unit dose or reservoir filling, as well as product shipping, can also affect the observed aerosol behavior of dry powders.

Because of their greater molecular mobility in the solid state, amorphous systems generally exhibit greater physical and chemical instability at any given temperature compared with their crystalline counterparts. Thus, DPI formulations are desirably prepared in a crystalline state. The low molecular weight of drugs in DPI products currently marketed supports their crystalline nature. Since the late 1980s, there has been increased interest in delivering drugs of biological origin, such as proteins for systemic uptake. These molecules typically do not crystallize and tend to remain amorphous. In freeze-dried and spray-dried biologicals for pulmonary delivery, excipients that act as protectants such as sugars must also remain amorphous to interact with the protein and/or provide a rigid matrix around the protein molecules to restrict and stabilize their motion. As with any amorphous product, physical change can be minimized by storage at temperatures well below the T_g and protection from moisture during handling and storage.

The chemical stability of an amorphous formulation also is usually a function of its storage temperature relative to T_g. The enhanced molecular mobility achieved near the glass transition translates into an increase in translational diffusion-dependent degradation pathways such as aggregation in proteins. It should be recognized that the reaction kinetics near the T_g do not obey Arrhenius kinetics and that extrapolation of the accelerated stability data generated near the T_g to stability at the storage temperature should be viewed with extreme caution. Amorphous materials must be stored well below the glass transition (at least 10°C and typically 40–50°C below T_g) to maintain their physical and chemical stability.

When dealing with partially crystalline materials such as those produced by milling, the impact of water uptake is exaggerated. The amorphous component likely absorbs greater quantities of water than its crystalline counterpart, leading to reduced T_g, increased molecular mobility and both physical and chemical instability.

Bulk Powder Properties

The respirable powders of a DPI cannot be characterized adequately by single particle studies alone; bulk properties must also be assessed because they contribute to ease of manufacture and affect maximal system performance. Primary bulk properties include particle size, particle size distribution, bulk density, and surface area. These properties, along with particle electrostatics, shape, surface morphology, etc., affect secondary bulk powder characteristics such as powder flow, handling, consolidation, and dispersibility.

The characterization and control of primary particle size and the particle size distribution of drug-containing particles are perhaps the most important factors in the design and manufacture of dry powders for inhalation. The size, density, and shape of a particle determine its aerodynamic behavior and therefore its likelihood of depositing in the desired region of the lung. The mean (average) or median (50th percentile) particle size may be based on the number of particles, the mass (or volume) of particles, or even the surface area of particles. The particle size distribution describes the range or frequency of particle sizes occurring in a sample or the width of the particle size distribution in a sample. The variation in these size parameters owing to sampling errors must be considered in characterizing blended powders, powders stored for prolonged periods, or powders that have been mechanically agitated.

Mass median diameter (MMD) is the most common descriptor of primary particle size and may be determined by sieving or centrifugal sedimentation. Volume median diameter, as determined by laser diffraction, may be used as an approximation of MMD provided the particle density is known and does not vary with size and the particle shape is near spherical. The MMD of a powder can be used as a predictor of aerodynamic diameter by:

$$MMAD = MMD \cdot \rho_{true}^{1/2}$$

where MMAD is the mass median aerodynamic diameter, and ρ_{true} is the true density of the particle, usually determined by helium pycnometry. Cohesion/ adhesion between particles normally results in the MMAD being larger than predicted. Values of MMAD less than 5 μm are considered necessary to facilitate airborne particle transit past the larynx and deposition within the lung. Powders intended for delivery to the deep lung, such as treatments for asthma or for systemic delivery, require aerodynamic behavior reflected by MMAD values between 1 and 3 μm. Particles of MMAD less than approximately 0.5 μm are likely to be exhaled.

Surface area is a bulk powder characteristic directly dependent on particle size distribution, porosity, and morphology. It is commonly determined by nitrogen adsorption, whereby the adsorption isotherm data are fit to a suitable mathematical model from which surface area is derived. If the particle size distribution is sufficiently narrow and the particles are not hollow or porous, the surface area can be used as a measure of change in average particle rugosity or shape. Surface area may be a more sensitive means of monitoring process control during fine particle manufacturing (jet milling or spray drying) than are particle sizing techniques.

Bulk powder density, porosity, and consolidation rate are used as characteristics of powder structure and ease of flow. These properties are typically more difficult to determine for fine respirable powders than for coarse particles owing to the formation of bridging structures caused by high interparticulate interaction. These forces must be overcome by introducing energy, such as ultrasonic vibration or mechanical agitation, to fluidize micron-sized powders in a controllable manner. Carrier-based powder formulations are designed in part to overcome the inherent cohesion of micron-sized particles. In these formulations, the microfine drug adheres to larger carrier particles, improving powder flow and metering capability. For effective delivery, the drug particles must, of course, separate from their carrier on aerosolization and/or inhalation. Pelletization is often used to improve the flow properties of micron-sized powders. Pelletization converts an ensemble of single particles into larger agglomerates through the formation of weak solid bridges between particles. This process also results in increased bulk powder density (ρ_{bulk}). The solid bridges formed during pelletization may aid powder flow and metering but must be overcome during aerosolization.

Bulk powder density must be distinguished clearly from the true density of particles. Bulk powder density is simply the mass of a powder bed divided by its volume. The volume of the powder bed includes the spaces between agglomerates, between primary particles, and the volume of micropores within the particles. These voids within the powder bed volume are collectively the powder porosity. Powder porosity (F) is calculated as:

$$F = (1 - \rho_{true} = \rho_{bulk})$$

The average number of contact points between particles increases as bulk density increases, and the inter- particulate forces at these contact points must be overcome to produce a dispersed aerosol cloud. Therefore, a powder of low bulk density may be more easily dispersed as an aerosol than an otherwise identical powder of high bulk density. However, a powder with low bulk density may be more prone to consolidation than a powder with high bulk density. Powder consolidation can be envisioned as a process of densification or packing of the particles. Consolidation occurs most rapidly during the powder agitation that accompanies powder filling or product shipping; even the imperceptible vibrations a powder experiences during seemingly static storage cause consolidation with time. The rate and extent of consolidation are dependent on particle size distribution and particle shape and can be used to describe the dynamic behavior of powder structures. The extent of powder consolidation, or compressibility, can be evaluated by performing tap density measurements, and using the following relationship:

$$100 \times (\rho_{tap} - \rho_{aerated})/\rho_{tap} = \%\ \text{compressibility}$$

where ρ_{tap} is the tapped bulk density, and $\rho_{aerated}$ is the aerated bulk density.

An understanding of the behavior of a powder during the manufacturing process, e.g., during blending, may aid in the identification of an optimal filling and packaging process. Blended powders may also undergo segregation of active particles from carrier particles concurrently with consolidation. Although segregation can lead to poor drug content uniformity, it is in fact desirable in the case of aerosolizing a powder composed of drug blended with a larger particle size carrier.

Powder Production: Formulation and Processing

The primary factor influencing the manufacture of DPI powders is the need to produce material that can penetrate into the lung. The manufacturing of fine particles is challenging, especially with regard to reproducibility. This challenge has resulted in the development of various approaches to the controlled production of fine particles, primarily depending on the nature of the drug. Of the processes described later, micronization and blending and, more recently, spray drying are used most often.

Once manufactured, small particles present another challenge. At small particle diameters, gravity ceases to be the major force exerted on the particles, and instead, interparticle forces become more prominent. The resultant increase in the cohesive and adhesive nature of the particles produces problems such as poor flow- ability, fillability, and dispersibility. These problems are typically minimized by blending with larger, less cohesive excipient particles such as lactose or pelletization of the individual drug particles. The cohesive nature of particles can be reduced further by modifying the particle surface, the goal of several emerging technologies. Secondary processing techniques are often employed in powder production to ensure that the stability of the manufactured drug product is ensured.

Formulation

Formulation of dry powders for inhalation must rely on a very short list of excipients to fulfill the customary roles of diluent, stabilizer, solubilizer, processing aid, and property modifier (e.g., flow sustain release agent). Only a few materials are approved in the United States for use in inhalation products, and of those (e.g., propellants, surfactants), many are of little help in dry powder formulation.

Where dose requirements and drug properties allow, drug may be processed in the absence of any excipient, e.g., Astra's Pulmicort Turbuhaler. Most DPIs marketed or under development, however, rely on the addition of lactose as filler and flow enhancer. Given the proprietary nature of product development, it is not known what additional excipient materials will immerge in the future as safe for inhalation. It is likely, however, that the expansion of inhalation technology to systemic delivery will call for the addition of sugars, buffer salts, and other excipients common to parenteral dosage forms to the list of acceptable inhalation excipients.

Controlled Crystallization or Precipitation

Crystallization, or precipitation, is the process by which particles are produced from solution of the material in a suitable solvent. The level of control over this process determines the physical nature and size of the finished particles. Most pharmaceutical bulk material is produced through crystallization as the final stage of the manufacturing process. The formation of a stable, crystalline material is normally the target of this final step. In the production of materials for use in DPI products, however, the particle size of the crystallized product is normally too large. Subsequent reduction in particle size is then necessary and can significantly alter the physical nature of the material

Micronization

Micronization is a high-energy particle-size reduction technique that can convert coarse-diameter particles into particles of less than 5 μm in diameter. Different types of equipment can micronize particles, for example, jet or fluid energy mills and ball mills. Although the different equipment have different operating parameters, the fundamental method of reducing the particle size is the same. All techniques involve applying a force on the particle, typically in the form of a collision, either particle–particle or particle–equipment. The force acts at imperfections in the crystal surface, initiating crack propagation through the particle. As the size of the particle decreases, the number of imperfections decreases, thereby making the task of reducing particle size more difficult.

Micronization has been used for the past 50 years to produce small particles for inhalation therapy. However, only in recent years have batch-to-batch reproducibility and stability problems been associated with the technique. Batch-to-batch variations can be caused by morphological differences in starting material; thus, it is critical that a reproducible raw material supply be available. Stability issues typically derive from changes to the varying quantities of amorphous material that are produced by the micronizing process on the surface of the resulting particles. This can be minimized through careful control of the micronization process, including processing conditions, batch size, and feed rate, or by the addition of a secondary processing procedure. In addition, micronization can cause decomposition of some materials. The issues associated with micronization are forcing many companies to investigate alternative methods of producing small particles.

Blending

The most commonly used method for improving the flowability, fillability, and dispersibility of small cohesive particles is blending the drug with excipient particles, most commonly lactose, of considerably larger particle size. Typically, these large excipient particles are greater than 60 μm, and the small drug particles are less than 5 μm. The objective of the mixing process is to produce an ordered powder in which the small particles attach themselves to the surface of larger "carrier" particles. The challenge is to ensure that the force of adhesion between the drug and carrier is strong enough to withstand segregation during blending and product storage and weak enough to allow separation of the drug particles from the carrier surface on aerosolization. During formulation feasibility, the blends are made by mortar and pestle and/or geometric mixing in a tumbling blender. For high-volume production, the process generally involves a high-shear mixer.

The final product performance of a powder blend in a DPI is ultimately dependent on the individual drug and carrier properties as well on the process by which they are blended. Small changes in carrier morphology can result in significant variations in the dose received by a patient. Again, control of the raw material supply is critical to successful product development. Moreover, secondary processing may be required to ensure that carrier particles behave consistently from batch to batch. Steps that involve transport or storage of the finished blend should be monitored closely to avoid segregation, which occurs when the drug separates from the carrier or when carriers of different sizes separate. Segregation can be minimized by the careful selection of formulation and process equipment. For example, hopper design can play a significant role in minimizing segregation.

Pelletization

Pelletization, which often does not require the use of excipients, may offer an alternative to blending for high-dose therapeutics. The process involves deliberate agglomeration of the fine drug material into less cohesive, larger units. Pelletization is usually achieved by vibratory sieving or any process that tumbles powder. All processes require particular attention to time and energy parameters to ensure a consistent product. The resultant pellets must be used in a system capable of deaggregating to an appropriate particle size for aerosol drug delivery.

Secondary Processing

As discussed, materials used in dry powder inhalation are predominantly crystalline in nature, with varying degrees of amorphicity. This typically results from the high-energy milling process, which introduces regions of amorphous material within a crystalline material. Occasionally, however, the converse is true. Minimizing any change over time and ensuring that the material is physically stable before final packaging are major formulation challenges. These stability issues tend to be physical in nature, but occasionally chemical changes such as impurity formation also occur.

The technique generally used to minimize the degree of change in crystallinity of the milled product is to eliminate the water or other solvents from the product, usually by packaging the material within a suitable barrier (for example, aluminum foil laminate). Other techniques include the production of a 100% crystalline material, which may eliminate the effects of moisture. This technique, however, may require a secondary production stage of annealing or a quarantine period to allow the product to equilibrate under controlled storage conditions.

The final measure of crystallization effects is assessed by appropriate rigorous stability data [for example, 6 months accelerated stability at 40°C/75% relative humidity (RH)]. This may seem excessive, but measuring the degree of crystallinity is inherently difficult because of low analytical sensitivity (for example, amorphous components below 5 wt%), and pure single-phase standards are difficult to prepare and, subsequently, to measure.

Spray Drying

Spray drying, a process typically used in the production of coarser (up to 500 μm) food, pharmaceutical, and industrial powders, can also be used to prepare microparticulate powders for DPIs. A typical first step involves creating a solution of the excipients and drug. Dissolving the excipients and drug ensures a uniform distribution of all the excipients and the active drug in the finished powder in contrast to the heterogeneous nature of blended powders. The solution is then atomized and mixed with a drying medium, usually air, or an inert gas if the feed consists of an organic solvent. The solvent is evaporated and removed from the drug solids.

Each spray-dried droplet forms a single particle whose size is determined by the droplet size, the dissolved solids of the feed solution, and the density of the resulting solid particle. For a given formulation and process, both the solid content and density of the powder remain constant within a batch and from batch to batch. Therefore, the distribution of the primary particle size is determined by the droplet size distribution. A narrowly distributed particle size can be achieved with a well-designed atomizer and well- controlled atomizer process parameters.

The droplet has a relatively short residence time (on the order of seconds) in the spray dryer, which minimizes the degradation of heat-sensitive components. In addition, the drug is exposed to a temperature much lower than that at the drying inlet owing to the cooling effect of the solvent evaporation. Control of droplet residence time and the lower temperature defines the amorphous versus crystalline nature of the material.

A spray dryer consists of a feed tank, a rotary or nozzle atomizer, an air heater, a drying chamber, and a cyclone to separate the powder from the air. A rotary atomizer uses centrifugal energy to form the droplet. Pressure nozzle atomizers feed solution to a nozzle under pressure, which forms the droplet. Two fluid nozzles feed solution separately into a nozzle head, which produces high-speed atomizing air that breaks the solution into tiny droplets. Both the feed solution and the drying air are fed into the drying chamber in a standard cocurrent flow.

Lyophilization

Lyophilization, although a relatively expensive process, can be a good process for relatively unstable compounds. In lyophilization, the solvent (usually water) is frozen and then removed by sublimation in a vacuum environment. The low temperature maintained during the entire process minimizes thermal degradation of the drug compound.

Typically, the drying process can be divided into primary and secondary phases. During the primary phase, the drug solution is filled into vials and then placed within a temperature-controlled drying chamber. There, the solution is frozen according to physiochemical principles as the shelf temperature is lowered to below freezing. The shelf temperature is subsequently increased but maintained below the freezing point. A vacuum is applied to the chamber to sublimate the solvent. This phase of the drying process extracts the majority of the solvent (50–80%).

During the secondary drying phase, the remainder of the solvent is removed at an elevated but still subfreezing temperature. During freezing, supercooling is necessary to encourage crystallization of the drug compound. The extent to which the compound is supercooled depends on the nature of the compound, the temperature program of the shelf, the heat transfer properties of the container, and the presence of particulates in the solution. The degree of supercooling determines the size of the solvent crystal and, subsequently, the size of the channel formed during primary drying. Consequently, the degree of supercooling affects the rate of sublimation, the rate of secondary drying, and, eventually, the surface area of the finished powder. A goal of secondary drying is to minimize product moisture content.

Therefore, it is most important to select a cooling temperature profile to achieve the desired objective(s). The objective could be simply to achieve a uniform degree of supercooling and freezing or to add an annealing process to allow the solute to crystallize or the ice crystal to grow. The possibility of allowing a long annealing process gives great flexibility to achieve the desired solid-state property for the powder.

The lyophilized cake must then be milled. Compared with particles generated by spray drying, the particle size of milled lyophilized powders generally has a broader distribution than does spray-dried powder, which is formed one particle at a time in a continuous process. Despite the longer processing time necessary to create a dry powder through lyophilization (and the consequent economic implications), this process can provide the formulator with better control of the powder in its solid state.

Supercritical Fluid Technology

Extraction by supercritical fluids, carbon dioxide and propane in particular, is currently being investigated as a means of controlling the size and shape of particles for inhalation. Supercritical fluids are liquids above their critical pressure and temperature. Under these conditions, the molecules exhibit the flow, polarity, and solvency properties common of liquids but have the diffusivities and reactivities characteristic of gases.

Precipitation of the particles occurs by two methods involving atomization of a feed: (1) rapid expansion of supercritical solutions containing dissolved drug, and (2) gas antisolvent recrystallization, the supercritical fluid acting as an antisolvent for dissolved drug contained in droplets of another miscible or partially miscible liquid (for example, ethanol, methanol, and acetone).

The second technique, sometimes described as SEDS (solution-enhanced dispersion by supercritical fluids), has been scaled up successfully for an inhalation application to pilot plant manufacture. As with spray drying, this technique is a single-step process. The drug material must show solvency in the cosolvent but complete insolubility in the supercritical carbon dioxide. The resultant solvent-free particles are less cohesive than micronized material as high crystallinity is achieved, leading to decreased charging effects. Particle size distributions for these powders are reported to be narrow, with small median aerodynamic diameters (<2.5 μm). In addition, regular particle morphologies are obtained for these thermodynamically stable powders, making them amenable to further processing steps and handling.

Filling and Packaging

The primary consideration when developing systems for packaging dry powders for dose delivery is the goal of delivering the correct drug dosage to the patient. When dealing with drug powders intended for use in DPIs, some basic issues must be considered—specifically, that the drug usually must be delivered in a small volume, which is often difficult to handle owing to small particle size.

The greatest challenge faced in developing packaging systems for dry powders relate to maintaining dispersibility in packaging, which can be affected by compression and electrical charge. Compression of the drug powder, which can be a consequence of excessive handling, can result in an unintended increase in drug concentration. The small drug particles are also vulnerable to alteration in electrical charge, which can result from the motion of particles, against both themselves and the packaging equipment, and from the unintended absorption of water by the drug powder.

Package dose metering can be accomplished by weight or by volume. Dry powders developed for DPIs are formulated to deliver a specific dose of drug per a given unit of drug powder. Drug powders can be packaged either in unit dose or in reservoir systems, each of which has certain advantages.

Unit-Dose Systems

Unit-dose systems package drug powders into individual-use packages that contain a known quantity of drug. Patients may use single or multiple units of the drug to obtain a given dose. The greatest advantage of unit-dose systems is that a greater degree of control at the manufacturing level can be maintained. Individual drug doses can be metered by weight or volume. Although metering by weight results in a high degree of accuracy, it is a slow process. Thus, more commonly, unit-dose packaging is metered by volume.

Metering by volume, although offering a reliable means for high-volume production, has disadvantages related to the dispersibility of the drug powder, which in turn can affect the accuracy and precision of the drug dose. Dispersibility can be managed by devising filling processes that optimize powder flow, which will vary by drug compound; by minimizing handling and thereby compression of the drug powder; and by minimizing the relative motion of drug particles against other drug particles and against the filling equipment. Minimizing drug powder motion can reduce electrostatic charging of particles and consequent equipment malfunctions and problems with packaging, which include dose-extraction difficulties and particle dispersion at the time of drug administration.

Unit-dose systems typically rely on blister packaging or capsules to contain the drug until it is dispersed by the delivery device. Blister packages have several advantages over capsules. Those constructed of aluminum are generally impervious to moisture. Inner linings of either polyvinyl chloride or polypropylene create means for sealing the package. Gelatin capsules generally contain approximately 12% water under ambient conditions and thus are a potential source of moisture to powder not equilibrated to ambient relative humidities.

Reservoir Systems

Reservoir systems offer the advantage of variable dosing, generate less waste, are less expensive to manufacture, and are simpler to use than unit-dose systems. Relying on a metering system contained within the delivery device, they may be less precise in their drug delivery. Because the drug reservoir must be accessed repeatedly, these systems encounter an increased difficulty in maintaining moisture level. Maintaining a highly flowable drug powder in this system may also lead to greater drug formulation challenges.

Devices: Forming the Dry Powder Aerosol

Design Objectives and Constraints

The ultimate goal of all pulmonary delivery devices is to reproducibly deposit the required quantity of drug in the target lung tissues. Many factors influence the selection of a particular DPI design, including the characteristics of the drug to be delivered, its powder formulation, and its associated therapeutic regime. Other factors that must be considered include drug cost, desired dose, market factors, and expected degree of patient compliance.

Drug cost plays an important role in determining the economic feasibility of a device by determining how much of a drug may be lost in administration and routine device use. Drug dose and side effects may determine the reproducibility bounds of particle size and mass of drug delivered that are necessary for effective therapy. The drug target tissue may determine the importance of achieving a very small particle size; local delivery of drugs to the upper airway may allow for a larger particle size than delivery of particles to the deep lung for systemic absorption. The degree of cohesiveness of the powder particles will determine how much energy the device must transfer to produce a particle of a given size. The therapeutic regime and a range of market factors, such as degree of convenience and cost of other available drugs and/or therapies, may determine how portable or inexpensive the device must be. The anticipated degree of patient compliance may favor some technological solutions over others.

DPIs cannot be considered devices alone but must be considered as components of a larger delivery system, which also includes the formulation of the drug powder, its manufacturing processes, and packaging.

Functional Description

Several DPI designs have been proposed, developed, and successfully marketed in the past 3 decades. Although these devices vary widely in characteristics and operation, they all perform certain basic functions. A DPI must extract the dose from the bulk powder drug package, generate a fine cloud of drug particles by deagglomerating the powder and diluting it with air, and deliver the drug cloud to the patients' airways.

Bulk Powder Drug Package

The first task for a device in delivering a dose is extracting the dose from the drug package. As addressed earlier, two primary alternatives are available: (1) a number of doses may be stored in a powder reservoir, and (2) each dose may be individually packaged as a unit dose. Reservoir systems are inherently multidose. With unit-dose systems, the device may require individual loading of a unit-dose package before inhalation or loading of several unit-dose packages into the device for multidosing.

Energy Sources

Energy input is required to extract the powder from its packaging, generate the fine particle cloud, and dilute it with air. Historically, this energy comes from the patient's inhalation effort. In some cases, the energy for extracting/metering the powder comes from the mechanical manipulation of the device by the patient. More recent designs use concepts borrowed from the MDI industry or novel approaches involving other technologies.

Uncontrolled vs. on-demand aerosol generation

DPI devices that rely on patient inhalation are inherently on-demand, that is, only when the patient inhales is the aerosol delivered. In contrast, MDIs are inherently uncontrolled, and the patient's breathing maneuver has to be carefully synchronized to the aerosol generation event for effective dosing. DPI devices that rely on sources of energy other than patient inhalation effort may face similar problems as MDIs. Devices may "trigger" the aerosol generation event, which then follows uncontrollably. Alternatively, the delivery of energy to the powder may be modulated by the device and controlled based on monitoring of the patient inhalation maneuver.

Homogeneous Powders and Blends

Dry powders must be able to flow readily to leave the capsule or powder reservoir but also must generate a fine aerosol so that the patient can inhale a proper dose. These two requirements are often difficult to achieve simultaneously. Fine powders tend to be cohesive and have poor flow properties. Blending with a carrier phase, pelletization, and other approaches have been used to overcome these limitations.

Performance and Regulatory Requirements for DPIs

Performance Characterization

Two critical attributes characterize the performance of DPIs: the uniformity of the delivered dose and the aerodynamic assessment of particle size distribution. To determine delivered-dose uniformity, an apparatus capable of quantitatively retaining the delivered dose leaving the device is used. For aerodynamic particle size assessment, a multistage liquid impinger or cascade impactor is used. All aerosol performance testing must be conducted under defined temperature and humidity conditions.

Performance Specifications

Currently, the United States, European, and British pharmacopoeias specify different requirements for delivered-dose uniformity. The Japanese Pharmacopoeia does not specify a delivered-dose uniformity requirement. Of the four pharmacopoeias, the U.S. Pharmacopeia (USP) has the strictest requirements for delivered-dose uniformity. Although the British Pharmacopeia (BP) allows the same performance range, the USP defines the range around the label claim, and the BP defines the range around the average value. FDA expectations for delivered-dose uniformity is currently tighter than those specified in all the pharmacopeias.

The various pharmacopoeias outline appropriate methods for aerodynamic assessment of particle size distribution. The USP defines the size distribution through mass median aerodynamic diameter (MMAD) and geometric standard deviation (GSD). None of the pharmacopoeias specify a requirement for particle size. However, the particle size specifications that are set should be appropriate for the intended use of the product. For example, if the particles are intended to reach the deep lung, the MMAD of particles exiting the device should be less than 5 *mm*. In general, the smaller the aerosol MMAD, the greater the deposition in the lung.

Two recent trends originating with the FDA may influence the assessment and reporting of aerodynamic particle size distribution. The first is determining the particle size distribution from a single or unit-emitted dose. This may pose an analytical challenge in some cases because the amount of active ingredient in each stage may be present only in trace amounts. The second is setting a drug quantity specification for each stage of the impinger or cascade impactor.

Release and Stability Testing Parameters

Various dry powder attributes are assessed at release and on stability. These include physical characteristics such as powder appearance, content uniformity, delivered dose uniformity, and particle size distribution. Chemical attributes that may be assessed include drug content, purity, and identity as well as the water content of a powder. Dry powders may also undergo microscopic evaluation for foreign particulate matter, unusual agglomeration, and particle size. Microbial limits also should be examined, including the total aerobic, yeast, and mold counts. The presence of specific pathogens should be ruled out. The dry powders also may be dissolved to test for pH level. In addition, certain compendial requirements for content and delivered-dose uniformity should also be measured.

The USP and European Pharmacopoeia (EP) propose that the total aerobic count not exceed 100 CFU/g, that the total yeast count and mold count not exceed 10 CFU/g, and that no specific pathogens be detectable. Specifications for the other attributes should be based on the intended use and the historical performance of the product. As with other dosage forms, specifications must be met throughout the intended shelf life of the product.

The International Conference on Harmonization (ICH) has identified stability requirements for room temperature storage and testing intervals. It recommends that dry powders be stored at 25°C and 60% RH for real-time conditions; at 40°C and 75% RH for accelerated conditions; and 30°C and 60% RH if significant change is observed at accelerated conditions. The ICH recommends testing samples every 3 months for the first year, every 6 months for the second year, and yearly thereafter. In addition to these requirements, the FDA suggests a storage condition at 25°C and 75% RH if significant change is observed at the accelerated condition. Six-month data would be required at the time of the New Drug Application (NDA) submission, and the study must cover 1 year.

When an NDA is submitted, the FDA requires that 12 months of data be collected at real-time conditions and 6 months of data be collected under accelerated conditions. If significant change is observed at 6 months for the accelerated condition, 6-month data at the 30°C and 60% RH condition must be submitted, and the study must cover 1 year.

Role of DPIs in Therapy

Some direct comparisons of DPI and MDI for the same drug have been made in the interest of developing alternative but comparable products for patients. The therapeutic performance of inhalation delivery systems is as dependent on the patient as it is on the product itself. Therefore, some demonstration of clinical comparability is generally required to support product substitution.

The deposition pattern of the inhaled dry powder aerosol can be strongly influenced by the patient's inhalation dynamics and lung anatomy. At high inhalation flow rates, a given particle will have a greater tendency to impact the back of the throat or to deposit in the upper airways. For those delivery systems requiring high flow to deaggregate the powder particles, deep lung deposition is less accessible. The proliferation of device designs has been in part the result of attempts to minimize dosing variability regardless of source.

The target for lung deposition varies depending on the therapy under consideration. In the treatment of asthma by β-adrenergic agonists, the Central airways are generally targeted. On the other hand, therapies intended to treat alveolar disease, chronic obstructive pulmonary disease, or systemic conditions must reach the peripheral regions of the deep lung.

Among the pharmacokinetic advantages offered by delivery to the lung are fast onset of action and lack of first-pass effect. Doses to the lung can prove 10–20 times more effective than oral dosing and for local therapy can result in substantially reduced side effects.

In a study, three different fluticasone propionate products—an MDI and two DPI products, Diskhaler and Diskus—were directly compared in healthy volunteers and patients. The systemic drug bioavailability was highest for the MDI, whereas the bioavailability was similar for the two DPIs. The pharmacokinetic results are consistent with the in vitro evaluation in which the MDI gave the highest fine particle dose (FPD), whereas the two DPIs had similar FPD values. It was also reported that in a separate study using healthy volunteers, the pharmacokinetics of a non-chlorofluorocarbon formulation have been shown to be similar to that for the original chlorofluorocarbon formulation for a fluticasone propionate MDI product. Consistent with their similar pharmacokinetic results, the clinical performance of Diskhaler and Diskus is similar in both children and adults.

DPIs: A Burgeoning Industry

The first commercially available DPI system appeared on the market in 1949, developed and marketed by Abbott under the name Aerohaler. Like all pulmonary drug-delivery methods that existed before now, it delivered small molecule compounds (brochodilators or inhaled corticosteroids) to the airway (not necessarily to the deep lung) for the treatment of asthma or chronic obstructive pulmonary disease. New DPI technologies in development by Inhale Therapeutic Systems and Alkermes are enabling the delivery of macromolecules to the deep lung. Leading this field is Inhale's insulin product, currently in the phase 3 trials with Pfizer. In the next years, it is expected that dry powder inhalation will become a broadly accepted and effective means of delivering a wide variety of therapeutics–antibiotics, analgesics, antibodies, hormones, proteins, and perhaps gene therapeutics. The potential of this technology continues to be explored.

16

LIQUIDS

Using the inhalation route to deliver therapeutic aerosols is a common practice in the treatment of patients with various airway diseases. Drug delivery via inhalation offers many advantages in the administration of pharmaceutical compounds, because the drugs are delivered directly to the site of action. Therefore, the required therapeutic dose for each treatment is lower than if the dose is administrated via oral or parenteral routes. As a consequence, the inhalation route reduces adverse effects due to systemic absorption and intensifies the amount of drug deposited to the targeted tissue. In the U.S. market, bronchodilator, anticholinergic, anti-inflammatory, and corticosteroid drugs are common inhaled dosage forms used for the treatment of respiratory diseases, such as asthma and COPD. Additional drug classes, such as antibiotics, antifungals, and antiviral compounds, are also used or under development for topical delivery via inhalation. Further, new inhaled applications are being developed for the treatment of systemic diseases. These products include both small and macromolecules. Pulmonary delivery of peptides and proteins is a rapidly growing area of inhaled drug delivery, spearheaded by the development of inhaled insulin for treatment of diabetes.

An aerosol is defined in its simplest form as a collection of solid or liquid particles suspended in a gas such as air. Aerosols are two-phase systems consisting of the particulates and the gas in which they are suspended. Aerosol science has been studied for many decades in various disciplines, especially related to environmental sciences, to understand the health effects associated with exposure to air pollutants. These activities have improved our understanding of the dynamic behavior of aerosol particles and their relative effects on human health, but also laid the foundation for the pharmaceutical industry to use inhalation of aerosols for therapeutic purposes. Pharmaceutical aerosols deliver therapeutically active drug compounds to the human respiratory tract for local orsystemic actions. This dosage form is intended to be inhaled through either the mouth or the nose. The increasing use of inhalation therapy has been mainly driven by the confluence of three factors:

1. Advances in aerosol generation technology, which provide more efficient and controlled delivery of aerosolized pharmaceutical compounds into the human respiratory airway;
2. Advances in biotechnology, with the development of new therapeutic agents that are often difficult to deliver by other routes of administration;
3. A better understanding of the pathophysiology of disease, which allows physicians and scientists to envision a broader range of therapeutic options.

Those involved with the pulmonary delivery of therapeutic agents are challenged in all three areas, especially the first two. We can now develop new therapies, but we must be certain that we can reproducibly deliver those therapeutic agents to the desired site, in the dosage and form in which they will be most effective. The benefit of using the respiratory airways as a route for drug delivery has been increasingly explored over the last 10 years. The large surface area of the human respiratory system, sometimes compared to the size of a tennis court (~ 100 m^2), is an attractive target site for pulmonary delivery of drugs intended for absorption into the blood. Drug administration via inhalation has many advantages for the systemic delivery of pharmaceutical compounds such as proteins and peptides, which are often degraded when delivered through the GI tract and avoid the need for repeated injections.

Inhaled aerosols also provide high drug concentrations in the respiratory tract. The treatment of airway diseases by aerosol inhalation is beneficial because of intensified localized drug deposition and fewer side effects. Consequently, smaller doses are needed to achieve the therapeutic level in the lungs via inhalation thereby avoiding high systemic levels of the drug. Therefore, inhaled drug aerosols have become the standard clinical approach for managing asthma, respiratory distress syndrome (RDS), chronic obstructive pulmonary disease (COPD), cystic fibrosis, and other respiratory tract diseases. Despite the spectrum of opportunities that now exists for new inhaled therapies, successful development of pulmonary drug products is a challenging task. The problems and barriers are multidisciplinary in nature, perhaps explaining why this field has not accelerated faster. Using aerosolization to administer drugs to the respiratory airway dates back to the early part of the 20th century, when the pneumatic nebulizer was used as a drug delivery device.

The nebulization principle for the squeeze-bulb nebulizers is the same as many conventional nebulizers. Liquid is forced through a small critical orifice. The particle size of aerosol generated from the early squeeze-bulb nebulizers was generally large (due to the inability to accurately machine small holes) and, therefore, largely unsuitable for human inhalation. However, the concept of delivering drug products via inhalation was an important milestone that established the foundation for developing better pulmonary drug delivery technology.

The modern pressurized metered dose inhaler (pMDI) was developed between 1955 and 1956. However, the pMDI had its roots in research carried out many years before. During the 1930s and 1940s, the discovery of liquefied propellants (chlorinated-fluorocarbons or freon propellants) such as CFC12, CFC114, CFC11, and CFC22 was a major step in the realization of a portable inhaler. However, the first pMDI was not invented until 1956, when the metering valve used in the device was developed and patented. The invention of the first pMDI by Riker Laboratories was described in detail recently, and was approved by the FDA in March 1956. The Medihaler-Ept and Medihaler-Iso were launched at the same time. The Medihaler-Iso was changed to accommodate suspension formulations during 1957. This proved particularly useful for formulating difficult to solubilize drugs, such as many of the steroids later developed for the treatment of asthma. The successful innovation of the pMDI established the foundation for the development of drug delivery via respiratory airways and remained the primary small volume nebulizer for the next 40 years.

Successful administration of any pharmaceutical compound to the human respiratory airway requires the generation and delivery of the drug in the form of an suitable for human inhalation. The human airway is a very complex structure that has evolved to serve two purposes: (1) exchanging gases vital to metabolism (O_2 and CO_2) and (2) defending against foreign particulates from entering the lungs. The generation of drug aerosols and their site of deposition in human lungs are dependent on many factors, such as the physical and chemical properties of aerosol particles, the mechanism of action and quality of performance of the drug delivery device, the patient's breathing pattern, and the morphometry of the human lungs. These factors are significant because:

1. Aerosol properties, such as particle size distribution, aerosol velocity, and hygroscopicity, affect aerosol deposition in the human lungs. Aerosol size distribution, including mass median aerodynamic

diameter (MMAD) and geometric standard deviation (GSD), is one of the most important variables in governing the site of droplet or particle deposition in the lungs.

2. Device characteristics play an important role in the delivery of pharmaceutical compounds to human lungs. The mechanism by which aerosols are created affect particle size distribution, kinetics of aerosol delivery, and the reproducibility of drug dosing from the delivery device. These factors are key to controlling the delivery of a constant amount of drug aerosol across a diverse patient population.
3. The breathing patterns or maneuvers of a patient can also significantly affect the site of aerosol deposition in the human lungs, even of aerosols with similar characteristics (e.g., MMAD and GSD). Aerosol deposition mechanisms in the airway mainly consist of sedimentation, inertial impaction, and diffusion. Pharmaceutical aerosols deposit mainly by sedimentation and impaction. Therefore, aerosols delivered under high velocity conditions, either due to high ballistic velocity produced by the device or due to high patient inspiratory flow rates, result predominantly in deposition due to inertial impaction, markedly enhancing conducting airway deposition. Conversely, deposition in the peripheral lung can be promoted by decreasing the velocity of an aerosol during inhalation. Further, deposition of these particles that reach the deep lung can be enhanced by a post-inspiratory pause (i.e., breath-hold), allowing particles to settle more completely.
4. Morphometry of the upper and lower airways will also affect the drug deposition in the lungs. Anatomical conditions such as airway size, disease status, and degree of obstruction are different from patient to patient; thus there will be variability in the site of drug deposition between patients.

The inhalation drug delivery devices currently available commercially consist of metered dose inhalers (MDIs), dry powder inhalers (DPIs), and nebulizers.This article will focus on the inhalation of aerosols generated from liquid systems using either small volume inhalers, or larger home or clinical nebulizers. Various drug delivery devices, including those available commercially and those under development, will be discussed in detail, so that the reader will have a better understanding of the advantages and disadvantages of those devices for pulmonary drug delivery. An emphasis will be given to new pulmonary drug delivery device technology in development, and its potential application to deliver pharmaceutical compounds for both local targeting and systemic absorption of drugs intended to act outside the lung. Over the last 10 years, many innovations have occurred in the area of inhalation drug delivery stimulated by advances in aerosol generation technology and the demand created by new biopharmaceuticals.

Commercially Available Pulmonary Delivery Technology

The inhalation drug delivery devices currently available commercially consist of metered dose inhalers (MDIs), dry powder inhalers (DPIs) and nebulizers. The effective performance (or lack thereof) of the inhalation devices is well recognized as being crucial in how effective a pulmonary delivered drug is in the treatment of diseases, both topical and systemic disorders. In order for a drug to be effective by inhalation, the generated aerosol must be of proper size to be deposited in the targeted location. The patient needs to inhale the drug formulation properly, and the drug must be deposited with sufficient quantity at the action site so that it can be absorbed or distributed effectively. The drug delivery devices available commercially have been used widely for the treatment of airway diseases such as asthma and chronic obstructive pulmonary diseases (COPDs). Such treatment is effective mainly because of the wide therapeutic index of the drug compounds. It is useful to review the advantages and disadvantages of current device technologies to provide a better understanding of how the devices are used by patients and what kind of improvements are needed to deliver various drug compounds by inhalation. This article is limited to discussion of devices that generate liquid drug aerosols as solutions, suspensions, and emulsions.

There are several ways to categorize drug delivery devices. The inhalation drug delivery devices discussed in this article are categorized according to their operating principles or fundamental mechanism of generating aerosols.

Pressure-Driven Devices

Jet nebulizers

The jet nebulizer has been used for many years to treat airway diseases both in the clinical setting and in home use. The jet nebulizer utilizes compressed gas from an air source either from a hospital air line or from a portable compressor to convert the liquid drug solution into small droplets by forcing the liquid through a small hole known as a critical orifice. Atomization occurs as a result of the disruption of the surface tension holding the liquid together by the action of internal and external forces. In the absence of such disruptive forces, surface tension tends to pull the liquid into the form of a sphere, since this has the minimum amount of surface energy. The droplets produced by atomization contain many large drops, which will undergo further disruption to form small particles. The particle size of the droplets will depend not only on the kinetic energy used during the nebulization, but also the pore diameter of the critical orifice and on the physical properties of the liquid formulation.

The jet nebulizer is driven by air pressurized typically at 20–40 psi. The compressed air accelerates through an arrow orifice to break the bulk liquid into sheets, jets, films, or streams. Those ligaments are accelerated to a velocity sufficient to impact on baffles or on the nebulizer wall. The outgoing air becomes saturated with water vapors derived from the liquid retained in the nebulizer, and this has two important consequences:

1. The nebulizer is cooled and reaches an equilibrium temperature approximately 10°C below ambient, so that the patient inhales a relatively cool aerosol cloud.
2. The evaporation of water causes the concentration of solutes to increase with time as the vehicle carrier evaporates.

Droplet formation

A general theory for the formation of droplets by nebulization has not been fully developed, although the understanding of the nebulization principle has been improved with mathematical modeling. A rigorous mathematical description of droplet formation requires knowledge of distribution of aerodynamic pressure on the droplet surface and the interaction of this pressure with internal forces acting on the droplets. Therefore, before further discussing of the effect of various parameters on the nebulization performance, it is beneficial to consider briefly the various ways in which a single droplet of liquid can break up under the action of aerodynamic forces. Once the droplets are generated using a compressed air source during the primary atomization, unstable droplets experience further disintegration to form smaller particles, which is referred to as "*secondary atomization.*" The formation of a single droplet under the aerodynamic forces exerted by the external sources, together with the internal forces of the liquid formulation, such as surface tension and viscosity, dictate the formation of the droplet. The relationship between these forces was described by Klusener, who offered the following equation:

$$P_1 = P_a + P_\sigma = \text{constant} \qquad \text{...(1)}$$

where P_1 is the internal pressure at any point on the droplet surface, P_a is the external aerodynamic pressure due to the compressed air source, and P_σ is the pressure caused by the surface tension. From the equation, it is observed that a droplet can maintain its stability as long as the change in the air pressure, P_a, is balanced by a corresponding change in the pressure caused by surface tension, so that the internal pressure remain constant. When the aerodynamic pressure is greater than the pressure due to surface tension, the external pressure will deform the droplet in order to reduce the pressure by surface tension to maintain the constant internal pressure. This deformation will continue to break up the droplet into smaller particles. For a formulation with low viscosity, such as aqueous formulation, the viscous force is relatively small compared with the surface tension force. Under such relative conditions, a dimensionless parameter can be obtained, as shown in Eq. (2). For a given liquid with low viscosity, the critical condition for the droplet to break up occurs when the aerodynamic force equals the surface tension, expressed as

$$C_D \frac{\pi d^2}{4} 0.5\rho V^2 = \pi d\sigma \qquad \ldots(2)$$

where C_D is the coefficient of drag, d is the diameter of the droplet, ρ and σ are the density and surface tension of the liquid, respectively. From the above equation one can calculate the maximum stable droplet diameter,

$$d_{\max} = \left(\frac{8\sigma}{C_D \rho V^2}\right) \qquad \ldots(3)$$

and the critical velocity at which the droplet will disrupt

$$V_{\text{crit}} = \left(\frac{8\sigma}{C_D \rho d}\right)^{0.5} \qquad \ldots(4)$$

The equation can also be expressed as the dimensionless parameter called the Weber number, as

$$We_{\text{crit}} = \left(\frac{\rho V^2 d}{\sigma}\right)\text{crit} = \frac{8}{C_D} \qquad \ldots(5)$$

which is the ratio of external aerodynamic force to surface tension force. Using the above equations, the maximum diameter at a particular critical velocity can be estimated. However, it should be noted that the estimated diameter results from only the process of primary atomization. Secondly, atomization will generally decrease and exaggerate the particle size distribution. Additionally, when a droplet impacts a baffle immediately after the primary atomization, the droplet diameter drops sharply. Baffles are used in nebulizer systems to help control the particle size distribution of the droplets so that generated aerosols are within a desired particle size range, usually with mean values that are less than 10 μm and preferably less than 5 μm, for effective deposition in the human lungs.

Effect of physical properties of formulation

The physical properties of the formulation, such as viscosity and surface tension, are important parameters that affect the process of nebulization. Surface tension can be considered as a consolidating influence that attempts to minimize the production of increased surface area, and the liquid viscosity exerts a stabilizing influence by opposing any change in the shape of droplets as they are produced. Studies have shown that the droplet size is proportional to the liquid surface tension for low-viscosity liquids, while the density has only a small effect on the droplet size. The effect of viscosity on the droplet size seems to be complex. Research by Searls and Snyder showed that high- viscosity liquids not only have increased nebulization time (decreasing the mass output), but also reduced mean particle size. However, Hinds, Macher, and First reported little change in droplet size with viscosity ranged from 17 to over 100 cP using a Laskin aerosol generator operated at 20 psi.

An extensive study was conducted by McCallion et al. investigating the effects of different physicochemical properties on the performance of the jet nebulizer. Materials with different viscosity and surface tension were nebulized using three different nebulizers, Pari LC, Sidestream, and Cirrus. However, only data from the Pari LC nebulizer were presented in the paper. The particle size distribution of the aerosols was quantified using laser diffraction, which has been shown by Clack to be a robust and reliable technique having good correlation with in vivo deposition data. The mass median diameters were obtained using two nebulization flow rates, 6 and 8 L/min, respectively. The authors concluded that the more viscous fluids tended to produce smaller droplets. Within a specific range of the surface tension, of approximately 70 dyne/cm (70.0–72.9 dyne/cm), the mass median diameter decreased from 3.2 to 2.5 μm as the viscosity increased from 1.0 to about 6.0 centipoise. The same was true for surface tension of approximately 20 dyne/cm: as the viscosity increased, the particle size decreased. The effect of surface tension on particle size distribution was not as clear. However, the authors pointed out that a correlation between surface tension and mass median diameter appeared to exist when the fluid systems were analyzed separately. In glycerol and propylene glycol solutions, surface tension was directly proportional to droplet size, while the converse was true for silicone fluids. A trend was reported for the other two nebulizers tested, but no data were presented.

Drug concentration effects

Because of the large volume of air used during nebulization, there is continuous evaporative loss of any solvent, such as water. This phenomenon has been described in several studies. Theoretically, the increase in drug concentration will continue until the solute concentration in the reservoir reaches the limit of drug solubility, at which point precipitation may occur. In practice, many drugs used in nebulizers (such as bronchodilators) are very hydrophilic, and the nebulizer solutions are formulated at concentrations well below the solubility limit, so there is little issue with precipitation. However, this results in changing particle size distribution with variable deposition patterns, and a change in the unit dose given per unit time. Collectively, this produces variable and unpredictable deposited doses for many drug products. The magnitude of the change in solution concentration is difficult to quantitatively predict and depends strongly on the formulation, nebulization condition, and type of nebulizers. Niven has recently derived a mathematical equation based upon the early work by Mercer to describe the relationship of drug concentration in the nebulizer as a function of time. The drug concentration obtained by Mercer was expressed as

$$C(t) = C_0\left(\frac{V_0}{V_0 - (W+S)Ft}\right)^{(W/W+S)} \qquad \ldots(6)$$

where W and S are the solution output and solvent output per liter of air (ml/L air) respectively. V_0 is the initial fill volume into the nebulizer, and F is the nebulization flow rate. A more user-friendly version of the equation was derived and expressed in terms of drug mass output that might be of more practical use in predicting drug output from a nebulizer for a range of operation conditions as claimed by the author:

$$M_{out} = M_0\left[1-\left(\frac{V}{V_0}\right)^{(W/W+S)}\right] \qquad \ldots(7)$$

where M_0 is the initial amount of drug in the solution, and V is the solution volume at any time, t, expressed as

$$V = V_0 - [W+S]Ft \qquad \ldots(8)$$

Newman et al. evaluated the concentration change using four different jet nebulizers, with a gentamicin solution, which is used to treat patients for cystic fibrosis. The types of nebulizers used were the Bird micronebulizer, DeVilbiss 646, Bard Inspiron mini-neb, and Medic-Aid Upmist. All were operated at four different air flow rates: 6, 8, 10, and 12 L/min. Nebulization time was defined as 30 s after the last visible release of aerosol. The concentration of the drug solution left in the nebulizers was then measured using an Osmometer. The initial drug concentration was 40 mg/ml for both fill volumes. Table 16.1 shows the final concentration of gentamicin solution at different nebulization flow rates.

It was found that the ratio of final to initial drug concentration ranged from 1.35 to 1.70 for the 2 ml fill volume, and from 1.45 to 1.96 for the 4 ml fill volume. The ratio did not vary significantly between the four different nebulization flow rates, but was significantly higher ($p < 0.01$) for the 4 ml fill volume than for the 2 ml fill volume, indicating that the larger volume allowed more time to concentrate the reservoir drug solution. The same phenomenon was observed using a albuterol solution, and the drug concentration increased after the nebulization. It was also found that the concentration ratio decreased with the increase in solution fill volume, which is different from the results. However the discrepancy may result from the different nebulization sources, where dry oxygen vs. an electric powered air compressor were used in the experiment.

Table 16.1. Final drug concentration (mg/ml) in the nebulizer reservoirs

	Nebulization flow rate			
Nebulizer type	*6L/min*	*8 L/min*	*10 L/min*	*12 L/min*
Solution fill volume: 2 ml				
Bird	54.4	62.0	57.2	58.4
DeVilbiss	55.6	60.4	56.0	65.6
Inspiron	58.4	65.2	68.0	68.0
Upmist	64.4	58.0	58.0	58.0
Solution fill volume: 4 ml				
Bird	59.2	65.6	58.0	64.0
DeVilbiss	78.4	77.2	71.6	75.2
Inspiron	71.2	69.2	74.0	74.8
Upmist	76.8	75.6	62.8	62.8

Temperature effects

It is well known that the nebulizer solution cools during nebulization, because a large amount of compressed air is used to generate aerosol particles. The temperature of the nebulizer solution decreases several degrees (5–10°C) due to the evaporation of solvent in the solution during the first several minutes of nebulization until a new heat balance is established. Some cooling of the solution in the nebulizer due to adiabatic expansion of the compressed air source may be absorbed by the thermal energy released by break-up and impact of the liquid. The magnitude of temperature change in the nebulization solution depends on many factors, such as heat capacity, properties of nebulizer material, ambient conditions, and the humidity and temperature of the compressed air. Four different types of nebulizers were used together with different air compressors to aerosolize a sodium chloride solution. The solutions in the nebulizers were initially at ambient temperatures (approximately of 23°C). Different nebulizers had different temperature reduction profiles, depending on the compressed air flow rate applied during the nebulization. as pointed out by the

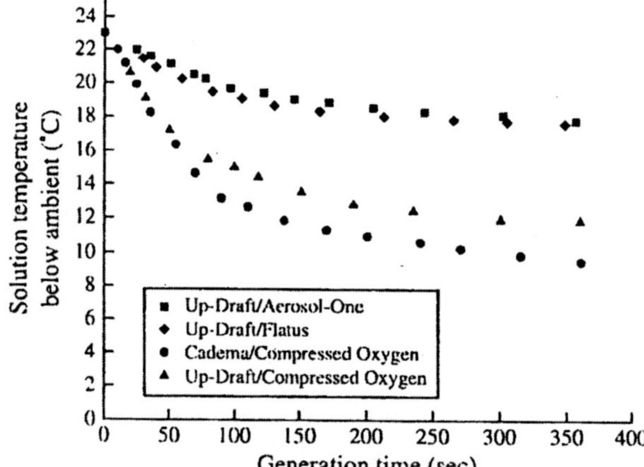

Fig. 16.1. Nebulizer solution temperature below ambient (23°C) vs. nebulization time.

authors. The solution temperature falls to a steady value, T_s, which is 5–6°C below the ambient temperature at the nebulization flow rate of 6.3–5.0 L/min, and 11–15°C at 8 L/min air flow rate.

Drug aerosol delivery efficiency and particle size distribution

Delivery efficiency of aerosolized drug product and particle size distribution are the two most important parameters in assessing the performance of a nebulizer for aerosol therapy. The aerosol output from the nebulizer depends mainly on the nebulizer type, drug formulation, solution volume placed in the nebulizer, and the applied air pressure (and hence the airflow through the nebulizer). The simplest method to calculate the output from a nebulizer is to weigh the nebulizer before and after the nebulization, often expressed as the solution volume output per unit time (i.e., mg/min). However, this method of calculation is subject to at least two possible error sources: (1) neglecting the change in solution density when it is used to transfer the mass output per unit time to volume output per unit time and (2) neglecting the change in solution concentration as discussed previously. The delivery efficiency of the nebulizer can be expressed simply as

$$E = \frac{M_p - M_d}{M_p} \qquad ...(9)$$

where E represents the nebulizer delivery efficiency, M_p is the drug amount loaded into the nebulizer before nebulization, and M_d is the drug amount left in the nebulizer after the nebulization. Nebulizers are often operated until there is no visible aerosol or "*sputtering*," and a significant reduction in the nebulizer output occurs when the solution volume in the nebulizer reservoir becomes so low that it fails to maintain a continuous liquid supply to the nebulizer orifice. However, these are very crude measures and provide no indication of the amount of aerosolized drug a patient inhales.

The delivery efficiency, or the nebulizer output, can be expressed in many different ways, as widely documented in the literature. Sometimes it is represented as the volume output, or solution mass output. However, it is more practical to use the drug mass emitted from the nebulizer at or near the mouthpiece to estimate the nebulizer output, because the amount of aerosolized drug mass at this point in the system is the best measure of how much drug the patient has available to inhale.

Nebulizer output depends mainly on three variables: the type of the nebulizer, the operating conditions during nebulization, and the solution to be nebulized. Although solution density and viscosity play minor roles in nebulizer output for the majority of aqueous formulation, viscosity becomes an issue when aerosolizing highly viscous solutions. For any given solution and nebulizer, the operating pressure primarily determines the nebulizer output. Increasing the nebulization pressure usually increases nebulizer output. Increasing nebulizer output typically has a clinical benefit: it can reduce the time required to nebulize an effective dose, particularly for young patients who are less tolerant of the treatment procedure. As drug mass delivered per unit time is increased, treatment time is reduced leading to better acceptability and improved clinical outcome.

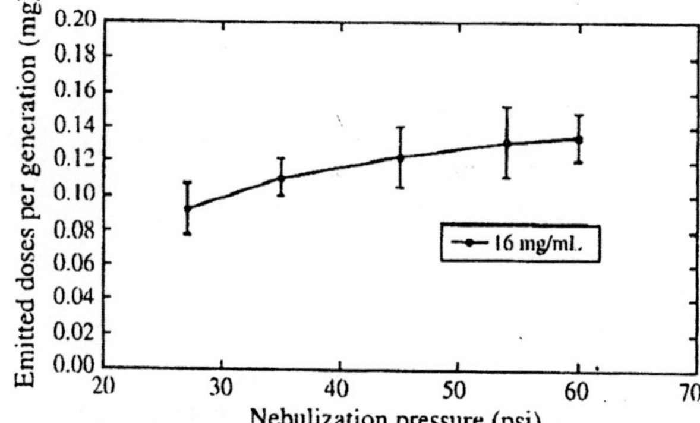

Fig. 16.2. Emitted dose per generation from the nebulizer vs. the nebulization pressure.

A Pari LC Plus jet nebulizer was used in the study. The nebulizer was operated using a specially designed electronic unit to regulate the compressed air supplied to the nebulizer. The nebulizer was operated in a pulse mode, in which the time of nebulization was set at 3s for each aerosol generation.

The drug output was generally greater with each incremental increase in operating pressure. These increases were significant ($p < 0.05$) over a range of nebulization operating pressures of 27–45 psi. Additional increases in operating pressure of 45 to 60 psi did not significantly increase aerosol drug output. Finlay, Stapleton, and Zuberbuhler recently tested 15 different jet nebulizers available commercially to investigate the performance of nebulizers. The drug compound used in the study was a 2.5 ml unit dose of Ventolin (containing 1 mg/ml of salbutamol sulfate), which corresponds to a 2.5 mg in nominal dose per drug container.

Nebulizers fitted with a T-mouthpiece have an unrestricted flow of ambient air passing through the nebulizer output, supplying inhaled air flow, which effectively increases drug output. In vented nebulizers, the inhaled air must flow through the droplet production region. Therefore, the breathing pattern of the patient has an effect on the aerosol characteristics produced by such devices. The delivery efficiency of the commercial nebulizers tested ranged from 6 to 30% of the nominal dose loaded into the nebulizers. For conventional nebulizers, the inhaled dose is approximated by the amount of drug leaving the nebulizer divided by 2, since inhalation is assumed to occupy half of the breathing cycle. However, this remains a very crude measure of delivered or inhaled dose.

The importance of particle size distribution in determining the site of the deposition of pharmaceutical compounds within the respiratory tract has been discussed extensively in the literature). For any given inhaled dose of aerosolized drug, the particle size distribution of drug aerosol, aerosol velocity, the breathing pattern (inspiratory flow and volume), and lung morphology, determine the location the aerosol is deposited in the respiratory airways. It is generally well accepted that the particle size of drug aerosols generated for inhalation should be within 1–5 μm in diameter. Because of polydispersity of the aerosol, the mass median aerodynamic diameter (MMAD) and geometrical standard deviation (GSD) are often used to describe the distribution of aerosol particles. The MMAD is defined as the mass median of the distribution of mass with respect to aerodynamic diameter.

The size distribution of aerosols generated using most commercial nebulizers is typically highly variable with somewhat large mean diameters. This not only results in poor transfer efficiency but poor and highly variable respiratory deposition patterns between and within patient populations.

Metered dose inhalers

Pressurized metered dose inhalers (pMDIs) have been widely used in the treatment of asthma and COPD. These devices are more popular than nebulizers and dry powder inhalers. The popularity of the pMDI has steadily increased since the 1950s due mainly to its compact and portable size, self-contained power source, and other rapid therapeutic effects in the use of bronchodilators. pMDIs appear to be simple to use, although this appearance is in fact deceptive. Many patients are not adequately trained to correctly use pMDIs or find it nearly impossible to effectively coordinate their breathing with the high velocity release of the aerosol. High ejection velocity of the aerosol at the mouthpiece (usually near 30 m/s) is the single largest deficit of pMDIs. At these high ballistic velocities, most of the drug aerosol impacts in the mouth or throat and can not be readily entrained within the respiratory flow (even when coordinated with aerosol release). Typically, about 60–90% of the emitted drug will be deposited in the oral-pharyngeal region. This not only reduces the amount of drug that reaches the intended action site, but often contributes to unwanted systemic side effects due to oral absorption. Spacers have been developed that help mitigate this problem. The spacers are placed in front of the pMDIs actuator to reduce the aerosol velocity, and reduce the number of large diameter droplets before entering into the airway. However, this occurs at the expense of delivery efficiency, further reducing the dose of drug inhaled.

A typical pMDI consists of a drug reservoir containing the drug compound suspended or solubilized in liquefied propellant, a metering valve, and an actuator that connects with the metering valve through a stem. The propellants historically have been chlorofluorocarbons (CFCs) which have high vapor pressures and are generally biologically inert. The pMDI delivers a metered dose of active drug compound using the propellants as a power source. In the rest position, the metering chamber is connected with the formulation reservoir. Depressing the drug canister activates the metering chamber and the formulation reservoir is then closed. Simultaneously, a connection is opened between the valve stem orifice and the metering chamber. The formulation contained in the metering chamber quickly escapes through the stem valve and spray orifice, atomizing the formulation. As the liquid CFCs vaporize, they generate sufficient energy to produce efficient two-phase atomization, without the need for an external power source. The primary factors that will influence the performance of the pMDI are the propellant used, the physical properties of drug formulation, which partially governs droplet formation and drug uniformity, and the device itself.

Propellants

The propellants used in the pMDIs consist of CFCs with different molecular formulas. The propellants commonly used in inhalers to disperse the liquid into aerosols are CFC-11 (CCl_3F), CFC-12 (CCl_2F_2), and CFC-114 ($CClF_2$-$CClF_2$). These three propellants have been used for decades in pMDI products because of their unique properties, which include low toxicity, excellent physical and chemical stability, ideal vapor pressure, and generally good compatibility with drug compounds and surfactants. These propellants possess an appropriate degree of solvency that solubilizes the surfactants typically used in pMDI systems such as oleic acid, sorbitan trioleate, and soya lecithin, yet dissolve low quantities of most drugs. This combination of surfactant solubility and drug insolubility in the pMDI formulation is essential for maintaining uniform suspensions of appropriate particle size.

The vapor pressure of the formulation in a pMDI can be adjusted to a targeted value by mixing propellants with different vapor pressures. Propellants offer the additional advantage of having a narrow density range that may be adjusted to balance the density of the drug particle in suspension.

Moren investigated the influence of vapor pressure on the characteristics of aerosols generated using pMDIs. In these studies, nine healthy volunteers inhaled eight doses at one-minute intervals coordinated with the dose firing, and the amount of drug deposited in the actuator, extension tube, and mouth was determined spectrophotometrically. It was found that an increase in vapor pressure results in higher initial velocity of the aerosols, smaller initial aerosol particle size, and more rapid propellant evaporation. The amount of drug deposited in the actuator increased at the higher vapor pressure of 502 kPa, which was likely due to the high velocity of the aerosol exiting the spray nozzle and a wide spray angle.

Aerosol formation

Aerosol formation from pMDIs is a complex process influenced not only by the propellant as discussed above, but also by properties of the formulation and device design (e.g., valve volume and orifice size). After aerosol droplets form at the exit of the spray nozzle, an aerosol plume begins to expand, and large particles travel along the axis of the actuator.

Most large droplets fall out from the aerosol cloud, and those droplets are deposited in the mouthpiece or in the oral-pharyngeal region of the respiratory airways when the inhaler is used by a patient. When spaces are used, many large particles are collected within the spacers. The remaining aerosol cloud continues to evaporate, and the velocity of the aerosol reduces dramatically from about 35 m/s at 5 cm from the spray orifice to about 10 m/s at 20 cm. During aerosolization, surfactant molecules, used as dispersing agents and valve lubricants, will influence the evaporation rate of the propellants. The dimension and shape of the aerosol cloud significantly influence the transport efficiency of aerosol to the respiratory tract.

Physical stability of drug suspension

The physical stability of the non-polar drug suspensions formulated in pMDIs again depends on many parameters, such as propellant type, chemical properties of the drug compounds, and the surfactants used in the formulation. A suspension is a liquid system in which insoluble solid particles are dispersed in a liquid medium. Suspensions can be divided into colloidal suspensions, in which the solid particles are less than 1 μm, and coarse suspensions, where particles are larger than 1 μm. The physical stability of a suspension can also be classified according to whether the formulation is flocculated or deflocculated. In a deflocculated system, the solid drug particles settle down slowly and form irreversible aggregates. As a result the particles form a distinct cake on the bottom of a container. The deflocculated system is impossible to redisperse by simple shaking, and the suspension is unlikely to be of use after caking. Therefore, it is necessary to develop the flocculated formulation systems for pMDIs. In flocculated systems, the particles form large aggregates, so that the solid particles can be resuspended upon shaking. The formulation of a flocculated system requires reducing or neutralizing the zeta potential around the drug compound. This means that repelling forces between the particles are neutralized and the particles can then interact with each other to form large aggregates which rapidly settle but, can be easily redispersed. In formulating a suspension for pMDI use, the drug particles are usually less dense compared with the suspension media. Therefore, in an unshaken inhaler the drug gradually separates as a layer, which floats on the propellant and surfactant mixture, and is resuspended immediately after shaking. The solubility of the drug compound in the propellant also plays an important role in the physical stability of the pMDI formulation. An extremely low solubility of drug compound is required in the non-polar system. Therefore, pMDI formulations usually require a polar salt to be incorporated, because significant drug solubility in the propellant can lead to crystal growth, often associated with the caking of the suspension and a reduced amount of fine particles.

Sedimentation ratio is often used to assess suspension stability. Byron reported the sedimentation ratios for a 1% sodium fluoresein suspension formulation with different amounts of surfactant (sorbitan trioleate) after standing for 20 days at room temperature. The suspension formulation with the lowest sedimentation ratio had the best-flocculated system. However, all formulations were easily redispersible: one complete revolution of the container was sufficient to produce a homogeneous dispersion. There was no clear difference in the times taken to reach apparent sedimentation equilibrium. Physical stability of the formulation was determined according to:

1. Whether the drug material was adequately deaggregated during manufacture,
2. Whether redispersibility was easy and allowed doses to be metered reproducibly,
3. Surfactant concentration-drug combination gave the greatest respirable fraction of the aerosols.

Determination of dose and particle size distribution

The amount of drug reproducibly delivered from pMDIs per actuation is one of the most frequently reported performance parameters of these products. Several experimental configurations are used to characterize the pMDI' s emitted dose. One of the most commonly used experimental protocols is described in the Official Compendia of Standards published by U.S. Pharmacopeia. The pMDI device is fitted with a sampling tube at one end, and a vacuum pump is connected with a filter holder at the other end. A continuous airflow is drawn through the sampling tube to avoid the loss of the drug material into the atmosphere. The active compound delivered from the pMDI is recovered from the filter and the sampling tube to determine the mass output from the device. There are no universal definitions for different terminologies used to express dosages provided by pMDIs, and the labeling requirements for pMDIs differ among nations. In the United States, the emitted dose (label claim) is defined as the amount of drug leaving the device, excluding the drug mass left in the actuator and valve stem of the device. However, in other nations, the metered dose is often used, which includes the amount left in the actuator but not that retained in the valve stem. Descriptions of the emitted dose often use different terms, which are often used for different purposes. Because of the lack of consistency in the terminology used in the literatures and by regulatory agencies, it is often difficult to compare the experimental results between different research groups, devices, and experimental methods and procedures. Therefore, it would be beneficial to harmonize the terminology commonly used to describe drug doses from different parts of the pMDIs, and efforts are currently underway to standardize the way delivered dose and device performance are measured and reported.

However, even with a clear understanding of the dose delivered by a pMDI, there is no direct or consistent correlation to the amount of drug delivered to the patient's lungs. The table is based on an experiment conducted on healthy volunteers with an average FEV_1 at 105% of predicted (range 92–119%). A terbutaline formulation was labeled with ^{99m}Tc and administrated to patients using a pMDI. The average inspiratory flow rate was 33.8 L/min, (SD = 6.7), and the total inspired volume averaged 2.86 L (SD = 0.87), with an average of (SD = 0.7) 9.1s breath-hold. The inter-subject variability in the patients' breathing patterns was relatively small, contributable to on-line monitoring of breathing patterns using a spirometer. The amount of drug deposited in the lungs expressed as percentage of emitted dose (including drug left on actuator) was about 16.7% (SD = 9.6), and the percentage of emitted dose deposited in the oral- pharynx was 68.3% (SD = 10.2). The percentage of emitted dose deposited in the actuator was 13.4% (SD = 2.1). The intersubject variability for the percentage of emitted dose found in the actuator and oral-pharynx was 15.3 and 14.9%, and the variability for the total lung deposition was 57.7%. These large variations in the total lung deposition are typical of clinical results when inhaled drugs are given using pMDIs.

The particle size distribution of drug aerosol generated from the pMDI is another important performance parameter of the drug delivery device, which depends on the combination of the propellants and surfactants, the original size of the drug particle, and the design of the device (metering valve, orifice, actuator). The initial atomization process and subsequent spray evaporation govern the amount of drug aerosol deposited both in the oral-pharyngeal and pulmonary regions. Aerosol particles ejected from the pMDI experience constant changes in size due mainly to the drug formulation. The experiment was conducted using a pMDI obtained commercially, and a laser diffraction instrument was used to determine the size of drug aerosol. The device was mounted on a platform, and the distances between the actuator and the center of the laser beam were chosen to be about 5, 10, 15, 20, and 25 cm. The pMDI was operated according to the instructions given by the manufacturer, and five measurements were repeated for each chosen distance.

The size of the drug particle was about 8 μm at 5 cm between the actuator orifice, and gradually decreased to about 2.5 μm at 35 cm from the actuator orifice due to the evaporational shrinkage. The particle diameter was about 6.5 μm at a distance of 10 cm, which was about the distance to the oral-pharyngeal region from the actuator orifice. The amount of drug deposited in the oral-pharyngeal region is mainly due to the inertial impaction; therefore it depends more on particle size than on particle velocity. The inertial impaction is proportional to the square of the particle diameter, and is linearly proportional to the particle velocity. The decreases in particle diameter followed exponentially with the distance from the actuator orifice. The exponential decrease rate of particle diameter differs with different drug formulations (vapor pressure, nonvolatile concentration, etc.).

High Frequency Oscillating Devices

Ultrasonic nebulizer

Ultrasonic nebulizers utilize high frequency sonic energy to convert liquid drug formulations into aerosol clouds. Although these devices have been used in clinical settings since the 1960s, they are not as widely used as the jet nebulizer and pMDIs. Ultrasonic nebulizers typically have higher drug mass output and significantly larger particle size distributions at the point of aerosolization compared with jet nebulizers. The output of drug compound leaving the ultrasonic nebulizer is at a relatively slow velocity compared with the jet nebulizer. Therefore, less patient coordination is required during treatment. The reservoir temperature in the ultrasonic nebulizer increases rapidly during operation. In the study by Phipps, Paul, and Gonda the solution in the nebulizer increased from room temperature (~23°C) to greater than 30°C after about 5 min of operation, and exceeded 40°C after 30 min of nebulization. This significant temperature increase may cause some pharmaceutical compounds to be degraded during aerosolization. Changes in drug potency due to delivery by ultrasonic nebulizer have been reported in the literature, with degradation more profound for protein and peptide therapeutics compared to more stable small molecules.

Mechanism of aerosol generation

Ultrasonic nebulizers generate aerosols using a piezoelectric transducer that vibrates when subjected to high-frequency electric energy. When liquid is fed continuously through or over the vibrating surface, a wave pattern is formed as the liquid spreads over the liquid surface. Liquid droplets are formed when the amplitude of the vibrating surface increases to the point at which the capillary wave becomes unstable and collapses. An empirical equation to calculate the droplet diameter (*D*) produced from an ultrasonic nebulizer was described by Lang. The diameter is approximately proportional to the capillary wave length (λ), density (ρ) and surface tension (σ) of the liquid, and the excitation frequency (F).

$$D = 0.34\lambda = 0.996\frac{\sigma}{\rho F^2} \quad \ldots(10)$$

As with jet nebulizers and pMDIs, the formulation characteristics include liquid density, surface tension, viscosity, and vapor pressure. Many of these that effect nebulizer performance of formulation properties are described in the above equation. The configuration of the device, such as the location of the baffles, mechanisms in the transport of the liquid formulation to the piezoelectric transducer, and the size of medication chamber, also affect the performance. The units frequency and amplitude of vibration, control the mass output and the particle size distribution permitting some adjustment in aerosol characteristics.

Performance characteristics

Greenspan summarized the performance of commonly used ultrasonic nebulizers. The excitation frequency ranged from 1.3 to about 2.6 MHz, and the MMAD of the produced aerosols was approximately 1–7 μm. Several ultrasonic nebulizers generated relatively large aerosol particles, which were usually associated with low excitation frequency. Hager, Gober, and Löhr characterized the performance of two ultrasonic nebulizers using a pentamidine solution, which is used to treat Pneumocystis carinii pneumonia associated with acquired immunodeficiency syndrome. The ultrasonic nebulizers used in the study were Fiso Neb and Porta-Sonic. It was found that the mass output for FISO Neb at airflow rate of 6 L/min were 201.4 and 36.7 mg for drug concentrations of 50 and 10 mg/mL, respectively. Corresponding outputs decreased to 85.2 and 23.6 mg for Porta-Sonic nebulizer. However the MMD of aerosol generated from the Fiso Neb was 5.8–6.93 μm, and 1.96–3.04 μm for Porta-Sonic nebulizer. The higher mass output from the Fiso Neb compared to the Porta-Neb was due to the presence of larger aerosol particles produced by the Fiso Neb nebulizer. However, these larger droplets are typically non-respirable, if they are transported at all to the patient inhalation port. Therefore, the overall dose efficiency of ultrasonic nebulizers tend to be poorer than jet nebulizers.

Advanced Drug Delivery Technologies

Using the various drug delivery devices, such as pMDIs, nebulizers, and DPIs, discussed in the first half of this article, has had an enormous impact on patient quality of life, as inhaled drugs play an important role in the management of airway diseases. However, past successes in topical delivery of drugs to the lung owe more to the therapeutic properties of the drugs used than to the delivery device itself. Currently used delivery devices tend to be inefficient, with small amounts of drug delivered to the site of action, with a large portion of the drug compound lost in the device or deposited orally, often causing unwanted side effects.

The shortcomings described for the current devices limit their ability to meet the demands created by advancements in more potent small molecules and biotechnology therapies. More and more new drugs are potential inhalation candidate therapies to treat various diseases, including non-airway diseases such as diabetes. There is an urgent need for more advanced drug delivery technology, which can deliver the drug more precisely to the targeted area for action, with better efficiency and improved reproducibility. Over the last 10 years, many innovations have occurred in the field of inhalation drug delivery with advances in aerosol technology and electronics, spurred by the demand created by new drug compounds. Most of the technologies have tried to tackle problems such as reducing the ballistic velocity of aerosol released from pMDIs by breath activated functions and developing new propellants with lower ejection pressures. Focus has shifted to defining and developing a more "ideal" inhaler to administering various pharmaceutical compounds for different diseases. The following describes many of the features these new pulmonary drug delivery devices are designed to include.

1. Aerosol generation independent of the patient's inhalation.
2. Duration of aerosol dose generation should occupy a substantial part of a slow inhalation cycle. A generation time of greater than 1 s will permit the patient to better coordinate aerosol delivery effectively during inhalation.
3. The aerosol cloud should consist largely of particles of less than 5 μm in size. Fine aerosols are necessary for delivery to the lung periphery if this is the site of action or if systemic delivery is the objective. The ability to vary and then control the mean particle size distribution of the aerosol would be an added advantage for targeting deposition within different regions of the respiratory tract.
4. The velocity of the aerosol should be minimal to reduce oral-pharyngeal deposition and provide maximum delivery to the lungs.
5. The inhaler should be simple to use, require little patient coordination and preferably should be breath-actuate.
6. The inhaler should have dimensions similar to those of the pMDIs, fitting the pocket or the handbag and permitting discrete use.
7. The inhaler should contain a large number of doses (>50 doses).
8. A dose counter should be included.
9. The device should be easy to manufacture and reasonably priced.
10. The device should generate uniform doses through-out its life, be resistant to microbial and other contamination, and have a suitable shelf life.
11. Propellants should be avoided, or designed for low environmental impact.

Pressure Driven Devices

New generation pressurized metered dose inhaler

Asthma affects an estimated 100 million people worldwide, including over 15 million in the United States, and while the pMDI has many disadvantages, it still is the most prescribed drug product for the treatment of asthma. The long-term dominance of pMDIs in inhalation drug delivery is mainly due to its convenience. However, it is extremely difficult to use effectively. Everard pointed out that the pharmaceutical industry elected to perpetuate the failings of the pMDI and develop replacements for CFCs, rather than develop novel devices to meet current demands. Extensive resources have been invested to preserve the pMDI when the industry was challenged with phasing out CFC propellants, and to reduce the oral-pharyngeal deposition by methods such as using attached spacers and breath-actuated devices.

pMDIs with new propellants

Since 1974, the CFCs have been believed to contribute to erosion of the earth's stratospheric ozone. Coyne summarizes the history and progress of the Montreal Protocol negotiations and formation in great detail, and introduces the objectives and history of the Pharmaceutical Aerosol CFC Coalition (PACC) in the United States and the International Pharmaceutical Aerosol Consortium (IPAC) in Europe. The objectives of the organizations are to find replacements for CFC propellants that can be used in pMDIs.

Reformulation of drugs used in pMDIs to avoid CFC propellants presented numerous obstacles, because no approved alternative pharmaceutical propellants were available. Replacement of the propellants used in pMDIs requires changes in many fundamental aspects of formulation, device design, device components, and manufacturing. Several classes of propellants have been considered as alternatives for use in pMDIs, but each has its disadvantages, as shown below, in a listing based on Leach.

Alternative propellant	*Disadvantage(s)*
Dimethylether	Flammable
Hydrocarbons	Flammable, high volatile organic compound content
Hydrochlorofluorocarbons	Some ozone depleting potential
Compressed gases (e.g., carbon dioxide and nitrogen)	Inconsistent pressure throughout the product life

So far, two alternative propellants, tetrafluoroethane (HFA-134a, CF_3CH_2F) and heptafluoropropane (HFA-227, CF_3CHFCF_3), have been successfully tested and developed as propellants in pMDIs. There are many similarities between pMDIs formulated with CFCs and HFAs, such as the operating principles and basic components. However, due to differences in the physical properties such as vapor pressure, density, and solvency characteristics, the pMDIs powered with HFA propellants encounter complex formulation challenges and the need for new hardware designs. The surfactants commonly used in the CFC-based pMDIs are oleic acid, sorbitan trioleate, and soya lecithin, which not only help to stabilize the formulation, but also help lubricate the metering valve system. These surfactants exhibit lower solubility when formulated with HFAs compared to CFCs. Therefore, sometimes a cosolvent will be added to the HFA formulation. New surfactants may need to be identified for drug formulations when using HFAs as propellants. However, with each change in product formulation, extensive testing is required before the product is approved for general clinical use.

Therefore, the phasing out of CFCs in pMDIs has provided an opportunity to improve the performance of the pMDIs and address the shortcomings of pMDI technology. Keller compared the performance of three different active compounds, beclomethasone dipropionate (BDP), budesonide, and di-sodium-cromo-glycate (DSCG), formulated with both CFC and HFA propellants. The HFA formulations were compared with three types of commercial devices, Becotide 100, Pulmicort, and Intal. The amount of drug deposited on the mouthpiece and USP throat was measured, and particle size distribution and fine particle dose were also determined accordingly. For the BDP formulation, the fine particle dose increased from 27 to about 61 μg and the drug lost in the mouthpiece and USP throat was reduced from 17 μg and 55 μg to about 8 μg and 22 μg respectively, when using the non-CFC formulation. The increase in the fine particle dose resulted from the reduction in the MMAD, which changed from 3.1 to about 1.4 μm. The particle size distribution of a suspension formulation is expected to be controlled mainly by the drug powder particles used in the formulation. For a solution formulation, particle size distribution is dictated by other factors such as formulation and device configurations. The fine particle dose was also increased for the budesonide formulation associated with a decrease in the amount of drug deposited in the USP throat, and the particle size distribution of budesonide delivered from both pMDIs changed slightly since both formulations were suspensions. Similar results were achieved for the DSCG compared with the Intal pMDI, except that the increase in fine particle dose was likely due to the decrease in the drug amount deposited in the mouthpiece.

These performance changes typically reduce the drug deposition in the oral-pharyngeal region, providing an added advantage of producing fewer steroid side effects such as candida infection and hoarseness of the throat.

pMDIs with breath activated function

The firing of the pMDI and inhalation by the patient have to be coordinated or "synchronized," because the drug aerosol is produced by the pMDI for a very short time only, in the order of milliseconds. This presents a challenge for patients to inhale and capture the aerosol as it is generated. It has been estimated that more than half of the patients (47–89%) receive little benefit from their pMDIs because of failure to coordinate the firing of the pMDIs and inhalation. A breath-activated pMDI has been developed to minimize the need for the actuation-inhalation coordination. This device is intended to reduce the performance variability of the pMDIs caused by differences in use techniques. The Autohaler is triggered by the patient's inhalation flow rate. To use the Autohaler, the patient turns a level on the top of the device that engages a spring mechanism to load the canister against a vane mechanism that is used between the canister and the actuator. When the patient's inspiratory flow rate exceeds 30 L/min, the vane moves and allows the canister to be pressed into the actuator to deliver the drug.

Newman conducted a clinical study to compare the performance of conventional pMDIs with the Autohaler using a scintigraphic technique to measure the drug deposition in the different sites of interest. The patients who participated in the study were divided into two groups classified as good coordinators and poor coordinators. Initially, patients used their own inhalers as base-line deposition values. The depositions were then measured after those patients were instructed about the proper inhalation technique when using their own inhaler and after using the Autohaler.

For the good coordinators, the deposition patterns were very similar for the patients using their own pMDIs and Autohaler, in which about 18% of the aerosol dose was deposited in the lungs and about 60% of the dose was deposited in the oral-pharyngeal region. There was a trend toward less deposition in the lungs after the patients had been taught the proper pMDI technique. It was possible that the patients had different abilities to familiarize themselves with the new technique as instructed during the study. There was a clear improvement in the lung deposition for the poor coordinators after they were given instruction or when they used the Autohaler, in which over 20% of the aerosol dose was deposited in the lungs. The increased lung deposition contributed to the improvement in the pulmonary function parameter, in which the FEV_1 increased significantly from the baseline.

New Pressure Driven Devices

Respimat

The agreement to eliminate the use of CFCs in pMDIs for respiratory medication has stimulated interest in the development of propellant-free inhaled drug delivery technology. The Respimat developed by Boehringer Ingelheim is one of the technologies under development. The device consists of a Uniblock, spring, drug cartridge with a capillary tube, and a non-return valve. The Uniblock is the major component of the device, which contains two nozzles positioned at opposing angles. The spring is the power source. Turning the lower part of the device, the rotation movement is transferred to a liner movement, which simultaneously tightens the spring and pushes the capillary tube with the non-return valve to the lower position. During this movement, about 13.5 μl of drug solution is drawn through the capillary to a pump chamber. When the patients press the release button, the mechanical force stored in the spring pushes the capillary tube and non-return valve to the upper position, driving the metered volume of drug solution through the two jet nozzles in the Uniblock, which generates two jets of liquid. The two jets are directed toward each other at a carefully controlled angle, and aerosol is generated by the impaction of the two jets.

Newman examined the deposition profiles in patients of several developmental Respimat prototypes using gamma scintigraphic techniques. In these studies, the deposition of the bronchodilator fenoterol and the corticosteroid flunisolide were examined. Fenoterol in the Respimat was formulated in an aqueous medium, and flunisolide was formulated in 96% ethanol.

The performance of the Respimat was clearly improved for the final prototype compared with Prototype III. Drug deposition in the lungs increased from approximately 31% to 39% for the fenoterol, and from about 40% to 45% for the drug compound of flunisolide respectively. At the same time, the oral-pharyngeal deposition decreased from approximately 54% to 37% for the fenoterol, and from 40% to about 16% for the flunisolide. Comparing the deposition data for the aqueous and ethanolic formulations, it can be seen that the ethanolic formulation had better performance, which may be due to the different particle size distribution for the formulations. The MMADs of the aerosols used in the Respimat were 2.0 ± 0.4 μm for the aqueous formulation and 1.0 ± 0.3 μm for the ethanolic formulation. The overall deposition efficiency of this device was apperently two to three times better than typically seen with pMDIs.

AeroEclipse

The AeroEclipse is a nebulizer powered by compressed air, which can be operated in both continuous nebulization and breath-actuated modes. The nebulizer was characterized, in vitro, using different breathing patterns, with either continuous nebulization or breath- actuated nebulization. A piston pump was used to mimic a range of breathing patterns in pediatric patients.

The average drug mass for the three breathing patterns were $11.1 \pm 0.74\%$ (P1), $22.9 \pm 2.74\%$ (P2), and $36.3 \pm 1.22\%$ (P3). The average mass median aerodynamic diameter was 3.55 ± 0.07 μm with the geometric standard deviation of 2.55. The test was also conducted to compare the device performance with other small-volume nebulizers, and found to be more efficient in the delivery rate (mass out per minute) than that of other SVNs.

AERx

The AERx, developed by Aradigm, is a metered dose liquid inhaler designed to deliver various pharmaceutical compounds to the peripheral lungs. The system consists of a unit dose disposable container equipped with a nozzle array, a piston assembly, and electronics associated with breath actuation and compliance monitoring functions.

The unit dose package contains the unit dose reservoir and an array of laser drilled nozzles, and the reservoir and nozzle array are connected with a heat seal that allows the formulation to flow from the reservoir to the nozzle after the seal is ruptured. The piston assembly consists of a motor, a piston, and a cam, which compresses the unit dose packet to extrude the drug under pressure through the nozzle array to produce aerosols suitable for inhalation. The AERx also has internal electronic monitoring, which measures the patient's inspiratory flow rate as a function of time of inspiration and triggers the dispensing of the dose at a predetermined inspiratory flow rate and time for optimal delivery. The dosage administered is also logged, thereby providing a record of treatments and an indication of patient compliance with therapy.

The performance of the AERx has been characterized both in vitro and in vivo. Schuster et al. reported in vitro experimental data of emitted dose as a function of inhalation flow rates from 20 to 100 L/min, and the emitted dose expressed as the percentage of loaded dose at different inhalation flow rates. The emitted dose was consistent at inhalation flow rates ranging from 30 to 70 L/min, which averaged approximately 60–70% of the loaded dose emitted from the device. The percentage of loaded dose emitted from the device was about 51% at the inhalation flow rate of 20L/min. When the device was used at this low flow rate, the aerosol was not efficiently entrained into the air, which was confirmed by a large fraction of the drug compound recovered from the air channel opposite the nozzle. The emitted dose was also decreased with the increase in the inhalation flow rate, which may have been due to increase in turbulent deposition as explained by the authors.

A study was also conducted both in vitro and in vivo to compare the performance of the AERx with a pMDI device that was operated with a SmartMist system for in vivo study using the scintigraphic technique.

The in vitro data showed that the fine particle fraction for the AERx was approximately 91% of emitted dose compared with 71% for the pMDI at the comparable emitted dose. The mass median aerodynamic diameter was 2.6 μm for the AERx and 1.2 μm for the pMDI, with a slightly larger GSD An experiment was conducted to compare the in vivo performance of both devices using scintigraphy. The average depositions (expressed as the percentage of loaded dose for the AERx and percentage of ex-valve dose for the pMDI) in the oral-pharynx and stomach were 6.9% with a relative standard deviation (RSD) of 47% for the AERx and 42% with a RSD of 16% for the pMDI respectively. The average depositions in the lungs were 53.3% (RSD = 10.9%) and 21.7 (RSD = 30.9%) for the AERx and the pMDI, respectively. The experimental data also showed that uniform drug distribution in the lungs was achieved while using the AERx (c/p = 1.15) as compared with that of the pMDI (c/p = 1.66), where the c/p ratio is defined as the ratio of drug deposition in the central region to that of peripheral region.

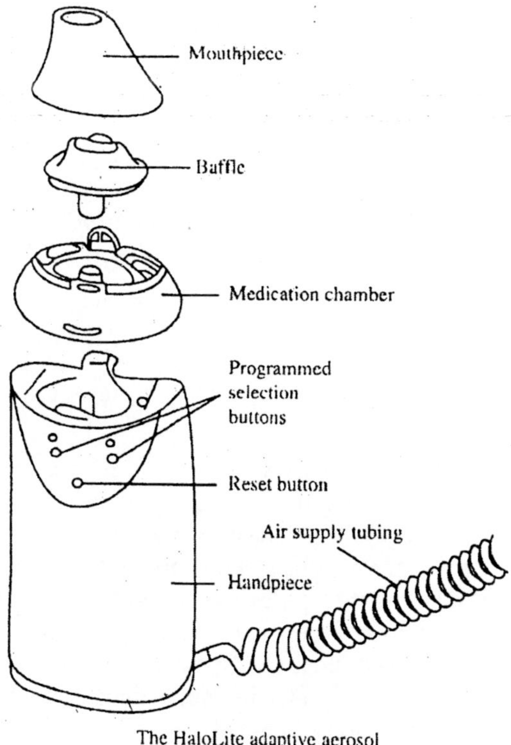

Fig. 16.3. The schematic diagram of the Halolite.

HaloLite

HaloLite is a hand-held drug delivery system developed by Medic-Aid. The device, which uses compressed air, consists of a medication chamber, a control unit, and an aerosol generation assembly that is operated by a portable, dedicated compressor. The aerosol is generated based upon conventional nebulization principles. The control unit allows the patient to select a budenoside nebulizing suspension, salbutamol, or terbutaline, since the device is calibrated to deliver preset doses of 50 μg of budenoside, 200 μg of salbutamol, or

500 μg of terbutaline from commercially available pre-mixed solution formulations of each drug. The device has the capability to analyze the patient's breathing pattern (flow rate, frequency, etc.) to determine (a) the aerosol pulse time for each inhalation; (b) whether the patient is inhaling or exhaling; (c) the start of inhalation; and d) trigger the aerosolization process.

In vitro experimental data show that the fine particle fraction (<5.0 μm) ranged from 70% to 80% of the device output, and the coefficient of variation for the dose output was 6% at a preset dose of 63 mg of 1% NaF solution. The device was also evaluated in vivo using healthy volunteers and asthmatics, and the coefficient of variations were 11% for the healthy volunteers and 21% for the asthmatics.

New High Frequency Oscillating Devices

AeroDose

The AeroDose is a battery-operated drug delivery device under development by AeroGen, Inc, which uses vibrating orifice technology to produce drug aerosols suitable for human inhalation. The device consists of a drug canister, aerosol generator assembly, and electronic control unit. The aerosol generator contains a dome-shaped aperture plate with 600 tapered holes that vibrate due to the attachment to a piezoelectric crystal. The piezoelectric material will undergo small physical displacement at ultrasonic frequency to generate aerosols with low velocity. During each use, a droplet of formulation (~15 μL) is dispensed from a multidose canister to an aperture plate by a metering pump, and an aerosol is then generated by breath activation.

Three AeroDose devices were characterized to determine the in vitro performance using albuterol sulfate with a nominal dose of 120 μg per actuation. The average liquid volume dispensed for three devices was 15.2 ml with a coefficient of variation (cv) of 2.7%. The emitted dose expressed as percentages of nominal doses were 80% (cv 5.9%), 81% (cv 3.7%), and 79% (cv 4.0%). The MMADs were 2.0 μm (cv 13%), 2.0 μm (cv 5.7%), and 1.9 μm (cv 21%), with GSDs of 2.1 (cv 7.2%), 2.2 (cv 4.5%), and 2.4 (cv 4.7%) for the three devices tested. A lung deposition study using ^{99m}Tc radiolabeled albuterol sulfate was also conducted to determine the amount of drug deposited in the lungs for both the AeroDose and the conventional pMDI. The average lung deposition was 18% (cv 32%) of the emitted dose for the pMDI and 70% (cv 28%) of the emitted dose or an overall delivery efficiency of approximately 56% for the AeroDose for the six volunteers who participated in the study.

Metered solution inhaler (MSI)

The metered solution inhaler (MSI), under development by Sheffield Pharmaceuticals, uses the same aerosolization principle as the AeroDose. Using a motorized pump, drug solution is delivered to the surface of a ultrasonic horn powered by a piezoelectric crystal upon actuation, and is then aerosolized in about 1 s.

The performance of the MSI was characterized in vivo using morphine sulfate for systemic absorption. A total of 1.25 mg of morphine sulfate was delivered in five doses of 250 μg per actuation to the healthy volunteers. The average amount of drug deposited was approximately 800 *pg* in the lungs and less than about 500 μg in the oral-pharynx; therefore the average respiratory deposition efficiency was approximately 64% of the inhaled dose. The average amount of drug deposited in the peripheral respire to region was slightly over 300 μg, a little less than 300 μg was deposited in the intermediate lung, and about 200 μg was deposited in the central region. The ratio of deposition in the peripheral to central regions ranged from 1.1 to 2.2. The morphine sulfate concentration in the plasma reached a peak within 3 min after inhalation, compared with 15 min for the subcutaneous injection. The peak plasma concentration level for the inhalation route was more than double compared to the subcutaneous route.

Vibrating membrane nebulizer

The vibrating membrane nebulizer is currently under development by Pari GmbH, which is based upon the TouchSpray technology developed by The Technology Partnership plc. The main aerosol generation principle is similar to that of AeroDose, which uses piezoelectric material as a power source to vibrate a surface having on it a droplet of drug solution. The membrane is a circular, wafer-thin metal plate with small holes. A ring-shaped piezoelectric actuator excites the membrane to vibrate, thus ejecting the fluid through the holes as droplets and creating aerosols. Unlike the AeroDose, which is a single-dose device, the vibrating membrane nebulizer is a continuous generation device similar to the conventional nebulizer, which produces aerosols during both inhalation and exhalation.

Experimental data obtained from in vitro testing using a functional model of the vibrating membrane nebulizer showed that the average percentage of emitted dose for a continuous aerosolization in approximately 8min was about 79% of dose loaded in the device, and the output rate of the delivery device was found to be about 238 μg/min. The mass median diameter measured by the Malvern Diffraction Sizer was 4.6 μm. It was also found that the cumulative output from the device was linearly proportional to the time of aerosolization, which implied a constant output rate throughout the entire aerosolization process. Experimental data obtained from a prototype device developed based upon the functional model showed a reduction from 79 to about 50% in the emitted dose of the device. The amount of drug left in the device increased from 477 to about 1060 mg, which changed from 19 to 43% in terms of percentage to the loaded dose. The increase in the drug amount left in the device reduced the delivery efficiency of the device. The delivery efficiency can be improved by redesigning the flow channel and incorporating a breath-activated function to eliminate the aerosolization process during exhalation, as suggested by the authors.

Novel Electrohydrodynamic (EHD) Devices

Electrohydrodynamic (EHD) aerosolization is a process of the disruption of a liquid surface into a spray of droplets when subjected to an electric field. The liquid meniscus at the outlet of a capillary tube takes a conical shape under the action of the electric field. The cone tip breaks up into a spray of fine, charged aerosol. The cone-jet mode offers the appealing feature of aerosol monodispersity. It can produce droplets/particles over a wide size range, from sub- micron to hundreds of microns in size, depending on liquid flow rate, applied voltages, and physical and chemical properties of the liquid. When considering the size range of interest to pulmonary drug delivery (1-5 μm), the production of monodispersed aerosols with relative ease by EHD aerosolization technology is unmatched by any other aerosol generation process.

Additionally, the aerosols are generated from capillary nozzles having relatively large diameters (e.g., 100 μm), which are therefore, unlikely to clog at the atomization site or during the metering of each dose. When considering the particle size range of 1–5 μm, the capacity to produce monodispersed aerosols with relative ease by EHD is also unmatched by any other aerosol generation process. The particle size distribution of the aerosol can be controlled by adjusting a number of variables, such as physical and chemical properties of drug formulations, operating conditions, and electric field. Another key clinical and technical attribute of the EHD technology is that it delivers a soft (isokinetic) aerosol cloud of nearly monodispersed particles to the patient, because aerosol formation does not require any liquid propellants or other pressurized systems. The EHD process can aerosolize a broad range of drug formulations, requires low precision manufacturing (i.e., low-cost production), and is amenable to miniaturization.

These fundamental features underpin the ability of EHD pulmonary drug delivery devices to aerosolize a wide array of drug formulations, and provide accurate, reproducible drug delivery with targeted dosing to the human respiratory tract. Battelle Pulmonary Therapeutics, Inc. (BPT) is currently developing an array of EHD pulmonary devices, ranging from small hand-held disposable units, home table-top aerosol delivery devices to large benchtop clinical devices designed to operate continuously with high outputs.

In vitro performance

Prior to clinical evaluations, comprehensive studies were conducted to characterize prototype EHD pulmonary drug delivery devices for emitted dose uniformity and reproducibility of particle size distribution. The nominal dose is defined as the amount of active drug metered as a liquid solution from the device. The emitted dose is the amount of aerosolized drug obtained at the exit of the mouthpiece, and the device delivery efficiency is the ratio of the emitted to nominal dose. The mean delivery efficiency was approximately 94% (SD = 3.2) with a 3.4% coefficient of variation. The delivery efficiency for the two devices tested was 93% (SD = 3.60, $n = 5$) and 95% (SD = 2.8, $n = 5$), respectively. The intradevice variation was 1.7% (coefficient of variation, n = 2 prototypes). There were no significant differences ($p > 0.05$) in the drug mass output within the device throughout its life cycle, nor between devices tested in the study.

The drug mass recovered from the various stages of the impactor and device at a nominal drug dose of 75 μg per actuation. The amount of drug deposited on each stage was used to calculate the MMAD and GSD. The calculated MMAD was 2.85 μm with a GSD of 1.6. The fine particle fraction (FPF) of the aerosol was 90% (<5.8 μm) of the emitted dose, and 95% (<5.8 μm) of the dose distal to the USP throat.

In vivo performance

A Phase I clinical study was conducted to evaluate the performance of the prototype EHD pulmonary drug delivery device in healthy volunteers. The EHD device was compared with a commercially available capsule dry powder inhaler (DPI). The NCE was prepared in two formulations. The first was a powder formulation specific for the DPI, and the second was formulated in a liquid solution for the EHD device. Each formulation was radiolabelled with ^{99m}Tc, and the amount of drug deposited in the lungs from each device was quantified using gamma scintigraphy. Each volunteer was administered one dose of drug using the DPI and three different doses using the EHD device. The nominal doses were 1000 μg for the DPI and 150, 250, and 400 μg for the EHD device. Multiple blood samples were collected from each subject up to 8 h after dosing to measure plasma drug concentration. An interval of 1 week was used between administration of the four doses.

The average whole lung deposition efficiency for the EHD device expressed as the percentage of the emitted dose was approximately 78% (cv 7.3%) for the 400 μg dose. It can be seen that the EHD pulmonary drug delivery device produced a uniform deposition distribution through the lung field with only ~16% deposition in the oral-pharyngeal region, and virtually no drug in the GI tract. However, the amount of drug deposited in the oral-pharyngeal region using the DPI averaged 67% of metered dose, which was nearly 6 times higher compared with that of the high dose delivered using the EHD device. The AUC for plasma drug concentration with the DPI was approximately 20% higher than that of the EHD device for a comparable deposited pulmonary dose. It appeared that the higher systemic exposure resulting from the DPI was likely due to absorption from the throat and GI tract.

Performance Comparisons

Comparison of the performance of various drug delivery devices based upon the data published in the literature is often difficult because of inconsistency in the experimental methods used in the characterization of those devices as well as differences in the devices. However it is also extremely important to understand the different features of the devices to help select the best device for a drug compound intended for delivery through the human respiratory tract.

The selection of a drug delivery system suitable for the administration of a particular drug compound to human respiratory airways depends not only on the device performance, but also on many other factors such as drug properties, formulation excipient, intended site of action, marketing preference, and regulatory requirements. It is important to fully understand the drug properties during the formulation development so that a proper excipient system can be identified. The selection of an excipient for a particular drug also influences the particle size distribution of aerosol generated from a drug delivery device. For example, increasing the volatile components in the solution formulation can reduce the diameter of aerosol particles because of solvent evaporation, which is another variable available to optimize drug formulation and device performance for either local delivery or systemic absorption. The stability of drug product in the long term (usually ~2 years) has also to be considered in the device selection process. Some drug compounds can only be packaged in a unit dose because of instability of the drug product in the multidose reservoir; therefore, a device that can be fitted with a unit dose package is needed for such purpose. The drug delivery devices mentioned above have different features and different requirements for the drug formulation, and there is no single delivery device that can meet all the needs for such requirements. To ensure a successful launch of a new inhalation drug product, it is necessary to conduct a comprehensive evaluation of a potential drug candidate for administrating via inhalation.

Liquid Oral Preparations

Various types of formulations, both aqueous and non-aqueous, have been placed under the rubric of "*liquid oral preparations*," including solutions, suspensions, and emulsions. These formulations are primarily employed to enhance the oral bioavailability of a therapeutic or eliminate the need for a patient to swallow a tablet or capsule. Compared with traditional solid-state dosage forms, a unique set of considerations is required during the design and formulation of oral solutions. The drug must first be rendered soluble, possibly requiring the use of solubility-enhancing additives. Once dissolved, care must be taken to limit the increased sensitivity of the solubilized drug to degradation and to prevent microbial growth in the aqueous, often nutrient-rich formulation. In addition, certain components are added to provide palatability. Here, the use of solutions for oral drug delivery is discussed with emphasis on application, design of formulations, stability, components, and manufacture.

Oral Solution Drug Delivery

Oral solutions are homogeneous mixtures of one or more solutes, dissolved in a suitable solvent or mixture of mutually miscible solvents. In pharmaceutical terms, solutions are defined as "liquid preparations that contain one or more soluble chemical substances, usually dissolved in water and they do not, by reasons of their ingredients, method of preparation, or use, fall into another group of products." Oral solutions are typically classified on the basis of their physical properties, method of preparation, use, and ingredient types or concentrations. Owing to the overlap in the definitions, distinctions among solution types can be ambiguous and hence, in some instances, definitions are irrelevant for commercial products. Solutions are marketed for oral delivery of many pharmaceutical agents including Amprenavir, Calcitriol, Cyclosporin A, Digoxin, Itraconazole, Lopinavir, Ritonavir, Loratadine, Risperidone, Ritonavir, and Sirolimus.

Applications

Liquid oral solutions are useful in oral drug delivery for a variety of reasons. Patient compliance is often problematic with oral solid dosage forms, especially with young children and the elderly. This refusal to accept medication may stem from difficulties experienced within these age groups in swallowing tablets or capsules. Such difficulties can be overcome by administering the active compound in a palatable liquid form. An oral liquid can be readily administered to children and the elderly who are unable to swallow. Furthermore, because solutions are homogenous mixtures, the medication is uniformly distributed throughout the preparation. The dose can be fractionally adjusted by simply diluting it to meet the needs of patients. Liquid extracts eliminate the need to isolate the drug in pure form, allowing several ingredients to be administered from a single source (e.g., pancreatic extract) and permit preliminary study of drugs from natural sources. In addition, some deliquescent and hygroscopic powders are easily dispensed as liquids.

The fact that drugs are rendered soluble in oral pharmaceutical liquids is advantageous in enhancing drug absorption. Because drugs are absorbed in the dissolved state, the rate and efficiency of absorption of oral dosage forms usually decreases in the following order: aqueous solution > aqueous suspension > tablets or capsules. A drug administered in solution is immediately available for absorption from the gastrointestinal tract and is more rapidly and efficiently absorbed than the same amount of drug administered in a solid dosage form such as tablets or capsules. Some drugs not tolerated in a concentrated form may be less irritating if dissolved in soothing liquid. Occasionally, solutions of drugs, such as potassium chloride, are used to minimize adverse effects in the gastrointestinal tract by avoiding longer transit times observed with solid formulations.

Limitations

Oral delivery of drugs via solutions is not free from limitations. Drug substances are generally less stable in liquid media compared with solid dosage forms. Furthermore, special techniques are often required to solubilize poorly soluble drugs. Masking the taste of inherently bitter drugs can be difficult. Also, improvements in the palatability or pourability of liquid formulations may require the addition of viscosity-increasing agents, which may themselves form complexes with drug molecules and hence result in undesired mitigations in drug activity. Extremely potent drugs with low-therapeutic indexes may be problematic when dosed in oral liquid preparations as the patients could easily err in dosage measurement. As with other oral dosage forms, liquid oral preparations cannot be administered to the unconscious patient.

Design and Formulation

Design of liquid oral solutions involves the combination of ingredients with therapeutically active agents to enhance the acceptability or effectiveness of the product. The formulation of pharmaceutical liquids requires several considerations: drug concentration; drug solubility; liquid vehicle selection; physical and chemical stability; preparation preservation; and appropriate additives such as buffers, solubilizers, sweetening agents, viscosity-controlling agents, colors, and flavors.

Pharmacists can handle liquid preparations in one of three ways: They may dispense the product in its original container; they may buy the product in bulk and repackage it at the time of dispensation; or they may compound a solution. Compounding may involve nothing more than mixing two marketed products in the manner indicated on the prescription or may require the incorporation of an active ingredient in a logical and pharmaceutically acceptable manner into aqueous or non-aqueous solvents forming the bulk of the product. Most prescriptions today are dispensed in their original containers. In these cases, the pharmacist depends on the manufacturer to provide a product that is efficacious, pharmaceutically acceptable, and stable when stored under recommended conditions.

Drug manufacturers attempt to guarantee efficacy by evaluating their products in a scientifically acceptable manner. However, in some instances, such efficacy is relative. For example, cough mixtures marketed by different manufacturers may contain active ingredients of the same therapeutic class and concentration. It therefore becomes difficult to assess the relative merit of the products. In such cases, the commercial advantages gained by one over another may be based on other product's characteristics. Thus, color, odor, taste, pourability, and homogeneity are important pharmaceutical properties. Hence, the successful design and formulation of liquids, as well as other dosage forms, require both scientific and pharmaceutical acuity.

Solubility

Solubility is of paramount importance when developing oral solutions. The drug and other dissolved substances should remain solubilized throughout the shelf life of the product. Therefore, the drugs are present in solution at unsaturated concentrations; otherwise, the drug may crystallize because of changes in temperature, by "*seeding*" from ingredients, or particulate matter present. Furthermore, the taste of organic drugs has been shown to be a direct function of aqueous solubility. For example, increasing the chain length of clindamycin esters reduces the aqueous solubility and dramatically improves the taste.

The solubility of most solids is temperature dependent, and the influence of temperature on solubility should be characterized for a given solute in a pharmaceutical liquid. In addition to room-temperature equilibrium solubility studies, it is important to determine solubility at refrigeration temperature (2–8°C) to establish the usable concentration in the range of 2–25°C without the risk of saturation and crystal growth. This procedure is necessary to cover wide temperature ranges that the product may be exposed to during normal the distribution process.

Effect of pH

Substances with acidic or basic functionality show differences in solubility characteristics with changes in solution pH in accordance with their ionization constants. These differences are often large and important in attaining desired concentrations in the formulation. Solubility-pH profiles can be established by conducting equilibrium solubility experiments covering the range of 3–4 pH units on both sides of the pK_a or pK_b; results are presented in the form of solubility as a function of pH.

The relationship between solubility of an acidic drug and pH is defined with respect to its pK_a as in Eq. (11):

$$pH = pK_a + \log\frac{[C_s]}{[C_a]} \quad ...(11)$$

where pK_a is the negative logarithm of the ionization constant of the acid, $[C_s]$ the molar concentration of the salt form in water, and $[C_a]$ the molar concentration of free acid in water. Thus, the total solubility S_T of a weak acid is given by Eq. (12):

$$S_T = [C_a] + [C_s] \quad ...(12)$$

Rearrangement and substitution of Eqs. (11) and (12) yields Eqs. (13) and (14), respectively

$$H^+ = K_a + \frac{S_T - S_o}{S_o} \quad ...(13)$$

$$S_T = S_o\left(1 + \frac{H^+}{K_a}\right) \quad ...(14)$$

where S_o is the solubility of the free acid.

Once the values of pK_a, $[C_a]$, and pH are known, the total amount of drug solubilized in water at a specific pH can be calculated. Substantial increases in aqueous solubility can be achieved simply by adjusting the pH. In fact, adjustment of greater than 3 pH units in the appropriate direction (weak bases solubilize at lower pH and weak acids at higher pH) away from the pK_a may result in more than 1000-fold increases over the intrinsic solubility of a drug. Analogous equations can be written for weak bases such as Eqs. (15) and (16).

$$S_T = [C_b] + [C_s] \quad ...(15)$$

$$H^+ = K_w + K_b + \frac{S_o}{S_T - S_o} \quad ...(16)$$

where S_0 is the solubility of free base and pK_w is the ionization constant of water.

Effect of temperature

For the majority of solids, solubilization is temperature dependent and increases in elevated temperatures as heat is absorbed during solubilizing. The degree to which temperature can influence solubility is dictated by the differential heat of solution, ΔHS, which represents the rate of heat change of a solution per mole of solute dissolved. The higher the heat of solution, the greater the influence of temperature on solubility, as shown by Eq. (17).

$$\frac{d \ln S}{dt} = \frac{\Delta H_S}{RT^2} \quad ...(17)$$

where S is the solubility of concentration of a saturated solution, often expressed in terms of molality, molarity, or mole fraction; R is the gas constant; and T is the absolute temperature. Eq. (17) can also be written as in Eq. (18).

$$\log S = \frac{-\Delta H_S}{2.303R} \frac{1}{T} + \text{constant} \quad ...(18)$$

By plotting the logarithm of the solubility in moles per liter vs. the reciprocal of the absolute temperature, the differential heat of solution can be calculated as the slope (-ΔHS/2.303 R). A positive heat of solution indicates an endothermic solubilization process (i.e., absorbs heat). Therefore, an increase in temperature increases solubility. A negative value indicates an exothermic solubilization process (i.e., emits heat) and a differential heat of solution near zero indicates that solubility is not significantly influenced by temperature.

Effect of solvent polarity

The solubility of the drug substance is attributable in large part to the polarity of the solvent, often expressed in terms of dipole moment, related to the dielectric constant. Solvents with high dielectric constants dissolve ionic compounds (polar drugs) readily by virtue of ion-dipole interactions, whereas solvents with low dielectric constants dissolve hydrophobic substances (non-polar drugs) as a result of dipole or induced dipole interactions. The former is classified as polar solvents, with examples such as water and glycerin; the latter are non-polar solvents, with example such as oils. Solvents with intermediate dielectric constants are classified as semipolar.

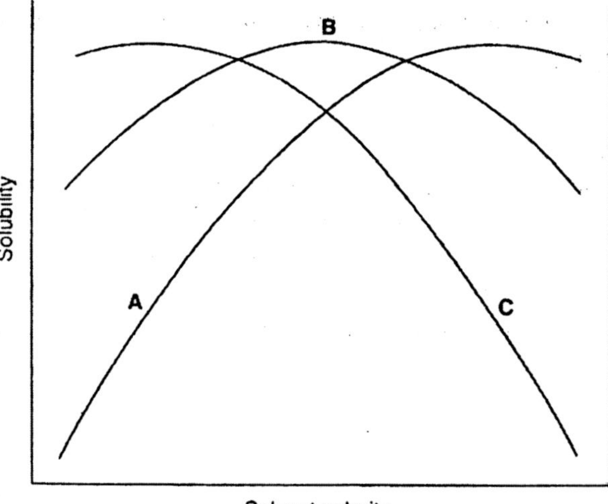

Fig. 16.4. Influence of solvent polarity on the solubility of drug: (A) Polar drug; (B) semipolar drug; and (C) nonpolar drug.

Effect of molecular structure

Variations in lattice energies between amorphous and crystalline forms can significantly influence a drug's aqueous solubility, and increases of several hundred-fold were observed for morphine and benzimidazole derivatives. Furthermore, a substance may exist in more than one crystalline form, such as chloramphenicol, dehydroepiandrosterone (DHEA), progesterone, sulfathiazole, carbamazepine, cortisone, or prednisolone, to name a few. Polymorphic transformations, routinely observed for pharmaceuticals, are structural differences resulting from different crystal arrangements of molecules in the solid state. Although thermodynamic differences between polymorphs disappear once dissolved, solid-state disparities in internal crystal structure between polymorphs may yield vastly different physicochemical properties; changes may include melting point, chemical stability, solubility, enthalpy, dissolution rate, and color to name a few. In fact, the Gibbs free energy difference (ΔG) between two polymorphs (A and B) is directly related to solubility of each polymorph (S_a and S_b) by Eq. (19).

$$\Delta G = -RT\ln\left(\frac{S_a}{S_b}\right) \qquad ...(19)$$

The most-stable crystal always possesses the lowest free energy (also the lowest solubility) and is the judicious choice when developing stable suspensions. Therefore, delineating the thermodynamic differences between polymorphs is of great interest for development of solid-state dosage forms and for predicting solubility of drugs to be delivered orally via solutions.

Solubilization Techniques

Often the desired drug concentration in a liquid dosage form cannot be reached because of the drug's low water solubility. In fact, poor aqueous solubility is observed in many drug candidates selected by high- throughput screening, as lipophilic moieties are frequently necessary for receptor binding. Solubilization is the process by which the apparent solubility of a poorly water-soluble substance is increased. Solubilization techniques include cosolvency, salt formation, prodrug design, complexation, particle size reduction, and the use of surface-active agents (micellization).

Cosolvency

Cosolvents are defined as water-miscible organic solvents added in liquid drug formulations to increase the solubility of poorly water-soluble compounds. Cosolvency, then, refers to the technique of using cosolvents to lower the free energy of a molecule in solution per number of molecules dissolved in solution (known as chemical potential). The need to use cosolvents in the formulation of new drugs as solutions remains high, especially with increasing structural complexity and lipophilicity of new therapeutic agents. Molecules lacking ionizable groups (or with ionizable groups too low or high for pH adjustment) cannot be rendered more water soluble via pH adjustment, and cosolvency is frequently employed for solubilization.

Cosolvency is highly effective in increasing drug solubility. Advantages include large increases in drug solubility and simplicity. Previously, ethanol was the most commonly used solvent in oral preparations because of its excellent solvent properties for many non-polar drugs, as well as its favorable taste. Its use is often undesirable, however, in preparations intended for pediatric patients. Ethanol may also accentuate the saline taste of ionic solutes. Sorbitol, glycerin, propylene glycol, and several polyethylene glycol polymers are cosolvents that are both useful and acceptable in the formulation of oral liquids. Cosolvents are used not only to affect solubility of the drug but also to improve the solubility of volatile constituents used to impart a desirable flavor or odor to the product. The primary limitation of cosolvency is toxicity of many water-miscible solvents, having high potential for increasing drug solubility. Toxicological properties of solvents limiting or eliminating their use in drug formulations include general toxicity, target organ toxicity, or tissue irritation. Even if found relatively non-toxic, a cosolvent is rarely administered neat (100%) because of poor taste or objectionable odor. Although a cosolvent may increase the solubility of the drug, it may also affect the solubility of other polar or ionic components of the formulation such as buffer materials.

Early formulation work on cosolvency involved an empirical approach for choosing the type and amount of cosolvent for a liquid vehicle. An improvement in the purely empirical approach was the introduction of alligation methods that could be used to reformulate vehicles based on experimental formulation or solubility data. Moore, reported a method using approximate dielectric constants of the pure and mixed solvents. The basic assumption is that all vehicles with the same dielectric constant solubilize a given drug to the same extent. However, the dielectric constant alone is a poor predictor of the degree of drug solubility. Rubino has described various mechanisms and equations that were derived with the objective of establishing a basic understanding of and developing a mathematical approach for interpreting and predicting drug solubility behavior.

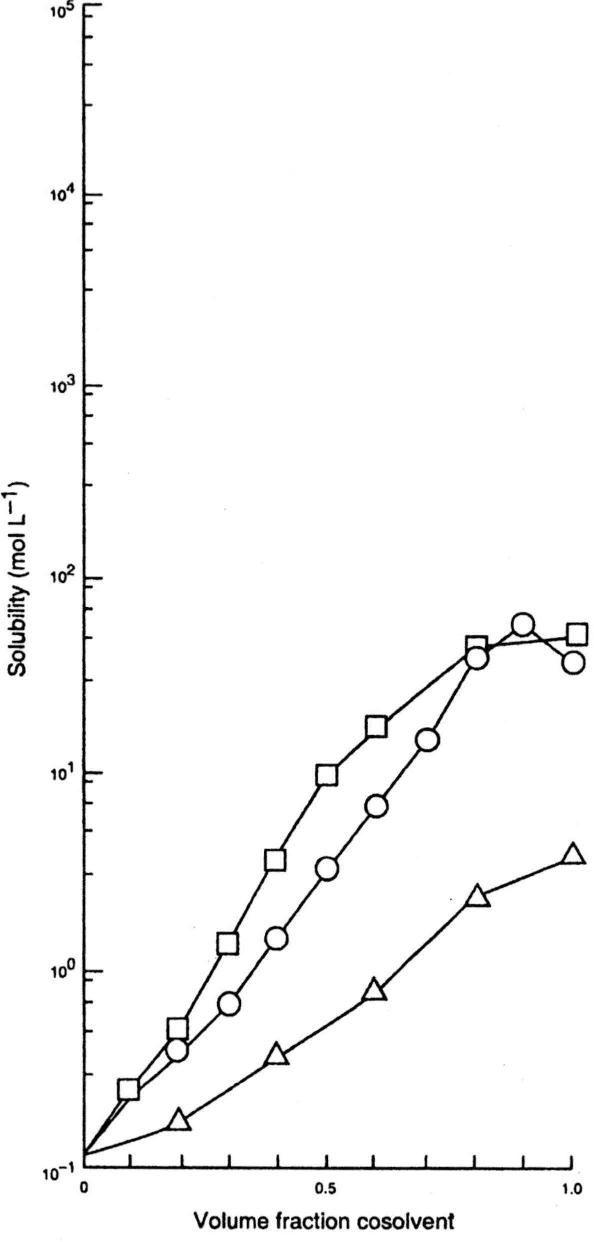

Fig. 16.5. Solubilization of alprazolam by ethanol, propylene glycol, and glycerin.

Salt Formation

Many poorly soluble, ionizable drugs can be readily solubilized through salt formation. Salt forms are regularly selected to serve as self-buffers and enhance the dissolution rates over the cognate conjugate acids and bases by altering pH of the diffusion layer. In fact, salt formation can drastically alter the physicochemical properties of a drug in the solid state, which govern solubility. For example, the compound α[-(2-Piperidyl) β-3,6-bis-(trifluoromethyl]-9-Phenan-threnemethanol, an antimalarial agent, and its hydrochloride salt are both only slightly soluble in water. However, its lactate salt is approximately 200 times more soluble than the hydrochloride. This enhanced aqueous solubility is attributed in part to the decrease in crystal lattice energy, as indicated by a reduction in the melting point. Furthermore, if a particular salt form cannot be isolated because of its high solubility, the same end result (i.e., desired aqueous solubility) can be achieved by in situ salt formation. This is accomplished by using an appropriate acid or base to adjust the pH level while formulating the drug product solution.

Prodrug Method

The solubility characteristics of a drug can be altered by chemical modification; this is referred to as the "prodrug" approach. The term was first used by Albert in 1958 for a compound that undergoes biotransformation before eliciting a pharmacological response. This method has been successful in the case of corticosteroids and recent prodrug blockbusters including omeprazole, simvastatin, lovastatin, and aciclovir to name a few. The addition of a cleavable moiety (known as a promoiety) can help to overcome carriers to bioavailability caused by undesirable physicochemical properties inherent to a drug.

Specifically, the addition of charged groups (including esters, aminoacetyl, and acetates) or neutral polyethylene glycol moieties has increased the aqueous solubility of drugs. For example, the solubility of betamethasone in water is 58 μg/ml at 25°C. The solubility of its disodium phosphate ester (a charged ester promoiety) is more than 100 mg/ml, an increase in water solubility greater than 1500-fold. Also, an acetylated sulfonamide moiety enhanced the aqueous solubility of the poorly water-soluble sodium salt of the COX-2 inhibitor Parecoxib ~300-fold. Further examples of drugs with promoieties added to increase the aqueous solubility include celecoxib, fosphenytoin, and paclitaxel. Although methods such as salt and prodrug formation can result in high increases in aqueous solubility, they require synthesis of essentially new drug entities, and additional animal studies to confirm their efficacy and safety. Thus, an undertaking of this magnitude can be justified when no other reasonable approach is available.

Complexation

Complexation is another means of improving the aqueous solubility of insoluble compounds; it is described by Eq. (20)

$$\mathrm{n}[D]_s + \mathrm{m}[L]_s \rightarrow [D_n : L_m]_s \qquad \ldots(20)$$

where $[D]_s$ = concentration of drug in solution; $[L]_s$ = concentration of ligand in solution; and $[D_n : L_m]s$ = concentration of the drug–ligand complex solution.

A complex is an entity formed when two molecules, such as a drug and a solubilizing agent (ligand), are bound by weak forces (e.g., dipole–dipole interaction or hydrogen bonding). For complex formation to occur, drug and ligand molecules must be able to donate or accept a pair of electrons. Complexation can drastically alter or mask the physicochemical properties of a drug substance. Cyclodextrins are commonly employed as ligands to mask undesirable properties of drugs by forming inclusion complexes. In essence, an equilibrium process dictates complex formation where the drug complexes with a methylene- rich hydrophobic cavity inside the cyclodextrin ring. In addition to increasing aqueous solubility, cyclodextrins have been shown to enhance taste, bioavailability, safety, and other undesirable properties of liquid oral formulations.

In general, complexation has several advantages such as reversibility of these interactions. Complex dissociation to individual reactants occurs rapidly and spontaneously on dilution. Consequently, the biological effects of complexes can be predicted based on knowledge of the pharmacological properties of each of the reactants. Another advantage is the predictability and physical stability of these systems. Because complex formation involves equilibrium attainment, once the necessary data defining the system parameters such as stability constants and solubility properties of the complexes have been gathered, the behavior of the system is reproducible and predictable. This contrasts with polymorphs and other crystal modifications, which can be thermodynamically unstable; they may also undergo unpredictable time-dependent changes leading to changes in solubility behavior.

The disadvantage of complexation is the requirement for ligands to be present in molar ratios equivalent to or higher than those of the drug. The ligand could have sensory or pharmacological effects deemed unacceptable. The formulator must also take into account detrimental interactions of the ligand with the excipients. Furthermore, the apparent solubility increase realized by complexation compared with other techniques is usually less by an order of magnitude. Therefore, complexation is usually employed when pH adjustment and cosolvents fail to provide adequate aqueous solubility.

Micellization

Micellization has been defined by McBain as the spontaneous passage of poorly water-soluble solute molecules into an aqueous solution of a soap or a detergent in which a thermodynamically stable solution is formed. Mechanistically, this phenomenon has been extensively investigated and surface-active agents have been shown to form colloidal aggregates, known as micelles. When surfactants (amphiphilic polymers containing hydrophobic and hydrophilic moieties) are initially added to liquids at low concentrations, they tend to orient at the air–liquid interface. As additional surfactants are added, the interface becomes fully occupied, and excess molecules are forced into the bulk of the liquid. At still higher concentrations, molecules of surfactant in the liquid bulk begin to form oriented aggregates or micelles; this change in orientation occurs abruptly, and the concentration of surfactant in which it occurs is known as the critical micelle concentration (CMC). Solubilization may occur by virtue of solute entrapment in or absorption onto the hydrophobic interior of the micelle. Thus, the ability of surfactant solutions to dissolve or solubilize water- insoluble materials initiates at the CMC and increases with the concentration of the micelles. One obvious caveat in utilizing micelles for drug solubilization is that exposure to biological fluids may dilute the surfactant below the CMC causing drug precipitation.

It has been observed that lyophilic surface-active agents with hydrophilic–lipophilic balance (HLB) values above 15 are the best solubilizing agents. Commonly used solubilizing agents in pharmaceutical systems include polyoxyethylene sorbitan fatty acid esters (Tween series), polyoxyethylene monoalkyl ethers (BRIJ and MYRJ series), and sorbitan fatty acid esters (Span series). The choice of solubilizing agents is based on phase-solubility studies in which drug solubility is determined as a function of surfactant concentration; several surfactants are often included in these studies. The appropriate surfactant can then be selected based on its efficacy as a solubilizer and effect on other product characteristics and formulation adjuvants.

Stability

Drug substances are generally more susceptible to degradation in liquids than in solid dosage forms. As a class of formulations, oral liquids are more complex in composition than parenterals, and more interactions may occur affecting the stability of the product. It is necessary to not only consider the solution stability of the drug, but also the stability of excipients such as colorants, flavors, preservatives, solubilizers, thickening agents, and sweetening agents.

Chemical Stability

The techniques for predicting the chemical stability of homogeneous drug systems are well defined. The formulation chemist should consider both the pH-solubility profile and the pH-stability profile when selecting the optimum pH for formulation of the liquid oral dosage form. The optimum pH for formulating an acetazolamide liquid dosage form would be at approximately pH 4, the pH of optimum stability, although the solubility above pH 7 is better because of sodium salt formation.

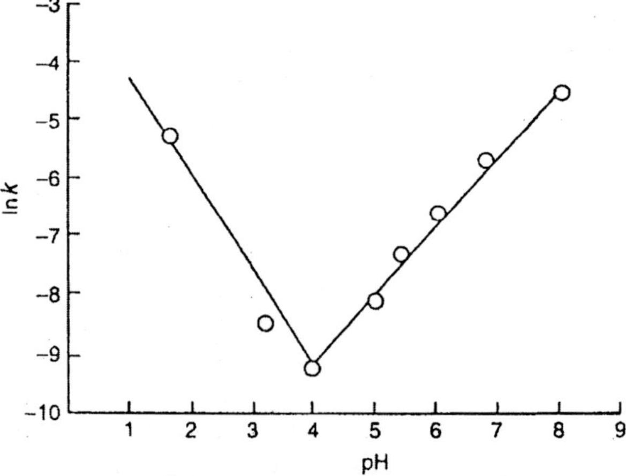

Fig. 16.6. pH-stability profile of acetazolamide.

Physical Stability

Physical instability of liquid formulations involves the formation of precipitates, less-soluble polymorphs, adsorption of the drug substances onto container surfaces, microbial growth, and changes in product appearance. Evaluation of product acceptability is subjective and includes properties such as color, odor, taste, and clarity. Dye stability depends on the excipients used in the formulation. For example, Food, Drug, and Cosmetics (FD&C) Blue No. 2 has been found to fade more rapidly in the presence of several sugars (sorbitol, mannitol, dextrose, sucrose, and lactose). In addition, trace amounts of impurities and non-ionic surfactants such as pluronic F-68 contribute to fading.

Certain preservatives are physically unstable with certain macromolecules. For example, adsorption of methyl *p*-Hydroxybenzoate to nylon was found to be dependent on nylon membrane size and the concentration of free methylparaben. The complexation of methyl *p*-Hydroxybenzoate with Tween 80 depends on the amount of free methylparaben and the concentration of Tween 80. Similar results have been reported for propyl *p*-Hydroxybenzoate.

Components and Additives

Sweetening Agents

Sweeteners are indispensable components of many liquid oral dosage forms, especially those containing bitter or other unacceptable tastes. In fact, sweetening agents may comprise large portions of solid content in most liquid oral dosage forms. Sweeteners are often classified as either nutritive (caloric) or non-nutritive (non-caloric). Non-caloric sweetening agents are preferred for diabetic patients, as ingestion does cause increases in systemic glucose concentrations. Some of the most commonly used sweeteners include sucrose, sorbitol, mannitol, liquid glucose, honey molasses, saccharin, aspartame, sucralose, and acesulphame-K. The types and concentrations of sweeteners for common prescription liquid medications are reported by Hill, Flaitz, and Frost.

Sucrose is the most widely used sweetener, with a long history of use. It is a white crystalline powder, soluble in water and alcohol. It inhibits the growth of microorganisms in solution at sucrose concentrations above 65 wt% by reducing the water-activity coefficient. Official simple syrup is an 85% w/v solution of sucrose in water. During the preparation of sucrose solution, care should be taken to avoid charring and caramelization caused by heat. Sucrose is chemically and physically stable in the pH range of 4.0–8.0. It is frequently used in conjunction with sorbitol, glycerin, and other polyols, which reduce its tendency to crystallize. One of the manifestations of the sucrose crystallization is "*cap-locking*," which occurs when sucrose crystallizes on the threads of the bottle cap and interferes with opening.

Liquid glucose is an extremely viscid substance that imparts both body and sweetness to liquid formulations. It is obtained by the incomplete hydrolysis of starch and consists chiefly of dextrose, dextrins, maltose, and water. It imparts a characteristic odor and flavor to the formulation in similar fashion to honey and molasses, but to a lesser degree. Although liquid glucose is not a pure chemical entity, its method of manufacture can be well controlled, and batch-to-batch variability is usually not significantly problematic. The same is not true of honey and molasses, in which quality depends on uncontrollable natural factors.

Saccharin is a non-nutritive synthetic sweetening agent. It has approximately 500 times the sweetening power of sucrose, depending in extent on the strength of the solution. The relative sweetening power is greatest in dilute solution. Saccharin is a sucrose substitute for diabetics, the obese, and others who do not wish to ingest sucrose. It is commonly found in its sodium salt form, which is more palatable than saccharin and comparatively free of unpleasant aftertaste. Sodium cyclamate is another synthetic sweetening agent that is approximately 30 times as sweet as sugar. However, its use as an artificial sweetener is banned in the U.S.A. because of the possible toxicity of its metabolite cyclohexylamine.

Aspartame, N-L-α-Aspartyl-L-Phenylalanine methyl ester, is 200 times sweeter than sucrose and, unlike saccharin, has no aftertaste. Its aqueous solubility is adequate for formulation purposes. It is stable in the solid form, but its stability in solution depends on temperature and pH. It hydrolyzes to aspartylphenylalanine and diketopiperazine, with a loss in sweetness by aspartame synergistic with saccharin, sucrose, glucose, and cyclamate. In addition, its taste can be improved by adding sodium bicarbonate, gluconate salts, and lactose.

Newer non-caloric sweetening agents have come to market in the last decade. Sucralose (Splenda) is approximately 600 times sweeter than sucrose and differs from sucrose by the substitution of three chlorines for hydroxyl groups. Sucralose is heat-stable and stable over a wide pH range affording its utility in formulations prepared at high temperatures. Acesulphame-K is approximately 200 times sweeter than sucrose and is commonly used concomitantly with aspartame to synergistically enhance overall sweetening. This sweetener is also heat stable. Furthermore, Monoammonium glycyrrhizinate has even been used in liquid oral preparations.

Flavoring Agents

The flavoring of pharmaceuticals is of great importance in liquid dosage forms intended for oral use as they mask the disagreeable tastes of drugs. Furthermore, flavoring agents are regularly exploited for taste masking in clinical trials where it is essential for subjects to lack differentiation between placebo and drug-containing formulations. Flavoring agents are thoroughly reviewed in an entry in this series.

Coloring Agents

Although the use of colorants in medicinal products affords no direct therapeutic benefit, the psychological effects have long been recognized. The appearance of clear liquid products depends primarily on the color and clarity of the solution. Many patients rely on color to recognize the prescribed drug and proper dosage. Unattractive medication can be made acceptable to the patient by careful selection of color. Color is usually chosen according to the flavor of the product.

The current list of FD&C-certified colorants contains both dyes and lakes. The latter are pigments that are insoluble in water and that impart color by dispersing and reflecting light; they are not used for aqueous solutions. In contrast, FD&C dyes are water-soluble and exhibit color by transmitting light. Dyes should be used at the lowest possible concentration required to produce the desired color; higher concentrations can result in a dull color. Most liquid drug products have dye concentrations of less than 0.001%. Because dyes are usually present in trace amounts, they are dissolved before mixing with the bulk of the formulation, ensuring complete dissolution before further processing. If dye is added directly to the bulk mixing tank, the presence of small amounts of undissolved materials is difficult to determine and can cause problems later during the compounding. Factors influencing the shade and stability of dyes in liquid systems must be carefully considered. Among these are pH level, microbiological activity, final package exposure to light, and dye compatibility with other ingredients. Because color shades vary greatly at different pH values, pH control is extremely important. All soluble dyes contain reactive sites, and some dyes may be incompatible with compounds containing polyvalent cations (such as calcium, magnesium, or aluminum) and precipitate. Certain dyes, such as FD&C Blue No. 2 and FD&C Red No. 3, exhibit poor stability in aqueous solutions hence precluding their use for coloring aqueous liquid pharmaceutical products.

Preservatives

Liquid oral preparations are the most likely of all non-sterile pharmaceutical products to be contaminated by microorganisms. Most of these preparations are marketed in a multidose form, enhancing the risk of exposure to microbes upon repeat dosing. The inclusion of sugars and other excipients only enriches the preparation with growth-supporting substrates. The manufacturing process also may contribute to possible microbiological contamination. In addition to the risks associated with even purified

(USP) water, many raw materials of natural origin are used that may contain a large number of viable spores. Many over-the-counter pharmaceutical products have been prepared traditionally at low costs without sufficient care to prevent potential microbiological contamination. Therefore, it is essential that liquid preparations be protected against microbiological deterioration by adequate preservation.

Preservatives must fulfill certain criteria for acceptability. The major factors are those of safety and lack of toxicity after oral intake, particularly because liquid medications are often administered to children and the elderly. Preservatives must be soluble, stable, microbiologically active against a broad range of microbes, and compatible with the active ingredient as well as with other components of the formulation. Preservative efficacy can be modulated by factors such as preservative concentration, temperature, pH of the formulation, interactions with extraneous organic materials, and even by partitioning of the preservative away from the aqueous phase in a multiphase system.

An ideal preservative that meets all the requirements does not exist. The choice must be made on an individual basis, balancing antimicrobial efficacy against safety. The antimicrobial preservatives are classified into four major types: acidic, neutral, mercurial, and quaternary ammonium compounds. Frequently, a combination of two or more of these preservatives is needed to achieve the desired efficacy.

Acidic preservatives are the most widely used for oral preparations, such as the *p*-Hydroxybenzoic acid esters and salts of benzoic acid. These are adequately soluble in aqueous systems and possess both antifungal and antibacterial properties. Methyl and propyl *p*-hydroxybenzoic acid are often used together in a 10:1 ratio. Concomitant use of multiple esters makes possible a higher total preservative concentration owing to the independent solubilities of each and, according to some researchers, maximizes the antimicrobial effect.

The other three classes of preservatives have been widely used in ophthalmic, nasal, and parenteral products, but not frequently in oral liquid preparations. The neutral preservatives are volatile alcohols; their volatility introduces problems of odor and loss of preservative on aging in multidose preparations. The mercurials and quaternary ammonium compounds are excellent preservatives but are subject to incompatibilities. Mercurials are readily reduced to free mercury, and the quaternary compounds are inactivated by anionic substances.

The use of multiple preservatives in a liquid formulation can be extremely advantageous. Individual preservatives are able to interact synergistically or antagonistically with one another. Synergy in combination preservative systems is thought to occur by inhibition of preservative inactivation, increasing accessibility of a preservative to the target or by acting at different molecular targets. The advantages of achieving synergy in the selection of a preservative system can include increased antimicrobial activity over a broader range of microbes, enhanced efficacy in microbial killing concurrent with lower preservative concentrations (can mitigate potential toxicity of single preservatives in higher concentrations), and a longer duration of antimicrobial action and others.

Buffers

Changes in pH of a preparation may occur during storage because of degradation of the product, interactions with container components, or dissolution of gases and vapors. To avoid these problems, buffers are added to stabilize pH levels. A suitable buffer system should have adequate buffer capacity to maintain the pH level of the product during storage. It can be based on the pH profile of the drug in solution. Commonly used buffer systems are acetates, citrates, phosphates, and glutamates. Although buffers ensure pH stability, the buffer system can affect other properties such as solubility and kinetics. Buffers can act adversely as general-acid or general-base catalysts and cause degradation of the drug substance. The ionic-strength contributions of the buffer systems can also affect stability. Therefore, the effect of buffer species should be studied before selecting any buffer system.

Antioxidants

Many drugs in solution are subject to oxidative degradation. Oxidation is defined as a loss of electrons from a compound that results in a change in the oxidation state of the molecule. Such reactions are mediated by free radicals or molecular oxygen, and are often catalyzed by metal ions. Furthermore, oxidation often involves the addition of oxygen (or other electronegative atoms like halogens) or the removal of hydrogen.

Drugs possessing favorable oxidation potential are especially vulnerable to degradation. Agents with an oxidation potential lower than that of the drug in question are called antioxidants. They are added to solutions alone or in combination with a chelating agent or other antioxidants and function by being preferentially oxidized and gradually consumed or by blocking an oxidative chain reaction where they are not consumed.

Salts of sulfites are the most common antioxidants in aqueous solutions. Irrespective of which sulfite salt is added, the antioxidant activity depends on its final concentration and the final pH level of the formulation; commonly sodium metabisulfite is used at low pH, sodium bisulfite at near neutral pH, and sodium sulfite is used at basic pH. A single antioxidant may provide incomplete protection and hence combinations are often used. Certain compounds (e.g., ascorbic and citric acids) have been found to act as synergists, increasing the effectiveness of antioxidants, particularly those that block oxidative reactions. Frequently, chelating agents such as edetic acid derivatives (EDTA) are used in formulations containing trace amounts of heavy metals that would otherwise catalyze oxidative reactions. Additionally, synthetic phenolic compounds, such as butylated hydroxytoluene (BHT), serve as hydrogen atom donors and can successfully prevent oxidation of oils and fats in oral liquid formulations. Furthermore, certain properties of the selected primary packaging (such as oxygen transmission rates, polymer degradation, impurities, etc.) can readily lead to oxidation of drug molecules in solution and hence may require the addition of antioxidants to maintain product stability.

Viscosity-Controlling Agents

It is sometimes desirable to increase the viscosity of a liquid to provide or to improve palatability or pour- ability. This can be achieved by viscosity-controlling agents such as polyvinylpyrrolidones, carbomers, and various cellulose derivatives. Aqueous solutions containing these compounds are stable over a wide pH range. Methylcellulose and carboxymethylcellulose are available in a number of different viscosity grades. The latter may be used in solutions containing up to 50% alcohol without precipitating. However, precipitation can occur with the insoluble salts to a number of multivalent metal ions such as Al^{3+}, Fe^{3+}, and Ca^{2+}. Methylcellulose polymers do not form insoluble salts with metal ions but can be salted out when the concentration of electrolytes or other dissolved materials exceeds certain limits. These limits may vary from 2% to 40%, depending on the electrolyte and the type of methylcellulose involved. Viscosity-inducing polymers should be used with caution. They are known to form molecular complexes with a variety of organic and inorganic compounds. It is conceivable that highly viscid systems that resist dilution by gastrointestinal fluid may impede drug release and absorption.

Manufacture

The preparation of liquid drug preparations involves choosing the ingredients (using principles already addressed) and the manufacturing equipment. The basic principles involved are the same, regardless of the materials and the quantities involved. Carstensen and Mehta report the scaling-up of solution dosage forms, including heating, agitation, and clarification along with basic equations and calculations.

Liquid processing lends itself to computer-controlled automation. A few pharmaceutical firms have already instituted automated or semiautomated processes for several large-selling liquid products.

Raw Materials

Although purified water (USP) is required in all operations, it is particularly important in liquid manufacturing. If deionized and other water-treatment equipment is used, special attention must be given to routine microbiological and chemical testing. Storage tanks for glycerin and propylene glycol should be constructed to facilitate examination as well as cleaning.

Equipment

Simple solutions are most straightforward to scale up but require tanks of adequate size and suitable mixing capacity. Most equipment should have heating and cooling capabilities for rapid dissolution of formulation components. Adequate transfer systems and filtration equipment are required, but they must be monitored to ensure that they can clarify the product without removing active or adjuvant ingredients. All equipment must be made of suitable, non-reactive sanitary materials and be designed and constructed to facilitate easy cleaning. Liquid pharmaceutical processing tanks, kettles, pipes, mills, filter housings, and so forth are most frequently fabricated from stainless steel. Of the three types commonly used in the industry (304, 308, and 316), type 316 is most often used because it is the least reactive. Stainless steel is virtually non-reactive but may react with some acidic pharmaceutical liquids. This problem can be minimized by treating the stainless steel with acetic acid or nitric acid solution to remove surface alkalinity. This process, known as passivation, may be needed periodically. For example, if an alkaline cleaning agent is used between batches of a reactive product, passivation may be required before the subsequent batch can be prepared.

Interaction with metallic surfaces can be minimized by using polytetrafluoroethylene (Teflon) liners. Although Teflon is inert, these liners have the potential disadvantages of cracking, breaking, flaking, and peeling, with resulting product contamination.

A valuable and practical discussion on the design of piping, valves, mixers, pumps, and controls to produce high-quality liquid products is given by FitzSimon.

Methods of Preparation

Dilute solutions of rapidly dissolving materials are prepared by adding solute to the solvent and agitating until the solution in homogeneous. Heat may be required for more concentrated solutions or when the solute is slow to dissolve. Excipients are usually added in a specified order to increase the rate of dissolution and to facilitate a rapid approach to equilibrium. For this reason, menthol and flavors are charged as alcoholic solutions to the batch. Solutes present in small concentrations, particularly dyes and other intensely colored materials, should be dissolved before mixing with the main portion of the batch to ensure complete dissolution. If the solutes were charged directly to the bulk-mixing tank, detection of small amounts of undissolved material at the bottom of the tank is difficult. As a rule, complete solution should be confirmed at every stage in the manufacture of a homogeneous liquid. In the laboratory, liquids are usually measured by volume. However, in large-scale production, gravimetric means of measurement are used. For this reason, all liquids components of the formulation are expressed in units of both volume and weight.

Solutions must be filtered and clarified; this stage of the process is called "polishing." A highly polished solution requires the removal of particulate matter down to at least 3 μm. Filters used in the manufacturing, processing, or packing of liquid drug products intended for human use should not release fibers. If a fiber-releasing filter needs to be used, it must be followed by a nonfiber-releasing filter of optimum porosity. Filter aids are commonly used to improve clarity and increase the flow rate, thus decreasing filtration time. The amount and type of filter aid must be determined during the development of the product; the amount usually does not exceed 0.5 g/L. Examples of filter aids are diatomaceous earth, carbon, expanded perlite, and cellulose.

Filling and sealing

A liquid may be removed from a bulk container in portions to individual-dose containers more easily and uniformly than solids. Certain fundamental features are found on all machines used for filling containers with liquid. A means of agitation is used for repeatedly forcing a measured volume of the liquid through the orifice of a delivery tube designed to enter the constricted opening of a container. The size of the delivery tube is governed by the opening in the container, the viscosity and density of the liquid, and the desired speed of delivery. The tube must freely enter the neck of the container and deliver the liquid deep enough to permit air to escape without sweeping the entering liquid onto the neck or out of the container; the tube should have the maximum possible diameter. Excessive delivery force causes splashing and troublesome foaming, if the liquid has a low surface tension.

Small volumes of liquids (usually for pediatric use) are delivered by the stroke of the plunger of a syringe, which forces the liquid through a two-way valve that provides for an alternative filling of the syringe from a reservoir and delivery to a container. For heavy, viscous liquids, a sliding piston valve provides more positive action. A drop of liquid normally hangs at the tip of the tube after a delivery, which is removed by a retraction device. Filling machines are designed so that the parts through which the liquid flows can be easily dismantled for cleaning. These parts are constructed of non-reactive materials such as stainless steel. Small-volume filling machines are designed to deliver volume precisely. Syringes are typically also made of stainless steel. The stroke of the syringe can be repeated precisely; therefore, once a particular setting has been calibrated for a delivery, high precision is possible. The precision can be affected by certain operating factors such as the speed of delivery, uniformity of speed, expansion of rubber tubing connecting the valve to the delivery tube, and rapidity of the action of the valves.

Large-volume filling does not normally require as rigorous precision as small volumes. Therefore, bottles of solution are usually filled by gravity, pressure, or vacuum devices. Gravity filling is relatively slow but simple. The liquid reservoir is connected to a shut-off device at the filling line, which is usually hand operated; the bottles are filled to graduation marks. The pressure- pump filler is often operated semiautomatically, differing from the gravity filler principally in that the liquid is under pressure. It is usually equipped with an overflow tube connected to a receiver to prevent excess filling.

Vacuum filling is commonly used for large liquid volumes because of easy adaptation to automation. A vacuum is produced in a bottle when the nozzle gasket seals against the lip of the bottle being filled. The vacuum draws the liquid from a reservoir through the delivery tube into the bottle. When the liquid level reaches the level of an adjustable overflow tube, the seal is mechanically loosened, and the vacuum is released. Any liquid drawn into the vacuum line is collected in a receiver and returned to the reservoir.

Accuracy and precision of filling with liquids vary with the method. Therefore, a method is selected to provide the degree of accuracy and precision required. A slight excess is required in each container to compensate for losses that occur at the time of administration resulting from adherence to the wall of the container. Danger of overdose and economic factors limit the amount of excess desirable in a given container.

Highly viscous solutions require specially designed equipment. To obtain a reasonable flow rate, high pressure is applied, or containers with large openings are used to permit the entry of large delivery tubes. Jacketed reservoir tanks may be used to raise the product temperature to lower its viscosity.

A problem common to all types of machines that fill containers with liquid, particularly bothersome in high-speed automatic equipment, is excessive foaming. Foaming during the filling operation can be reduced by using filling equipment that minimizes product turbulence, closed-system filling to limit the introduction of air or other gases that cause foaming, mechanical defoaming devices, or reduction in the speed of the filling line. All these methods introduce considerable engineering and production difficulties. Careful consideration of the problems that might eventually be encountered in large-scale production and high-speed filling operations should be planned early in the product development process. Furthermore, a microbial survey should be performed on all packaging materials that come in contact with the product to ensure the absence of microbial contamination. Attention must also be given to details during packaging operations. For example, on small-volume orders, bottle closures, or tips for plastic squeeze-spray containers are often placed on the product by hand. This procedure can be a source of microbial contamination unless operators use gloves that are sterilized and disinfected periodically during use.

17

LOZENGES

Lozenges are solid preparations that contain one or more medicaments, usually in a flavored, sweetened base, and that are intended to dissolve or disintegrate slowly in the mouth. They can be prepared by molding (gelatin and/or fused sucrose and sorbitol base) or by compression of sugar-based tablets. Molded lozenges are sometimes referred to as pastilles, whereas compressed lozenges may be referred to as troches. They are intended to be allowed to dissolve on the back surface of the tongue to provide drug delivery locally to the mouth, tongue, throat, etc., to minimize systemic and maximize local drug activity. The USP currently recognizes Cetylpyridinium Chloride Lozenges and Nystatin Lozenges. However, more than five dozen over-the-counter (OTC) lozenge products are currently marketed. These contain a variety of active ingredients including antimicrobials and local anesthetics for throat pain; aromatics, herbals, zinc salts, decongestants, and cough suppressants for colds, allergy, cough, and congestion; and nicotine-like substances for smoking cessation.

HARD CANDY LOZENGES

Raw Materials

The types of raw materials used in medicated lozenges may vary according to a number of factors. Most medicated lozenges contain sugar, corn syrup, acidulant, colorant, flavor, and the medicament. Sucrose, a disaccharide of glucose and fructose, is obtained from sugarcane or beet. The choice of beet or cane sugar is based on availability and geographical considerations. Sucrose and sucrose products are used in medicated lozenges because of their value as neutral sweeteners, their ready solubility, and their function as a "*drier*" to reduce the weight of the confection through crystallization. Invert sugar, derived from sucrose, possesses the very desirable physical property of controlling the crystallization of concentrated sugar solutions and maintaining freshness of the finished product through its humectant properties.

Corn syrup is used in almost every type of confection to control sucrose and dextrose crystallization, which may lead to crumbling. Corn syrup in appropriate proportion with sucrose and dextrose allows the formation of an amorphous glass and produces a candy with the desirable appearance. The following physical properties of corn syrup are extremely important in the preparation of medicated candies: density, dextrose equivalent (DE), hygroscopicity, sugar crystallization, viscosity, freezing- point depression, and osmotic pressure. Colorants are incorporated into medicated lozenges for appearance, product identification, and masking of physical degradation. Dyes and other organic colorants may degrade by heat or light via oxidation, hydrolysis, photooxidation, etc., and their compatibility with drug, excipients, and process conditions should be studied before selection. Suppliers of colors are excellent sources of information on current regulatory status of colorants.

Acidulants are generally added to medicated lozenges to fortify and strengthen their flavor profile. Organic acids such as citric, malic, fumaric, and tartaric acids are most commonly used. Citric acid alone or in combination with tartaric acid is the most common. Another use of acids in medicated lozenges is to alter the pH to maintain the integrity of the drug. Regular conversion corn syrup has a pH of 5.0–6.0. Addition of a weak organic acid to improve flavor lowers it to 2.5–3.0, a pH at which some medicaments exhibit maximum stability. If necessary, some drugs can be stabilized by adjusting the pH to 7.0–8.0 with a suitable weak base such as calcium carbonate. Some research has shown that excessive use of acidic lozenges could have the potential to enhance existing dental erosion, and that low pH (2.6–3.7) leads to dissolution of calcium and phosphorous from hydroxyapatite. Others have shown that excessive use of citric and tartaric acids may effect bioavailability of zinc in zinc lozenges. Another report indicated that the activity of cetylpyridinium chloride in candy-base lozenges is influenced by pH, with >5.5 being most desirable.

Acceptable taste is necessary to ensure patient acceptability, and this can be the determining factor between commercial success and failure of an OTC product. Flavors used in medicated lozenges must be compatible with the drug and excipients and capable of withstanding the rigors of the manufacturing conditions. Flavors consist of numerous chemicals that may interact with excipients or medicaments and that degrade by heat and light. Aldehydes, ketones, and esters may react with drugs. A classic example of flavor–drug interaction is that of a primary amine drug (benzocaine, phenylpropanolamine) with aldehyde-containing flavor components like cherry, banana, etc., resulting in the formation of a Schiff base, drug decomposition, and loss of efficacy. Adjustment of lozenge base pH to accentuate certain flavors (e.g., citrus) may also result in incompatibility with some medicaments (e.g., benzocaine).

The last major ingredient in lozenges is salvage obtained from lozenge batches rejected because of imperfect shape or size, presence of air bubbles, or unacceptable drug concentration. Salvage, if properly heated, can be reused in finished products without altering color, texture, lozenge base composition, or drug concentration. Before any salvage can be used as part of a medicated lozenge base, it should be adjusted to a pH of 4.5–7.5 to prevent excessive and uncontrolled formation of reducing sugars, and the stability of the drug at cooking cycles should be determined.

Processing Methods

There are three types of candy-base cookers: fire cookers, high-speed atmospheric cookers, and vacuum cookers. Vacuum cooking is the process of choice for manufacturing hard candy lozenges. It is based on the principle that water boils at a lower temperature under vacuum, and can thus be removed. Sugar solutions and corn syrup are boiled at 125–132°C, vacuum is applied, and, due to the heat of the batch, additional water is boiled off without further heating. The resulting vapor is condensed and removed by the cooling water of the vacuum pump.

The continuous batch process cooker installation consists of an automatic sugar dissolver, a sugar solution and corn syrup storage unit, metering pumps, precookers and a holding tank, a vacuum pump, and a collection kettle. Precookers are standard steam-jacketed kettles equipped with an additional heat exchanger to provide better circulation in addition to more exchange surfaces. Each component (water, sugar, corn syrup, and salvage) is added by pumps and metering devices controlled by one gearing system, in order to bring the finished precooked syrup to the desired temperature (110–120°C) in 1 min or less. The short dwell time significantly reduces the Browning reaction and the amount (1–2%) of invert sugar developed. Cooking machines consist of a heating coil, intermediate chamber, vacuum chamber, flow metering valve, turning device that charges the receiving kettle, receiving kettle, kettle turning device, and rotary vacuum. In the standard procedure, a precooked sugar–corn syrup solution at 110–120°C is passed through a chrome–nickel steel cooking coil housed in a steam dome at a temperature of 135–150°C. The coil leads to an intermediate chamber that is vented to the atmosphere.

From the intermediate chamber, the syrup is sprayed into the vacuum chamber, which is regulated by a vacuum-actuated metering valve. This affects reevaporation of the sugar mass, further increasing the content of dry substance. An adjustable timing device charges the receiving kettle by opening an air valve the moment the batch is cooked. The filled receiving kettle drops from the vacuum hood and is held in front of the cooker by a spring-activated timing device; it is replaced by an empty one. The kettle is charged by the syrup pump, resulting in uniform weight of all batches. By selecting an appropriate model, more than 3000 kg of candy can be produced per hour.

Replacement of the collection kettle by a continuously moving stainless steel belt to carry the candy base away from the cooker at a predetermined rate in an unbroken stream has resulted in the continuous process cooker, which has some advantages and some limitations. Its advantages are high-speed production, improved organoleptic characteristics, extended shelf life for physical properties, and cost effectiveness. The disadvantages are reduced controls, the addition of flavor at very high temperature, and increased possibility of non-uniform candy-base production. Preparation of candy base from gear metering of sugar solution and corn syrup to vacuum drying is identical to the batch process described above. However, candy base is continuously drawn off in a thin ribbon. As it leaves the cooker the flavor, preheated to 50–60°C, is injected. The flavored candy mass is dropped onto a variable-speed rotary cone head where it is mixed. Medicament as a solution or dispersion, preheated to 110–120°C, can be metered into the candy mass through dosing pumps. The candy mass then slides down the delivery chute onto the stainless-steel belt where it is mixed and sized by plows and rollers. The temperature of the conveyor belt is controlled by a spray of heated water that can be adjusted as necessary. The acidulant may be deposited onto the candy mass via a vibratory dosing auger; the subsequent steps are identical to those of the batch process.

Candy-Base Manufacturing

The first step in the manufacture of medicated lozenges is the preparation of candy base, followed by the addition of medicament, flavor, acidulants, colors, etc., and finally by lozenge formation. Irrespective of process, the manufacture of medicated lozenges involves the cooking of candy base, mixing, batch forming, "rope" sizing, adjustment of weight, lozenge formation, cooling, and storage of lozenges. Candy base is prepared from liquid sugar (67% sugar) and corn syrup (liquid glucose 43°Be, 80% solids) in a ratio of about 60:40. Precooking is initiated under vacuum at controlled temperature. The precooked solution is transferred into the steam- heated coil, where it is boiled and from which it is moved to the intermediate chamber where final mixture is produced. The final moisture content of candy base should be about 1%, its temperature about 135°C, and its consistency plastic-like. The candy base is transferred into a kettle mounted on a suitable scale and, if necessary, batch weight is adjusted.

Heat-stable colors are added at this point as cubes or paste. The colored candy base is transferred to a cold stainless-steel cooling plate for the mixing operation. Mixing can be manual or mechanical, using a series of plows and rollers, or a mixer consisting of two arms, a plunger, and a slowly rotating table top. The temperature of the mixing table is maintained at 40–50°C. Flavor, medicament, acidulant, and ground salvage are added to the colored candy mass when mixing is initiated. After completion, the medicated candy base is transferred to a warm slab and allowed to equilibrate to a uniform temperature. The mass is cut into workable portions, properly tempered, and placed into batch-forming (holding) machines. For candy formers requiring a flat sheet, heated tables are used. For candies requiring cylindrical pieces to be fed into the batch formers, batch rollers are used. A plastic-like mass is formed into a sugar cone and transferred at a predetermined rate to the sizing roller. The operation of the batch former is synchronized with the rope sizer. In order to maintain a temperature at which the outer shell of the candy would not crack, the batch formers are kept at 80–90°C.

The height to which the batch formers are adjusted and the amount of material in them dictates the delivery rate of the candy flowing as a rope from the batch former to the sizing rollers. The sizers consist of sets of successively smaller forming rolls. The thickness of the rope is determined by the diameter of the sizing rollers and governs the weight and size of the candy. The sizers are generally heated to maintain temperatures of 50–60°C, preventing the candy from cracking by rapid cooling. For the formation of the final lozenge, the candy rope is discharged into a forming machine. The formed lozenges are then fed onto the distribution belt, which provides intensive cooling and shaking to prevent deformation of the still plastic lozenge. The formed candy must be cooled as quickly as possible to prevent loss of shape. The candy is usually cooled on a conveyor belt made of chain or canvas. Multibelt coolers are designed in such a way that the first narrow belt (15–20 cm wide) runs as rapidly as the candy-forming machine. At the end of the first belt, a breaker separates the candy and distributes the lozenges uniformly across a wider, slower-moving second belt. The third belt is still wider and travels even more slowly, allowing enough time to cool the lozenge to the desired temperature (below 35°C).

In the sizing operation, the medicated lozenges are collected as they leave the cooling belt and transferred to a series of counter-rotating rollers separated via caliper adjustment. The sizing operation removes all oversized and undersized lozenges, ensuring uniformity. The properly sized lozenges are collected and stored in a climate-controlled room at 15–20°C and a relative humidity of 25–35% until the product is cleared by the quality control unit for packaging. Recent technological advances in lozenge manufacture include a patent that teaches a continuous process for producing dextromethorphan lozenges. A new lozenge cutter apparatus consisting of a drum with an array of cutter elements is described in a 1997 patent. A distributing device for feeding lozenges (or other flat products) via a feed conveyor to a "user" machine, such as a packager, is described in a 1993 patent.

Compressed Tablet Lozenges

Commercially, the preparation of lozenges by tablet compression is less important than hard-candy manufacturing techniques. Essentially, lozenge tablets differ from conventional tablets only in their organoleptic and non-disintegrating properties and slower dissolution rate. The associated attributes of pleasant taste with or without matching color, smoothness, and mouth feel during prolonged dissolution on the tongue, and the physical consideration of holding the tablet in the mouth while swallowing its dissolved components, present unusual formulation requirements compared to those of tablets intended for swallowing or chewing. The commonly used drugs mentioned previously tend to be bitter, unpleasant tasting compounds. The desire to release these agents slowly in the mouth, in constant contact with the tongue, demands a formulation approach unlike that found in any other dosage form.

Processing and Excipients

Any of the common tablet-processing methods, such as wet granulation, dry granulation, or direct compaction, may be utilized in the production of lozenge tablets. However, because the tablets should dissolve very slowly without disintegration, wet granulation is preferable because it generally provides better control. Through the judicious use of wet binders that retard dissolution, it should be possible to design a formulation having the appropriate dissolution rate. Formulating for slow dissolution, plus smoothness and good mouthfeel, requires careful excipient selection and appropriate process development to ensure that the controlling variables are dealt with correctly. Several important aspects of lozenge tablet manufacture are critical to all of the desired performance attributes of the finished product. These include assurance of necessary particle size and distribution, maintenance of correct moisture content, and achievement of proper tablet hardness. Process development and scaleup considerations must be thoroughly explored to ensure the establishment of proper specifications for these parameters. As always when the process involves wet granulation, the extent of wetting and the rate and extent of drying must be defined. Overwetting almost certainly produces harder granules that may have poor compressional characteristics, resulting in softer and more friable tablets unacceptable for lozenge application. Because of the lesser degree of particle deformation, such granulations produce tablets having a gritty mouthfeel. Overwetting also leads to longer drying times in order to achieve the desired moisture level or, to a higher moisture level due to failure to compensate through adjustment of the drying cycle. Lozenge tablets are generally formulated as relatively large-diameter (>12.5 mm), flat-faced (beveled edge), heavy (>700 mg) tablets with high hardness (>15 kp). These physical attributes lead to ease of use in the mouth and contribute to the desired slow dissolution. The formulation factors primarily responsible for controlling dissolution, hardness, and mouthfeel are the presence of a high strength, dissolution- retarding binder and the absence of a disintegrant. Several commonly employed binders meet these criteria and provide the added benefit of delivering a demulcent-like action in the throat.

Gelatin (in the form of a warm 10% aqueous solution) and acacia gum (in the form of an aqueous mucilage) in wet granulation form very hard tablets with slow dissolution. Guar gum, used as an aqueous thixotropic mucilage, exhibits behavior similar to that of acacia gum. The sugar bases frequently associated with lozenge tablets are sucrose or compressible sugar, dextrose, mannitol, and sorbitol, which are available in special tableting grades from a variety of excipient manufacturers. Generally intended for direct compaction applications, they may also be utilized with the above binders in wet-granulation systems. Lactose, because of its extremely low sweetness (15% of sucrose), is limited for use in lozenges because it would require the addition of an artificial sweetener of sufficient potency to overcome its blandness. Xylitol is relatively sweet and has an advantage in lozenge formulation with respect to its lack of caries production. Artificial sweeteners are of significant importance to lozenge tablet formulations. As noted above, some sugars may not be sweet enough to mask the bitterness or sourness of many drugs. Presently, there is considerable regulatory disagreement worldwide concerning these materials; some are approved for use in certain countries but not others. Aspartame, asulfame-K, cyclamate, saccharin, and sucralose appear to be technically usable, but their selection requires care from the regulatory perspective. All have potency (sweetness) levels orders of magnitude higher than that of sucrose, permitting the use of very low concentrations (less than 1%) to cover most bitter drugs. Semisynthetic sweeteners, derived from glycyrrhiza, have enjoyed some degree of popularity over the years. They are much sweeter than sucrose, but less sweet than saccharin. It is strongly recommended that the formulator validate the current regulatory acceptance of the intended sweetener prior to its use for a particular product and market country. In addition, a recent report suggests that the common lubricant, magnesium stearate, reduced the effectiveness of cetylpyridinium chloride in compressed tablet lozenges, and that the concentration of this ingredient in such a formulation should be maintained at not more than 0.3%.

Quality Control

Lozenges require the same quality assurance and control measures as any pharmaceutical dosage form. Because of their unique composition, however, certain additional methods are necessary.

In-Process Testing

In addition to all of the common in-process tests used for all dosage forms, certain specialized procedures are necessary for hard candy lozenges. These include checking the corn syrup and sugar delivery gears, temperature, steam pressure, and the cooking speed of precooker and cooker; analysis of the candy base and its moisture content, and determination of the sugar-to-corn syrup ratio using the dextrose equivalent method, percent-reducing sugar (by reacting candy with copper sulfate and alkaline cupric tartrate and titrating with dextrose solution), pH, cooked candy batch weight, lozenge weight, and lozenge size. The usual in-process tests for compressed tablets apply to lozenge tablets, including particle-size distribution, moisture content, flow, blend uniformity, tablet weight and thickness control, hardness, etc.

Batch-Release Testing

In addition to the usual quality control procedures and the above in-process tests, batch-release testing includes dosage uniformity and a test for grittiness, performed by partially dissolving lozenges under running tap water until one-third to one-half has been removed. No grittiness must be felt when rubbed between thumb and forefinger. Test procedures that are ordinarily applied to compressed tablets are also employed for lozenge tablets. However, because the lozenge is intended to dissolve slowly in the mouth, typical disintegration and dissolution testing is inappropriate. Lozenges should be non-disintegrating; therefore, there is no need for disintegration testing. Dissolution specifications should be developed on the basis of aminimum and maximum time to physically dissolve, rather than on the basis of minimum percent drug released in the maximum time interval. As with hard candy lozenges, microbial testing may be appropriate, especially when wet granulation has been used in processing the materials and high concentrations of carbohydrates are present.

Stability

For both hard candy lozenges and compressed tablet lozenges, stability considerations extend to areas not usually of concern with other types of tablets. These products should not only conform to chemical and physical specifications, but should also exhibit satisfactory stability of organoleptic attributes. Because lozenges are flavored, flavor stability is important. There is, however, no objective method for measuring flavor stability in a finished dosage form, although GC may be used for chemical analysis of flavor compounds. Even subjective methods such as tasting are difficult because formal taste panels are needed to acquire reliable data. Subtle changes in flavor with time, although not affecting product performance, may have a significant impact on product market acceptability. This could also be true of minor changes (increase or decrease) in tablet hardness, which could affect dissolution time and therefore acceptability.

PACKAGING

Medicated lozenges, especially those of hard candy base composition, are hygroscopic because of their unique ingredients. In order to be competitive in the marketplace, they need a shelf life longer than 3 years. For these reasons, they are usually packaged individually wrapped in polymeric moisture-barrier material. The wrapped lozenges are placed in a tight or moisture-resistant glass, polyvinyl chloride, or metal container that is overwrapped with cellophane or aluminum foil. This complex, multiple packaging is intended to provide the maximum possible protection from moisture in order to ensure the longest possible shelf life for the product. Lozenges are medicated confections designed to locally deliver drug to the mouth and throat. Very widely sold as OTC products, there are also prescription products marketed in the lozenge dosage form. Lozenges are used to deliver local anesthetics, cold and allergy treatments, antimicrobial drugs, antismoking drugs, and anticariogenic drugs. They are usually produced in the form of cooked, hard candies based on sugar and corn syrup or sorbitol. They are totally different from any other pharmaceutical dosage form in terms of ingredients and method of manufacture and, therefore, require specialized facilities. Compressed tablet lozenges differ from conventional tablets by requiring materials and methods that provide slow dissolution and drug release. For these and other reasons, lozenges are produced by few pharmaceutical manufacturers, and represent a very small percentage of total pharmaceutical sales. Nosignificant growth can be currently anticipated in these areas.

18

LENS CARE PRODUCTS

Contact lenses are made of polymeric materials designed and fabricated to correct vision. Because these lenses are removed from the eye after a prescribed wear time, lens care products are required to clean, disinfect and rinse them prior to reinsertion to avoid ocular infections and other complications. Lens care products are also required to enhance the comfort of lens wear.

HISTORICAL OVERVIEW

Lens care products are relatively new compared to many other pharmaceutical products. Leonardo da Vinci was the first to conceive the concept of the contact lens. In 1508 he illustrated the concept of vision involving "upside down" images with a water-filled sphere covering the eye. However, the actual development of contact lenses did not occur until about 100 years ago (1887–1888) when scleral contact lenses were fabricated. The three innovators credited for this are Dr. A.E. Fick, a physician in Zurich, F.A. Mueller, a maker of prosthetic eyes in Germany, and Dr. Eugene Kalt, a French physician. The earlier lenses were made of glass. In the late 1930s (1937–1939), Mullen, Obrig and Gyorrfy are credited with fabricating plastic contact lenses made from methyl methacrylate (PMMA). However, Kevin Tuohy, who filed a patent for contact lens design in 1948, is recognized as the "father" of modern day corneal contact lenses.

These early lenses were rigid and uncomfortable with very low oxygen transmission. Advances in rigid lens technology have provided materials capable of oxygen transmission required to maintain corneal health. In the 1960s Otto Victerle developed the hydrophilic soft contact lens from polyhydroxyethyl methacrylate (HEMA). Hydrophilic soft contact lenses are the primary lenses available today. Since then, significant technological advances have been made in contact lens material, designs, and manufacturing processes. In 1990, the estimate of contact lens wearers in the United States alone was around 30 million.

The commercialization of the first pharmaceutical quality lens care products occurred in the 1950s. Harry Hind, a pharmacist and founder of the Barnes-Hind Company, has been credited as one of the first to develop and commercialize a wetting and storage solution for the rigid PMMA plastic lenses. Prior to his efforts, the literature mentions formulation of a saline solution containing sodium bicarbonate to be used with scleral lenses made from glass.

CURRENT CONTACT LENS MATERIALS AND FUTURE DIRECTIONS

Most of the materials currently used in fabricating contact lenses have been available since the mid- 1960s with the exception of polymethyl methacrylate. Lens materials can be broadly classified as follows:

Rigid Gas-permeable lenses:

1. Cellulose acetate butyrate
2. Silicone
3. Silicone acrylate
4. Fluoro silicone acrylate
5. t-Butylstyrene
6. t-Butylstyrene-co-silicone acrylate

Soft hydrophilic lenses:

1. Polyhydroxyethyl methacrylate
2. Polyhdroxyethyl methacrylate-co-methacrylic acid
3. Polyglyceryl methacrylate
4. Polyhydroxyethyl methacrylate-co-polyvinylpyrrolidone
5. Polyvinylpyrrolidone-co-methyl methacrylate
6. Polyhydroxyethyl methacrylate-co-silicone (silicone hydrogel)

In addition to these materials, several others, such as polyurethanes, polysulfones, polyvinyl alcohol, and various copolymers, have been tried or are under development. Recently, silicon hydrogel lenses with high oxygen permeability were marketed. The future trends in material development will continue to include polymers which have a high degree of oxygen permeability, resist accumulation of metabolic products of the cornea, and materials that resist lens deposits and bacterial attachment on lens surfaces to minimize the potential for ocular infection.

Classification of Contact Lenses Currently Marketed

During a period beginning from mid-1970, numerous hydrophilic and rigid gas-permeable lenses were introduced into the market. Although many had similar basic chemical compositions, they contained different additives designed to achieve desirable properties or to avoid infringement of existing patents. Such a proliferation of contact lens materials created confusion regarding Food and Drug Administration (FDA) criteria for approval of contact lenses and their care products. In the mid-1980s, the FDA worked with the contact lens manufacturers and evolved a classification for soft contact lenses based on the ionic or non-ionic nature of polymers constituting the lens material and the water content. A classification was also worked out for rigid gas-permeable (RGP) lenses based on the chemical nature of the polymers. It is interesting to note that contact lenses and their care products were originally considered as drugs. However, upon passage of the U.S. Medical Device Act in 1996, contact lenses were reclassified as devices. Contact lenses and their care products were considered Class-III devices, which mandate the filing of a premarket approval application and obtaining FDA approval prior to marketing. Recently these products were reclassified as Class II devices and are currently cleared for marketing under the 510(k) premarket notification section of the regulations.

Lens Care Products by Functional Purpose

Marketed lens care products fall mainly into the following categories: cleaners, disinfectants, lubricants, and multipurpose products. Cleaners are subdivided into daily or weekly cleaners. Disinfectants comprise solutions containing chemical antimicrobial agents, which do not require heating the lenses, and preserved or unpreserved saline solutions, which are used with an electrical thermal device for lens disinfection. These products are also used to rinse contact lenses. Lens lubricants are intended to enhance the comfort of lens wear and are used prior to insertion and during wear. Multipurpose solutions are intended to accomplish two or more of the functions described earlier (cleaning, rinsing, and disinfection).

Rigid lens care also includes conditioning solutions to make the basic hydrophobic polymers wettable when placed on the eye.

PRODUCTS FOR CLEANING SOFT CONTACT LENSES

Lens Deposits

Composition

Basically there are two types of deposits: those resulting from tear components and those derived from other sources. Tear components especially proteins can accumulate on the lens surface. These proteins can denature or change conformations during absorptions on over tissue. Most deposits, with the exception of those that are tenaciously bound to the lens, can be cleaned easily with a surfactant-type of daily cleaner. Deposits resulting from tear components include proteinaceous deposits such as lysozyme, lactoferrin, albumin, globulins, etc. Proteinaceous deposits are present on all types of lenses. However, the amounts differ, depending on the number of ionic charges on and in the lens, the pore size, and the relative hydrophobicity of the polymers. For example, conventional non-porous and uncharged hard PMMA lenses with a hydrophobic surface attract very little proteinaceous deposits. Among the soft contact lenses with hydrophilic surfaces, the extent of deposits differs among various groups. For example, Group-4 lenses, which exhibit considerable negative charges due to methacrylic acid content, interact readily and heavily with a positively charged protein (lysozyme). Group-2 hydrogel lenses have no ionic charges, but can acquire substantial amounts of protein because of their large pore size. Besides protein deposits, lipid deposits are also found on contact lenses. These deposits are more common with rigid gas-permeable lenses because of their lipophilic nature. Such deposits may include cholesterol esters, wax esters, triglycerides, sterols, fatty acids, etc. Calcium present in tears results in calcium carbonate or phosphate-type of deposits as well as so-called mixed deposits (calcium bonded to organic compounds). Such deposits are common mainly in high water content soft contact lenses and are difficult to remove without damaging the contact lenses. Other deposits result from the patient environment These include deposits resulting from cosmetics, make-up, and hair-spray, as well as materials from the wearing environment such as pollen dust and debris.

Problems associated with lens deposits

Cleaning is one of the most important steps in contact lens care. It helps in the removal of surface debris and contaminating microorganisms, thus facilitating the disinfection process. Improperly cleaned lenses can cause discomfort, red eye, decrease in visual acuity, and giant papillary conjunctivitis (GPC). The last often requires discontinuance of lens wear, at least until the symptoms clear. The change from heat to cold disinfection technology and the introduction of disposable lenses may have reduced the incidence of GPC. However, since these lenses can be worn on an extended basis for up to seven days without cleaning, GPC can still occur, as has been noted in the literature.

Classification of Lens Cleaners

Daily cleaners vs. weekly cleaners

Daily cleaners generally contain surfactants and are used every day. They may also contain abrasive (deposit-shearing) particles, which enhance product performance. There are two types of weekly cleaners: those containing enzymes and those containing concentrated surfactants. Products containing enzymes for daily use are usually accepted by the patients and recommended by practitioners.

In-the-eye vs. out-of-the-eye cleaners

Most of the cleaners marketed are out-of-the-eye cleaners; however, in recent years there has been a trend to try to develop cleaners for use while the lenses are inserted. A specific instance where such products could be beneficial is the case of the extended-wear lenses, which are not removed daily but are worn up to a week at a time. Generally, these cleaners are less effective in removing deposits already formed on the lens surface. However, they may play a role in retarding deposit formation.

Consumer vs. professional use cleaners

Cleaners for lens wearers are used either on a daily or weekly basis and are fairly innocuous. Even upon gross misuse, they are not likely to be sight-threatening. Professional cleaners, however, are potent as well as toxic if not used properly. They are also more likely to damage the lens if used too frequently.

Active Components of Lens Cleaners

Surfactants

Surfactants are broadly classified into non-ionic, anionic, cationic, and amphoteric types. Non-ionic and amphoteric surfactants are most commonly used in contact lens cleaners, because strong anionic surfactants are generally toxic to the cornea. The recommended procedure by the manufacturer removes several types of deposits, except the most tenaciously bound and denatured proteins, lipids, and mucins. Surfactant-type cleaners are also effective in removing greater than 99.9% of microorganisms contaminating the lens. There are several mechanisms for their effectiveness, which include displacement of contaminants from the surface by mechanical force after the surface debris has been loosened as a result of a reduction in the interfacial tension. In addition, surfactants act by emulsification and micellar solubilization. They may also play a role in preventing or retarding deposition of contaminants.

Enzymes

Enzymes are biochemical molecules responsible for catalyzing reactions in which certain chemical bonds are broken. Their mechanism of action in cleaning involves attacking substrate protein, lipid, and mucin deposits, and fragmenting them into smaller molecules which are readily removed by the mechanical action of rubbing with the fingers and rinsing. Marketed products contain different enzymes, such as papain, pancreatin, and subtilisin. Papain and subtilisin are only proteolytic in nature, whereas pancreatin is a broad-spectrum enzyme containing protease, lipase, and amylase enzymes that digest proteins, lipids, and mucins. Enzyme cleaners are effective in attacking all lens proteins, including the removal of tenaciously bound and denatured deposits, that cannot be removed by surfactant cleaners. Traditional enzymatic cleaning of contact lenses is recommended usually once a week. The soaking time varies from 15 min to overnight, followed by a disinfection process. However, more recently products have been introduced that can be used simultaneously during disinfection on a daily process. Certain enzyme products are recommended for this single-step cleaning and disinfection, using a heat or chemical regimen that enhances convenience and increases user compliance.

Oxidizing agents

Oxidizing agents such as sodium perborate and sodium percarbonate have also been used in cleaning contact lenses. None of these products are currently marketed for that purpose in the United States. Products marketed earlier were withdrawn because of their deleterious effects on lens polymers.

Deposit-shearing particles

Deposit-shearing particles are incorporated in suspension form in some daily cleaners. These formulations are more effective than daily surfactant cleaners as they are capable of removing tenaciously bound and denatured deposits. Some of the marketed products contain polymeric beads or silica. When used as recommended, these products are very effective and do not scratch the lens surface.

Chelating agents

Chelating agents such as disodium edetate (EDTA) are commonly used in lens care products to enhance the antimicrobial activity of preservatives and remove calcium and magnesium from the lens.

EDTA is the most effective chelating agent known for calcium and magnesium. Other chelating agents have been used such as phosphonates, which are most effective against iron.

Solvents

Solvents such as isopropyl alcohol have been incorporated in daily cleaners to aid in removing lipid type of deposits. Such solvents have been reported to affect certain lens materials, especially silicone acrylate rigid gas-permeable lenses.

Accessory Cleaning Products

Hand soaps

In the daily care of contact lenses, wearers are instructed to clean their hands with soap and to dry hands their hands with lint-free towels prior to handling their lenses. Selection of the specific soap product is important. In addition, to cleaning the hands thoroughly, it should be rinsing and should not cause ocular irritation even if residual amounts are transferred to the lens. With these considerations in mind, some hand soaps have, therefore, been designed specifically for contact lens users.

Cleaning devices

The general method of daily lens cleaning involves rubbing lenses between the index finger and thumb or placing the lens in the palm of the hand and rubbing with the index finger after applying cleaning solution to the surface. However, there are also special devices available in the market for cleaning lenses. They are said to clean lenses more effectively and avoid potential scratching by the fingers. These devices involve mechanical agitation and are manually or electrically operated. Ultrasound devices have been used mainly by lens practitioners in their office. None of those devices per se are effective in removing tenaciously bound, denatured deposits.

Products for Disinfecting Contact Lenses

Disinfection of contact lenses is an important step in preventing ocular irritation, red eye, and potential loss of eyesight due to corneal ulcers resulting especially from *Pseudomonas aeruginosa* infections. The pore openings of hydrophilic soft contact lenses are estimated to be between 3.0 and 7.0 nm, and are considerably smaller than the average bacterial particle size of 0.2–1.0 μm or fungus particle size of 2–6 μm. Even viruses ranging in particle size from 25 to 200 nm are large in size compared to the pore openings of soft lenses. None of the microorganisms can penetrate an intact lens matrix. However, when lenses are not properly cared for, some fungus growth facilitates the penetration of fungal hyphae into the matrix.

Contact lenses and their cases are frequently contaminated by microbes. Although studies have indicated that as many at 30% of lens cases are contaminated, the incidence of permanent ocular damage due to this is very low. Nevertheless, it is critical to properly instruct lens wearers and emphasize the importance of disinfection in order to avoid the potential risk of ocular infection or damage to the eyesight.

Thermal vs. Chemical Disinfection

Both thermal and chemical methods are commonly used for the disinfection of soft contact lenses. With the former, a case containing the lenses immersed in saline solution is heated by an electrical unit with a predesigned heating cycle. The current FDA requirement for thermal disinfection by saline solution requires a minimum temperature of 80°C for 10 min within the contact lens case. This ensures elimination of vegetative forms of ocular pathogens but not the spores.

The chemical method involves antimicrobial compounds with an adequate antimicrobial spectrum and biocidal action. The FDA guidelines include the methods for determination of efficacy for all disinfecting solutions. The initial testing process is defined as the elimination or reduction of microorganisms achieved over the disinfection period. The FDA guidelines also provide a method for manufacturers to conduct use tests on purposely contaminated contact lenses, following a complete disinfection regimen, which includes cleaning and rinsing. This test is generally known as the FDA regimen test. The FDA guidelines specify the types and levels of organisms as well as the details of the test. Other methods using ultraviolet light, microwave, and ultrasonics, have been tried for lens disinfection but are not widely applied because of ineffectiveness or deleterious effects on lens materials.

The advantage of the thermal method is that it ensures complete elimination of vegetative forms of microorganisms, whereas chemical disinfectants may encounter some resistant organisms. Although the thermal method is preferable from the microbiological viewpoint, it has several disadvantages: It is a complex method involving the use of electrical devices. The failure of an electrical heating unit to perform properly presents a potential risk of ocular infection. Malfunctioning units and improper use may result in electrical shock to users and fires have been reported. If the saline solution in the lens container evaporates during the heating cycle as a result of carelessness in not properly tightening the lens case cap, the lens might be damaged. Thermal disinfection has been cited in shortening lens life and enhancing the formation of deposits on the surface. This occurs especially if the lens has not been properly cleaned prior to thermal disinfection. The method is not practical for campers who are frequently without an electrical outlet.

Chemical disinfection, on the other hand, is not as effective in killing organisms as thermal disinfection, but has several advantages: It is simple to use, thereby ensuring greater user compliance. Lens life is longer with chemical disinfection as lenses are not subjected to daily heat treatment. The method results in fewer deposit problems as surface debris left on the lens surface due to improper cleaning is not baked by heat.

The choice between thermal and chemical disinfection depends, to a large extent, on the recommendation of the lens practitioners. Factors involved include the wearer's sensitivity to preservatives, needs, personal hygiene habits, and product cost. Today fewer heat disinfection units are available.

Thermal Disinfection

Soft contact lenses were introduced in the United States in 1972. At that time, the thermal disinfection method was the only method available. It uses either preserved or unpreserved saline solution.

Unpreserved vs. preserved saline solutions

Prior to the commercial availability of pharmaceutically prepared saline solutions, they were prepared by the lenswearer using salt tablets and distilled water. This method was undesirable and created many problems as the pH and osmolarity of such solutions were not controlled, which often resulted in parameter changes in some soft lenses. The major problem stemmed from non-compliance. In order to reduce cost, tap water was often used instead of distilled water for preparing saline solutions, which resulted in mineral deposits on the lens surface. Microorganisms proliferated in non-sterile saline solution prepared with distilled water stored for a number of days and instilled in eyes directly to hydrate contact lenses while they were worn. Such gross misuses resulted in ocular infection affecting vision. By the mid-1980s products label and package inserts warned against the use of tap water for contact lens care. In the mid-1970s, pharmaceutically prepared sterile saline solution preserved with thimerosal was introduced to eliminate the disadvantages of home-made saline. However, thimerosal often caused a brownish and grayish lens discoloration and also led to red-eye and sensitization reactions in some patients. Soon after the introduction of pharmaceutically prepared preserved saline solutions, most salt tablets were withdrawn from the market. They were, however, reintroduced because of the red-eye and sensitization problems associated with thimerosal-preserved salines. In 1987, the FDA asked companies marketing salt tables for their voluntary withdrawal because of several incidences of keratitis caused by *Acanthamoeba* species, resulting in significant loss of vision or eyesight of several lens wearers. Most of these cases were associated with the use of salt tablets to prepare homemade saline solution.

In the United States today saline solutions are marketed in preserved and unpreserved forms; both are sterile and pharmaceutically prepared. The unpreserved solutions are available in unit dose or multidose plastic containers and multidose aerosols. In the latter instance, the pressurized container and the construction of the valve prevents innoculation of microorganisms into the container during its use, thus maintaining sterility more effectively in comparison to multidose non-preserved saline solution in plastic containers. Non-preserved saline solution in an aerosol container is, therefore, preferred over non- preserved saline solution because it eliminates the potential of irritation and sensitization reactions caused by thimerosal and sorbic acid preserved salines. Such reactions may result in considerable patient discomfort and require temporary discontinuance of lens wear. However, the newer preservatives Polyquad and Dymed do not cause significant levels of such reactions. The disadvantage of unpreserved saline solution in unit dose is higher cost. There is also a potential risk of ocular infection as it is a common practice among lens wearers to leave their lenses in a lens case containing an unpreserved saline for several weeks, often without appropriate disinfection. Unpreserved saline does not protect against proliferation of microorganisms.

In contrast, preserved saline helps to prevent microbial growth when lenses are not worn and stored in lens cases. They are also less costly in comparison to unit dose or multidose pressurized non-preserved saline solution containers. As already noted, the principal disadvantage of preserved saline solution is that some of the preservatives, such as thimerosal and sorbic acid, have the potential of causing irritation and sensitization in some patients. However, these reactions are not sight-threatening. In most instances these symptoms clear on discontinuance of the product without requiring any drug therapy. Again, this problem now appears to have been eliminated or greatly minimized with the introduction of newer preservatives such as Polyquad and Dymed.

Both preserved and unpreserved saline solutions are multifunctional solutions. In addition to thermal disinfection, they are also used to dissolve enzyme tablets in cleaning contact lenses, as a rinsing solution following cleaning and chemical disinfection, and as a lens storage solution.

Thermal disinfecting units

The FDA guidelines require that thermal disinfecting units must attain a minimum temperature of 80°C for 10 min in the saline solution, which is placed in the lens cases. There are several units on the market, which meet these requirements; they vary in their time–temperature profiles. Certain lenses such as those belonging to the FDA Group-4 classification (ionic, high-water-content lenses) do not withstand repeated heat treatment and tend to discolor. In general, FDA Group-4 lenses are not heat disinfected. Units on the market today have a thermostat, which cuts off the electrical current when a certain temperature is reached, eliminating the need for patients to switch it off. However, malfunctioning of units occasionally does occur.

Units on the market today are much different from those available earlier. The first unit was analogous to a "baby bottle warmer." Lenses were placed in a lens case, which was placed in a reservoir of water in an electrical heating unit. The temperature in the reservoir reached almost the boiling point of water and the time for disinfection was 30 min. To ensure not only disinfection but also sterilization of lenses, a unit was introduced capable of achieving 120°C for 20 min to ensure complete elimination of vegetative organisms as well as spores. This unit, however, was not successful since the high temperature was detrimental to many lens polymers. The current trend is toward developing a heating unit, which reaches temperatures below 80°C but ensures elimination of vegetative forms of ocular pathogens.

Chemical Disinfecting Agents (Oxidizing and Non-Oxidizing)

There are two categories of chemical disinfecting solutions: The first category comprises those containing non-oxidizing chemical antimicrobial agents, which are non-toxic at the concentration level used in the products. The second category constitutes those containing oxidizing agents, which are toxic at the level used for disinfection but are degraded to a non-toxic level during the disinfection process over a course of time or by use of a second step that involves a neutralizing ingredient. Disinfecting solutions containing oxidizing agents (specifically hydrogen peroxide) gained popularity among lens practitioners in the mid- to late-1980s because of the absence of traditional preservatives, which often caused red eye and delayed hypersensitivity. However, the neutralizing solution used with hydrogen peroxide often contains preservatives that can cause ocular reactions. Lens practitioners liked the concept of hydrogen peroxide decomposing to innocuous water and oxygen. Fewer reactions have been observed with such products, but the long term toxic effects on the eye of the free radicals which are generated by low concentrations of undergraded oxidizing agents are not well known. Hydrogen peroxide products can cause severe toxic reactions if the products are not used properly and the patient inserts a lens without neutralizing the hydrogen peroxide.

The ideal chemical disinfecting agent should possess the following properties: It should have excellent wearer's acceptance in terms of being non-irritating, non- sensitizing, and easy to use. It should be relatively non-toxic compared to the earlier preservatives in terms of cytotoxicity, including its effects on epithelial and endothelial cells as well as its ability to maintain mitotic activity of corneal epithelial cells. It must have an adequate antimicrobial spectrum and be able to eliminate ocular pathogens in short lens-soaking regimens. It should not bind or bind minimally to the lens surface. It should be compatible with the lens and not cause discoloration or alter the tint of colored contact lenses.

A hydrogen peroxide disinfection system for soft lenses was tried initially in the early 1970s. The system failed to gain FDA approval because of the potential toxic nature of the chemical, the complexity of several steps, and the cost. The system was approved by the FDA in the early 1980s after having undergone significant refinements compared to the original system.

All products currently marketed in the United States under the oxidizing agent category contain hydrogen peroxide. In the international market, products containing chlorine-releasing agents are also available. These products are generally indicated for the disinfection of hydrophilic soft contact lenses and are contraindicated for rigid gas-permeable lenses. Most of the hydrogen peroxide is decomposed by catalytic degradation (platinum ring); chemical neutralization using pyruvate, sodium bisulfite, or sodium thiosulfate; dilution and rinsing; and enzymatic neutralization (catalase).

Hydrogen peroxide, on degradation, forms water and oxygen and, hence, it is perceived by practitioners as a superior product. However, most of the neutralizers used in the second step contain preservatives such as thimerosal and sorbic acid, and stabilizers such as stannates or phosphonates. Consequently, they have the associated disadvantages of those ingredients. On the other hand, not having a preservative in a neutralizer makes these products vulnerable to microbial growth on accidental contamination. A single-step product containing hydrogen peroxide is also available on the market, which is convenient, but has the same disadvantage of not having any preservative effect at the end of the disinfection cycle. The disinfecting time recommended by various companies ranges from 10 min to an overnight soak. This category of disinfecting agents has a better antimicrobial spectrum and a faster kill rate. However, their shortcomings included toxicity if the regimen was not followed properly, complexity of use, and zero to minimal protection against microbial recontamination once the disinfection cycle was complete.

The first generation non-oxidizing chemical disinfection solution contained a combination of antimicrobial agents incorporating thimerosal with chlorhexidine or alkytriethanol ammonium chloride. These solutions are now not commonly used because of the thimerosal problems as discussed previously. The newer antimicrobial agents, Polyquad and Dymed, because of their molecular structure and large molecule size have a better profile. These antimicrobial agents were introduced in the late 1980s and their long-term use has not caused reactions similar to those observed for older antimicrobial agents. Products with these agents currently dominate the lens care market.

Products for Enhancing Soft Contact Lens Wear Comfort

Factors Contributing to Wear Comfort

It has already been noted that hydrogel contact lenses are inherently more comfortable that rigid (RGP or PMMA) lenses. This is related to the former's superior flexibility and hydrophilic character which permits incorporation of substantial amounts of water (38–74%) into the lens material. However, after periods of wear time, some lenses may experience changes in hydration, that may be related to deposits, environmental (e.g., temperature and humidity) changes and improper care. In particular, "dry spots" may become evident on the lens with attendant reduction in comfort and visual acuity. When this happens, the wearer may benefit from periodic administration of rewetting (or soothing or comfort) solutions onto the lens while being worn. These solutions are usually low-viscosity aqueous compositions containing polymers or surfactants, which enhance the wettability of the surface, facilitating the spreading tears, and enhancing the stability of the tear film. They may also provide cushioning and lubricating actions, lessening impact, and reducing the frictional forces of the eyelids as they move across the lens on the corneal surface. The frictional forces would be especially important in instances where deposits or debris on the lens are present in sufficient amounts to cause physical irritation to the ocular tissue. In addition to wetting, cushioning, and lubricating, the ability of the solutions to facilitate removal of contaminants and retard further soilage are also desirable attributes. It is also desirable, in terms of convenience to the lens wearer, that the frequency of administration of drops of the above-mentioned types be minimal. Therefore, the use of polymers and surfactants that associate with the (deposited) lens and resist removal by the rinsing action of the tears is called for (i.e., polymers and surfactants with good substantivity).

Although rewetting efficacy is usually the primary requirement for hydrogel lens wearers, all three actions (rewetting, cushioning, and lubrication) may be of considerable significance for RGP or PMMA lens wearers. The practitioner should seek to help the wearer find the product best suited for his or her specific comfort needs. Solutions designed for hydrogel lenses generally have lower viscosities, whereas solutions for rigid hard lenses usually have higher viscosities. Although high viscosities can be of distinct benefit in enhancing cushioning action, a solution that is too viscous can cause blurred vision and hinder normal lid movement to an undesirable extent.

Components of Lens Comfort Solutions

Among the polymers used in lens comfort solutions are polyvinyl alcohol, polyvinylpyrrolidone, dextran, and various cellulose derivatives such as hydroxyethyl cellulose, hydroxypropyl cellulose, and hydroxypropyl methylcellulose. Surfactants include certain poloxamer and poloxamine compounds. Other normal components comprise appropriate preservative(s) as well as buffering and tonicity-adjusting agents.

Lens Care Products for Rigid Gas-Premeable Lenses

Several types of RGP lenses are marketed and others are under development. Because of their rigid nature, they have certain characteristics in common with conventional hard PMMA lenses. In many cases, care products available for use with the latter have been found to be also suitable for the care of the RGP lenses. Although they may not have optimal characteristics, they are still preferred by many practitioners in comparison to products that were originally designed for use with soft lenses and were subsequently approved by the FDA also for use with RGP materials.

Most categories of products indicated for the care of soft contact lenses are applicable to rigid gas- permeable lenses. These include daily cleaners, wetting and cushioning drops, and weekly enzymatic cleaners. While disinfecting solutions are necessary for RGP lens care, they are often positioned as conditioning solutions. Conditioning is important in providing a hydrophilic lens surface during wear. Because RGP lenses do not withstand heat, saline solutions (both preserved and unpreserved) are not needed for these lenses, except for dissolving enzymatic cleaners for weekly cleaning or rinsing.

Because RGP lenses are not as porous or water absorbing as soft lenses, wearers do not experience the problems that are specific to soft lenses, resulting from preservatives penetrating and concentrating within the lens polymer matrix, which often cause toxic and hypersensitivity-type reactions. However, certain preservatives bind with RGP surfaces and can create clinical problems. Binding may involve ionic and/or hydrophobic interactions.

In addition to accumulation of proteinaceous deposits, such as those occurring on soft hydrophilic lenses, the molecular make-up of many RGP lenses also tends to attract lipid deposits, such as cholesterol esters, wax esters, triglycerides, etc. This is especially true of the more hydrophobic materials such as silicone acrylates with high Dk (oxygen permeability) values. Accordingly, more recent developments in material science related to contact lenses have resulted in materials such as fluorosilicone acrylates and fluorocarbons with purportedly less propensity for deposits.

Wearing rigid lenses is much less comfortable than wearing soft contact lenses. In fact, this is generally perceived to be the major factor limiting the growth of the RGP lens market segment. Consequently, the need for superior wetting, cushioning, and lubricating products is clearly recognized. Superior combination products are also required for RGP lenses, which provide convenience and enhance product performance.

Multipurpose Solutions

Multipurpose solutions are designed to increase wearer compliance and the convenience of product use. Such solutions are not commonly used for the conventional PMMA hard lenses and rigid gas-permeable lenses. They combine two or more basic functions of lens care, including cleaning, disinfection, soaking, wetting, and lubricating. Combination of these functions in a single product may compromise certain aspects of product efficacy. For instance, a solution designed to clean and disinfect may not clean as well the cleaner would alone. However, a combination cleaning and disinfection solution provides the convenience of a single step and would be particularly useful for wearers whose lenses do not attract deposits as readily because of their tear chemistry.

Multipurpose solutions for soft lenses are primarily limited to cleaning and disinfecting. Wetting and lubricating combinations are not a major need because of the inherent hydrophilic nature of soft lenses that makes them comfortable to wear. The technology advances made in identifying preservatives with broader spectrum and capacity along with the ability of chemicals to clean while disinfecting has further simplified care of lenses. Recently, a new product has been developed in a multipurpose solution format that has allowed removal of the rubbing step.

Packaging of Contact Lens Products

All lens care products are packaged in plastic containers or pressurized metal containers with the exception of enzymatic or disinfecting tablets. The tablets are generally effervescent and packaged in laminated foil or blister packs to ensure adequate shelf life. The packaging materials normally used by the pharmaceutical industry for effervescent tablets are adequate for this purpose. The plastic containers are usually fabricated from low-density polyethylene, high-density polyethylene, or polypropylene materials. Many of the containers are opaque for protection against light. Several types of colorant mixtures, which usually contain titanium, are used in squeeze bottles, and the composition and thickness of the container wall should be designed to allow easy delivery.

Another important consideration is the orifice at the tip, which allows the desired product to flow. For instance, a disinfecting or saline solution needs to be delivered in a large volume of 3 to 5 ml to fill the lens case. A steady stream is desirable and acceptable here, but not for products like wetting, lubricating, and cushioning drops, which are directly instilled in the eye. For these products, the tip has to be designed to allow drop-by-drop instillation. Formulation characteristics such as viscosity and surface tension determine the tip design. The tip must be smooth and rounded as it can come into contact with the eye. The caps for the bottle are normally constructed of polystyrene or polypropylene material.

Because all lens care products, with the exception of the tablet dosage form, have to be sterile, the containers must be sterilized prior to filling unless the process involves form, fill, and seal technology. Containers are usually sterilized by ethylene oxide or gamma irradiation. The latter method is preferred because of stringent government regulations and requirements regarding ethylene oxide residues and its degradation products. Recent years have also seen strict controls regarding the exposure of workers to ethylene oxide and its by-products. Terminal sterilization of the final product is normally not done for lens care products, with the exception of non-preserved saline solutions in aerosol containers, which are sterilized by gamma irradiation.

Accessory Contact Lens Products

Accessory contact lens products include cases and devices for cleaning contact lenses and facilitating insertion.

Lens Cases

Lens cases are utilized for disinfection and storage while the lenses are not being worn. Lens cases may have a single compartment with a barrel shape, generally holding 7 to 10 ml of solution, or they may have two compartments in a flat case design, each compartment holding 3 to 5 ml of solution. Lens cases are also used by lens manufacturers as mailers to ship RGP and PMMA lenses in the dry state. Recently, shipping the lenses in conditioning solution has been approved. On the other hand, hydrophilic soft contact lenses are generally shipped in sealed sterile glassvials containing buffered isotonic saline solution. Plastic lens cases are fabricated from polymeric materials such as polyethylene, polypropylene, polysulfone, or polycarbonate.

Devices Facilitating Cleaning

Cleaning devices are useful for lens wearers who lack the manual dexterity to clean lenses with their fingers. They are also used for cleaning lenses that could be scratched easily by fingertips. The consumer versions provide mechanical action by manual swirling or by agitation with the help of an electrical motor or sonication The professional versions are usually ultrasonic- type devices. None of these devices are capable of removing tenaciously bound protein. The reservoir of the cleaning device is filled with special cleaning fluid or a saline with a few drops of a surfactant-type daily lens cleaner. The device should allow easy lens placement and retrieval and minimize the potential of damage. Lens baskets that allow for rinsing after the cleaning regimen without additional handling are a desirable feature.

Devices Facilitating Lens Insertion

These devices are generally helpful to elderly patients, especially those wearing aphakic lenses. They consist usually of a rubber bulb with a suction cup. They can cause severe corneal damage if used improperly as well as ocular infection if they are not properly cleaned and disinfected.

Future Directions in Lens Care Products

Of the persons fitted with contact lenses (both soft and hard), 40% discontinue wearing them within the first three years. One of the reasons cited is the time and effort required in taking care of them. Therefore, lens care systems will be developed that are simple and more convenient to use, requiring fewer products, and less time. The new products will minimize patient problems through safer preservatives, which are nontoxic even on misuse and do not produce hypersensitization. More effective cleaners as well as products which minimize protein and microbial attachment to lens surfaces will also be forthcoming as well as cleaners that can be instilled in the eye during lens wear to retard deposit formation on extended-wear lenses or to clean lenses while they are being worn. Other future product types may include special artificial tears and comfort drops for older patients who are prone to dry eye.

There is also a need for diagnostic products that can detect potential problems before they are manifested clinically. Universal products that could be used with all contact lenses (i.e., hard PMMA, RGP, and soft lenses) may be desirable; however, it is unlikely that such products will be available as different contact lenses vary significantly in their chemical and surface characteristics. The main emphasis in the future will be on the development of convenient, easy-to-use products that can increase patient compliance and reduce the dropout rate, while ensuring desirable efficacy without compromising product safety. Products specifically designed for the care of disposable and frequent replacement lenses will also be forthcoming.

Components of Lens Care Products

Active Components

Active components play a primary role in the intended use of a product. The active components in lens care products are usually limited to either one or two chemical entities. However, a product may contain several active components if it is designed for multiple functions or indications.

Chemicals with disinfecting capability

Active chemical entities must have bactericidal and fungistatic properties. However, cidal properties for fungal organisms is preferable. The product performance criteria encompassing the types of organisms to be tested, levels of inoculum, and method of testing are defined by guidelines developed by the FDA. Current chemical systems have disinfection times of 4–6 h. This fits with most wearing schedules, because more than 90% of patients remove their lenses overnight between wear periods. Overnight removal seems to help the eye recover from the stress of lens wear. Recently, some efforts to move to shorter disinfection time are under way to increase convenience. The products will require dramatically enhanced disinfection efficacy than currently available or strict compliance to a regimen to achieve the required level of disinfection.

Surface-active and other agents with cleaning capability

Surfactants of various types have been traditionally used for cleaning conventional PMMA hard lenses. They are considered effective in removing surface deposits on these lenses, such as cosmetics, hair spray, mascara, etc. However, they are not effective in removing tenaciously bound deposits (e.g., proteins, lipids, lipoproteins, mucoproteins) that are commonly encountered with soft hydrophilic contact lenses and rigid gas-permeable lenses. Such deposits are more effectively removed by products containing enzymes, strong oxidizing agents, or suspended abrasive (deposit-shearing) particles. The types of surfactants used and representative products on the market are discussed later under Products for Cleaning Soft Contact Lenses. A few other agents such as citrate and some phosphates have been used as cleaning agents.

Components with wetting, lubricating, and cushioning capabilities

Polymers and surfactants are the two main classes of compounds used as wetting, lubricating, and cushioning agents. Contingent on the nature of the specified polymers, they are used in various combinations to achieve desired product characteristics.

Both synthetic and natural polymers are commonly used in lens care products. These agents can provide a cushioning effect as a result of increased viscosity. The need for products with such action is greater for the wearers of conventional hard PMMA lenses and rigid gas-permeable lenses, for these are inherently not as comfortable as soft contact lenses because of the lens design and the physiochemical nature of the polymers. Viscosity-building agents provide the necessary initial coatings on the lens surface before it is coated by natural tear components. Besides contributing to viscosity, the ability of polymers to adsorb on lens surfaces and to elicit surface-active (wetting) properties are important considerations.

Surface-active agents are adsorbed on the lens surface and allow ready spreading of tears when the lenses are inserted, thus making them more comfortable to wear. The use of surface-active agents to impart wettability to the lens surface is of lesser value for products used for hydrophilic soft contact lenses, which have built-in wetting characteristics because of their water content. Addition of surfactants may be of value, however, in retarding deposit formation or for cleaning while the lenses are worn. The methodology for measuring both advancing and receding contact angles, as an indication of wetting efficacy, has been standardized for contact lenses. Various polymers have different degrees of wettability as measured by contact angle using a goniometer. However, the in vitro contact- angle measurement of contact lenses made from various polymers is of little clinical value. No discernible differences in in vivo contact angle can be detected on insertion of a contact lens in the eye following a few blinks that result in coating the lens surface with tear components. Surfactants are usually combined with polymers to impart sub stantivity and cushioning characteristics. The types of polymers and surfactants used in representative products in the market are discussed later under Products for Enhancing Soft Contact Lens Wear Comfort. Again, the need for surface-active agents which can facilitate wetting of lenses and spreading of tears is greater for PMMA and rigid gas-permeable lenses because of their hydrophobic surface characteristics.

Ancillary Components

Preservatives

Preservatives are used in almost all multidose contact lens products. Because the potential for misuse of products by lens wearers is significant, preservatives prevent the potential proliferation of microorganisms. A contaminated product could ultimately lead to an ocular infection and possible loss of eyesight. Preservatives are considered active components when incorporated in products for the purpose of disinfecting contact lenses. The preservative must possess the antimicrobial activity described in the FDA guidelines for contact lens care.

The FDA has issued guidelines for preservative efficacy, which include an additional safety factor to compensate for potential misuse of products. These requirements are more stringent than the requirements of the United States Pharmacopeia (USP) for preservative efficacy. The FDA requires rechallenging the preserved products on day 14 with a defined inoculum of microorganisms; this is not required by the USP. The preservatives generally used are mainly the same as those used for thermal or chemical disinfection of contact lenses. The concentrations could be different than in the chemical disinfection of contact lenses. The concentration is generally higher in cleaners and comfort-enhancing solutions because of possible binding with polymer and surfactant components, which result in a decrease in preservative efficacy.

Different countries have different standards for preserving contact lens solutions; the requirements of the British Pharmacopeia are the most stringent. Many marketed products do not meet these requirements. The three major preservative efficacy tests, which must be considered in developing products, are delineated in the United States Pharmacopoeia (modified test to meet FDA guidelines), the British Pharmacopeia and the German Pharmacopeia (DAB). In terms of difficulty to comply, the British Pharmacopoeia test is the most stringent and the modified USP test the least stringent. The main differences among the test requirements are the exposure times and use of Escherichia coli as a challenge organism. The British Pharmacopeia utilizes a 6 h criterion for antimicrobial activity, whereas the USP uses a 14 day criterion. Recently, an International Standard has been approved which is comparable to the US FDA procedure. The types of preservatives used are described in the tables related to various product categories.

Buffers for adjusting pH

The use of buffers and pH adjustment is an important consideration in lens care products. It is a general practice that all products which are likely to come in direct contact with ocular tissues should be buffered for ocular comfort around physiologic pH and preferably in the range 6–8.0. The most commonly used buffers in contact lens care products are phosphates and borates. Buffers used occasionally are acetate, citrate, and others. Besides buffers, sodium hydroxide and hydrochloric acid are generally used to achieve a desirable pH in the final product. They are also used to adjust the final pH in products, which do not have any buffering system. The selection of an appropriate buffering system should consider the pH necessary for optimal performance of the product, as well as products stability and potential incompatibility with other components of the product.

Although it is desirable to have a product as close to physiologic pH as possible, it is often essential to formulate a product outside the physiologic pH range in order to achieve the desired stability of the product, optimal efficacy, or appropriate solubility of active and ancillary components. Products formulated outside the physiologic pH range should have low buffer capacity to allow quick equilibration to tear pH by the bicarbonate buffer system present in the tears. The maintenance of pH close to physiologic pH is essential for products intended for soaking and disinfection of hydrophilic soft contact lenses in order to maintain the parameters of some lenses, especially those belonging to FDA Group-4. Such changes in parameters can cause not only discomfort but can also produce blurred vision.

Tonicity-adjusting agents

Contact lens products should be formulated as closely as possible to the tonicity of tears. This is important for optimal comfort. Prolonged exposure to hypotonic solutions can induce edema in corneal epithelial cells, which can cause blurred vision and discomfort, whereas prolonged exposure to hypertonic solutions can cause corneal epithelial cells to shrivel and cause discomfort by exposing nerve endings. None of the currently available contact lens solutions have been responsible for such symptoms as most of them are formulated close to isotonicity and many contact lens products have minimal contact with the cornea. Nevertheless, maintaining the tonicity of products close to the isotonic value of 280 ($\pm$ 50) mOsm/kg is important for optimal comfort as well as for maintaining the integrity of certain hydrophilic soft contact lenses. The type of compounds commonly used for imparting isotonicity include buffering agents, sodium chloride, potassium chloride, propylene glycol, mannitol, dextrose, etc.

Viscosity-building agents

Viscosity-building agents such as synthetic and natural polymers are used as active ingredients in solutions providing comfort and rewetting products. However, they are also used as ancillary agents in contact lens cleaning products. These agents allow better cleaning of contact lenses by enhancing the contact of the cleansing agent with the soiled lens and by facilitating the process of rubbing the lens between fingers or between the palm of the hand and an index finger. Highly viscous or gel-type cleaners are also available. However, they are not very popular as they are difficult to rinse and may cause ocular irritation. The types of polymers used as ancillary agents are the same as those used for solutions providing comfort or rewetting solutions.

Pharmaceutical Technology Considerations in Product Design

With few exceptions, contact lens products are sterile solutions. The sterility requirements are important because of the potential of sight-threatening ocular infections. The sterility test procedures and pass–fail criteria as described in the United States Pharmacopeia must be met for FDA approval of contact lens products. The technology practiced in the development of pharmaceutical products, such as injectable and large volume intravenous fluids, is generally acceptable, with somewhat less stringent requirements for contact lens care products because most of these products do not come into direct contact with the eye (i.e., its interior cells and fluids). Products that are packaged in unit dose containers or multidose pressurized aerosol containers do not have to be preserved. However, multidose products other than aerosol containers should be preserved and should pass the FDA preservative efficacy test. Manufacturers intending to develop lens care products should consult with the FDA for the latest guidelines.

Apart from solutions, there are other pharmaceutical dosage forms for contact lens products that are less commonly used. They include gel- and suspension-type cleaners, powders, and tablet dosage forms for enzymatic cleaners or disinfectants. All of these products are formulated as sterile products with the exception of powders and tablets. These, however, must comply with USP requirements for bioburden with added specifications for absence of colony-forming units of *Staphylococcus aureus* and *Pseudomonas aeruginosa* among other organisms. The choice of components in formulating these products is much more restrictive in comparison to pharmaceutical products intended for systemic or topical use because of the potential of causing irritation to the sensitive ocular tissues.

Chemical components must be non-irritating and compatible with ocular tissue as well as with lenses. The choice of components for tablets, such as binding and lubricating agents, is much more restrictive, as these ingredients must be soluble and form a clear solution when dissolved in saline solutions. Formulation components generally used and acceptable for ophthalmic products may be unacceptable for contact lens products, as many contact lens materials can concentrate components used in contact lens products as much as several hundredfold. On insertion of the lenses, these ingredients are released in toxic levels to the cornea, causing minor to severe ocular reactions. The binding and release of ingredients can be further complicated by the condition of the lens. For instance, thimerosal and chlorhexidine, commonly used ingredients in contact lens products, concentrate differently in new, deposit-free lenses as compared to used lenses with protein deposits on the surfaces. Appropriate studies must be designed to address these issues to minimize the potential of ocular irritation. Certain ingredients such as thimerosal, when used initially are well tolerated. However, on prolonged exposure, some lens wearers develop hypersensitivity, resulting in intolerance of thimerosal products. Such intolerance is difficult to predict and currently no satisfactory method is available to predict delayed hypersensitivity-type reactions, which are modulated immunologically. The commonly used guinea pig maximization test is not predictive of delayed hypersensitivity reactions.

As noted previously, formulating products close to physiological pH is desirable. However, for optimal product performance or meeting regulatory requirements, it is sometimes necessary to formulate products outside the physiologic pH range. Sorbic acid, a commonly used preservative for lens care products, is a marginally effective antimicrobial agent with a pKa value of 4.8. A product fails the FDA preservative efficacy test if it is formulated around a physiologic pH of 7–7.4 at a concentration of 0.1 sorbic acid normally used in marketed products. To maximize its antimicrobial activity without compromising ocular comfort to a significant extent, it is necessary to formulate such products around pH 6.5–6.8. Thus, a consideration of the dissociation constants of preservatives is essential as the antimicrobial activity of many preservatives depends on the undissociated species, which should be present in an adequate amount at physiological pH without causing ocular irritation.

The product design should also consider the nature of the lens polymer and its surface charges. For example, FDA Group-4 lenses, which carry negative surface charges, can react with positively charged product components, resulting in severe ocular toxic reactions. Such toxic reactions can be prevented by incorporating non-ionic surfactants to form micelles with the cationic components, thus minimizing surface interactions and toxicity. If a cationic agent in the product is a primary disinfecting agent, efforts to minimize toxicity or surface interactions often result in reduced antimicrobial performance. It is, therefore, essential to minimize surface interactions and yet have a product, which meets the requirements for disinfection or preservation.

The hydrophilic–lipophilic balance (HLB) and molecular dimensions of a preservative should also be considered in the design of contact lens products. For example, chlorobutanol (a non-ionic preservative used in ophthalmic products) penetrates into the matrix of rigid-gas-permeable (RGP) lens materials because of the molecule's substantial lipophilic characteristics. The preservative present in the lens matrix may change the parameters or may be gradually released during wear, causing irritation and toxicity to the corneal cells. On the other hand, the molecular dimensions of a preservative are very important in designing a product for hydrophilic, soft contact lenses. Generally, preservatives with a high molecular weight and appropriate molecular configuration are less likely to penetrate the porous matrix of hydrogel lenses. Products containing preservatives like Dymed and Polyquad, with molecular weights above 1000, are currently available.

INDEX